Workbook and Review Guide
to accompany
Egan's Fundamentals of Respiratory Care

# WORKBOOK and REVIEW GUIDE
## to accompany
## EGAN'S Fundamentals
## of
## Respiratory Care SIXTH EDITION

Robert E. St. John, R.N., R.R.T., M.S.N.
Adjunct Assistant Professor
Jewish Hospital College of Nursing and Allied Health
Pulmonary Clinical Nurse Specialist
Jewish Hospital of St. Louis
St. Louis, Missouri

Craig L. Scanlan, Ed.D., R.R.T.
Professor
Department of Cardiopulmonary Sciences
University of Medicine and Dentistry of New Jersey
Newark, New Jersey

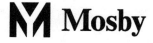 Mosby

St. Louis  Baltimore  Boston  Carlsbad  Chicago  Naples  New York  Philadelphia  Portland
London  Madrid  Mexico City  Singapore  Sydney  Tokyo  Toronto  Wiesbaden

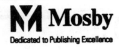

Mosby
Dedicated to Publishing Excellence

A Times Mirror
Company

*Editor: James F. Shanahan*
*Developmental Editor: Anne J. Gleason*
*Cover Designer: Susan Lane*
*Manuscript Editor: Susan Warrington*
*Interior Design and Layout: Chad Reidhead*

Printed in the United States of America.
Composition by Wordbench.
Printing and binding by Plus Communications.

Mosby-Year Book, Inc.
11830 Westline Industrial Drive
St. Louis, MO 63146

**International Standard Book Number 0-8151-7517-5**

95 96 97 98 99/9 8 7 6 5 4 3 2 1

# Preface

This workbook provides a comprhensive review of the content of the sixth edition of *Egan's fundamentals of Resiratory Care*. Students will be challenged with a series of **content exercises** presented in a variety of formats designed to reinforce basic comprehension, recall, and critical-thinking skills. Depending on the nature of the text material, these exercises will take the form of **diagram labeling, true/false** and **short answer** questions (fill-in-the-blank), **computations** and **multiple choice** questions (modeled after NBRC format).

Selected workbook chapters have a special section called **Problems for Thought and Discussion.** Although most of these exercises can be solved independently by the student, the instructor may wish to use them as the basis for group discussion. At the conlusion of the workbook, there is a list of **Recommended Readings** taken from each chapter in the *Egan* text which may be used for supplemental study. Last, in order to provide students with the opportunity to confirm their mastery of the material, a complete **Answer Key** is provided at the back of the workbook.

We gratefully recognize the work of the contributors to the previous *Workbook and Review Guide* and offer *this edition* to further build on its strengths.

**Robert E. St. John**

**Craig L. Scanlan**

**Acknowledgements**

I would like to thank the sixth edition contirbutors for their helpful suggestions and input and the people at Mosby—Anne Gleason, Susan Eriksen, and Jennifer Roche—for their support and cooperation during the revision process.

# Contributors

James R. Brennan, M.Ed., R.R.T.
Department Chair, Health Sciences
Program Director, Respiratory Therapy
St. Louis Community College at Forest Park
St. Louis, Missouri

Paul M. Reading, M.A., R.R.T.
Affiliate Program Director
St. John's Mercy Medical Center
University of Missouri at Columbia
St. Louis, Missouri

Edmond R. Smith, M.A., R.R.T., R.P.F.T.
Clinical Research Respiratory Care Practitioner
Cardinal Glennon Children's Hospital
St. Louis, Missouri

Kevin Thorpe, B.A., R.R.T.
Saint Luke's Hospital
Kansas City, Missouri

Joan Vernitte, B.H.S., R.R.T.
Director of Clinical Education
Respiratory Care Program
St. John's Mercy Medical Center
University of Missouri at Columbia
St. Louis, Missouri

## Contributors to the previous edition

William Carroll, B.S., R.R.T.
Director of Respiratory Care Services
Kessler Institute for Rehabilitation
West Orange, NJ

G. Woodard Gross, M.A.., R.R.T.
Program Director
Respiratory Therapy Program
UMDNJ/Camden County College
Blackwood, NJ

Alan M.Realey, B.A., R.R.T.
Director of Clinical Education
Respiratory Therapy Program
UMDNJ/Camden County College
Blackwood, NJ

F. Robert Thalken, M.A., R.R.T.
Clinical Assistant Professor
Respiratory Therapy Program
Department of Cardiorespiratory Sciences
School of Allied Health Sciences
Indiana University School of Medicine
Indianapolis, IN

Sharon Williams, M.A., R.R.T.
Program Administrator
Northwest New Jersey Consortium for
Respiratory Care Education
St. Clares-Riverside Medical Center
Denville, NJ

Kenneth A. Wyka, M.S., R.R.T.
Director of Clinical Education
Respiratory Therapy Program
Department of Cardiopulmonary Sciences
School of Health Related Professions
University of Medicine and Dentistry of New Jersey
Newark, New Jersey

# Contents

# Respiratory Care and the Health Care System

## CONTENT EXERCISES

**True/False:** For each of the following statements, indicate whether it is mainly true or mainly false by circling the corresponding letter (T=True, F=False):

1.1   T   F   The enactment of non–smoking laws is considered a type of health service.

1.2   T   F   The distribution of current spending for health services is about equal to the relative importance of the factors determining the population's health status.

1.3   T   F   The U.S. spends more money on national defense than on health care.

1.4   T   F   The majority of health expenditures are for hospital care and physicians' services.

1.5   T   F   All monies necessary to support the U.S. health care system ultimately come from the government.

1.6   T   F   Employment of health professionals in settings other than acute care hospitals is growing.

1.7   T   F   No major segment of the U.S. population has difficulty obtaining health care.

1.8   T   F   Most adults believe the U.S. health care system works pretty well.

1.9   T   F   In recent years, access to health care for the uninsured and poor appears to be improving.

1.10   T   F   Most Americans believe that health care costs are going up too fast.

**Short Answer:** Complete each statement by filling in the correct information in the space(s) provided:

1.11 Individual health activities such as promotion of health, prevention of illness, diagnosis, treatment, and rehabilitation are grouped together under the category of _____ services.

1.12 By the year 2000, health care costs are expected to be more than _____ % of the GNP.

1.13 All monies necessary to support the U.S. health care system ultimately come from the _____.

1.14 The process whereby individuals who have met certain predetermined standards attesting to their occupational skill or competence are recognized is called _____.

1.15 The process whereby the government grants permission to an individual to practice a given occupation after verification that the applicant has demonstrated the minimum competency necessary to protect the public health, safety, or welfare is termed _____ _____.

1.16 _____ is the voluntary process whereby a nongovernmental or private agency or association grants recognition to an individual who has met certain predetermined qualifications.

1.17 Voluntary certification in respiratory care is conducted by the _____.

1.18 A nursing home which provides continuous nursing service on a 24–hour basis is termed a _____ _____.

1.19 A _____ is a predefined category of patient illness which is used by the federal government to establish Medicare reimbursement rates.

1.20 Prospective reimbursement by DRGs has provided a powerful incentive for cost–efficiency in the provision of inpatient hospital services because it _____ _____.

1.21 The primary organization responsible for voluntary standard setting among health care organizations is the _____ _____.

1.22 The primary organization representing individual respiratory care professionals is the _____ _____.

**Listing:** Complete each list as directed in its statement.

1.23  List the four (4) primary factors affecting human health status:

1. _____

2. _____

3. _____

4. _____

1.24  List the four (4) primary ways we pay for personal health services:

1. _____

2. _____

3. _____

4. _____

1.25  List the three (3) major third–party payors for health services:

1. _____

2. _____

3. _____

1.26  List at least five (5) organizations responsible for the delivery of health care services directly to consumers, i.e., primary providers:

1. _____

2. _____

3. _____

4. _____

5. _____

1.27  List the four (4) basic health maintenance organization models:

1. _____

2. _____

3. _____

4. _____

1.28  List five (5) major issues facing the current health care system:

1. _____

2. _____

3. _____

4. _____

5. _____

## PROBLEMS FOR THOUGHT AND DISCUSSION

Although the U.S. claims to have the most sophisticated health care system in the world, it has one of the highest rates of infant mortality among all industrialized nations. What aspects of the current U.S. health care system are contributing to this continuing problem? How might this problem be addressed?

As a component of your benefits package, your employer offers you a choice between a standard Blue Cross/Blue Shield plan and enrollment in an HMO. Which would you choose and why?

Determine the status of licensure for respiratory care personnel in your state. If licensure exists, delineate the key administrative regulations governing respiratory care practice in your state and their implications for both practitioners and employers. If licensure does not exist in your state, determine what your state respiratory care society is doing to promote its implementation and why.

Rising costs are consistently cited as a major problem facing the U.S. health care system. In their role as professional providers, how can respiratory care practitioners help stem this growing problem? In their role as health care consumers?

When considering technological advances in health care delivery, most health care professionals consider only their positive aspects. What are some of the negatives aspects of technology?

# 2

# Modern Respiratory Care Services

## CONTENT EXERCISES

**True/False:** For each of the following statements, indicate whether it is mainly true or mainly false by circling the corresponding letter (T=True, F=False):

2.1  T   F   According to the JCAHO, respiratory care services must be available 24 hours a day, seven days a week.

2.2  T   F   According to the JCAHO, respiratory care services should be provided to patients in accordance with a written prescription by the physician responsible for the patient and documented in the patient's medical record.

2.3  T   F   Most hospitals are organized in a dual administrative and medical structure.

2.4  T   F   Final approval of departmental clinical policies and procedures is the responsibility of the technical director of respiratory care.

2.5  T   F   The medical director of the department is the individual ultimately responsible for the quality and appropriateness of respiratory care services.

2.6  T   F   The assistant director of a respiratory care department often functions as the chief clinician and first–line supervisor.

2.7  T   F   Technical proficiency and knowledge are all that is needed to deliver safe and effective respiratory care.

2.8  T   F   Respiratory care equipment aides commonly provide direct patient care at the bedside.

2.9  T   F   Failure to follow the specifications provided in the department policy and procedure manual can result in personal liability.

2.10  T   F   Diagnostic equipment capable of computerized computation and reporting can provide long–term cost savings to a respiratory care department.

2.11  T   F   The medical record of a patient is a legal document.

2.12  T   F   Ultimate authority for quality assurance within a respiratory care service lies with the medical director.

2.13  T   F   Respiratory care quality assurance procedures should give particular attention to evaluating services that have low utilization rates.

**Short Answer:** Complete each statement by filling in the correct information in the space(s) provided:

2.14  Minimum basic standards for respiratory care services in hospitals are provided by the _____ _____.

2.15  Typically, overall policy–making responsibility for a community hospital is vested in a _____. _____.

2.16  Overall responsibility for the daily operation and management of the respiratory care service falls on the _____.

2.17  _____ is an ongoing program designed to ensure the safe and effective operation of vital life support and monitoring equipment.

2.18  The scope and conduct of patient care services provided by a respiratory care department are formally described in the _____ _____.

**Listing:** Complete each list as directed in its statement.

2.19  List at least four (4) general therapeutic services offered by a typical respiratory care service department:

1. _____

2. _____

3. _____

4. _____

2.20  List the two (2) key diagnostic services that must be available wherever respiratory care is being used to its maximum potential:

1. _____

2. _____

2.21 List at least four (4) therapeutic and diagnostic support services that a comprehensive cardiopulmonary service may provide in addition to traditional respiratory care:

1. _____

2. _____

3. _____

4. _____

2.22 In light of the rapidly changing face of health care delivery, many respiratory care departments are now providing many "nontraditional" services for health care consumers or the community at large. List three (3) such nontraditional services:

1. _____

2. _____

3. _____

2.23 List at least three (3) operating principles that underlie the operation of the patient–focused hospital:

1. _____

_____

2. _____

_____

3. _____

_____

2.24 List at least four (4) elements of an acceptable protocol:

1. _____

_____

2. _____

_____

3. _____

_____

4. _____

_____

2.25 List, in order, the nine (9) key steps necessary to systematically implement a quality assurance plan for a respiratory care service:

1. _____

2. _____

3. _____

4. _____

5. _____

6. _____

7. _____

8. _____

9. _____

**Multiple Choice:** Circle the letter corresponding to the single best answer from the available choices:

2.26 Which of the following are examples of educational services offered by a comprehensive respiratory care department?
I. patient and family education
II. in–service education (staff, physicians, nurses, etc.)
III. clinical education for students
IV. community education

a. II and III     c. I, II, and III
b. I and III     d. I, II, III, and IV

2.27 Which of the following are required when describing a procedure in a respiratory care department procedure manual?
I. who may perform the procedure, with what supervision
II. under what circumstances the procedure is to be performed
III. the steps to be taken in the event of adverse reactions
IV. how to respond to situations lacking explicit instructions

a. II and III     c. I, II, and III
b. I and III     d. I, II, III, and IV

2.28 The primary technical and legal guide to service provision in a respiratory care department is the:

a. hospital library
b. department book collection
c. policy and procedure manual
d. department journal collection

2.29 The most expensive major capital equipment items maintained by a respiratory care service are:

a. oxygen therapy devices
b. bedside oxygen monitors
c. mechanical ventilators
d. incentive spirometers

2.30 Which of the following is not a component of a typical patient medical record?

a. history and physical
b. nursing notes
c. patient charges
d. admitting data

2.31 Implementation of the prospective payment system has resulted in which of the following changes for respiratory care services?
I.   an increased length of patient stays
II.  a greater intensity of services provided
III. a greater emphasis on documenting the need for and impact of respiratory care services

a. I and III          c. I only
b. II only            d. II and III

2.32 In regard to respiratory care services, the patient's medical record must document which of the following?
I.    the origination of prescribed treatments
II.   respiratory–related consultations
III.  actual service provided
IV.   evaluation of the results of intervention

a. II, III, and IV       c. III and IV
b. I, III, and IV        d. I, II, III, and IV

2.33 An ideal prescription for respiratory care services should include which of the following?
I.    the type of treatment
II.   the duration of treatment
III.  the type and dosage of medication
IV.   the goals and objectives of the therapy

a. I, III, and IV        c. II and III
b. II, III, and IV       d. I, II, III, and IV

2.34 The documentation of respiratory care provided by a practitioner in the patient's medical record should minimally include which of the following?
I.    the date and time of administration
II.   the effects of the therapy
III.  any adverse reactions exhibited by the patient
IV.   the type of therapy provided

a. I, III, and IV        c. II and III
b. II, III, and IV       d. I, II, III, and IV

## PROBLEMS FOR THOUGHT AND DISCUSSION

Compare the services offered by one of your program's clinical affiliate respiratory care departments with those listed in the boxed material on page 21 of the text. Which of the listed services are and are not provided? If a listed service is not provided by the respiratory care department, determine what, if any, other hospital department provides that service and why.

Get permission to review the procedure manuals for two (2) of your program's clinical affiliate respiratory care departments. What essential elements are similar? What are the differences? Who is responsible for maintaining and updating the procedure manuals?

Obtain a report of patient care services provided to one of your program's clinical affiliate respiratory care departments categorized by DRG. Which diagnostic groups appear most frequently? Least frequently? Not at all? Which groups have the longest length of stay? The shortest? Of what importance is this information in running the service department?

Get permission to sit in on a respiratory care department or hospital continuous quality improvement (CQI) committee meeting at one of your program's clinical affiliates. What area of quality assurance was the focus of the meeting? Who was responsible for gathering pertinent information? For taking appropriate actions? How are records maintained?

# 3

## Patient Safety, Communication, and Recordkeeping

## CONTENT EXERCISES

**True/False:** For each of the following statements, indicate whether it is mainly true or mainly false by circling the corresponding letter (T=True, F=False):

3.1  T  F  The importance of communication in both patient and professional interaction is underestimated.

3.2  T  F  Cultural and ethnic differences have little impact on the process of communication.

3.3  T  F  Effective health communication is a two–way process.

3.4  T  F  Symbols used in human communication may be verbal or nonverbal in nature.

3.5  T  F  For effective communication, the symbols used must have the same meaning to both sender and receiver.

3.6  T  F  Courteous listening can serve as a therapeutic tool.

3.7  T  F  The importance of family members in improving and maintaining a patient's health is overestimated.

3.8  T  F  The most critical factors required for ambulation are stable vital signs and absence of severe pain.

3.9  T  F  Infrequently, shock hazards are due to inappropriate or inadequate grounding.

3.10  T  F  Fire hazards are unusual in respiratory care areas in which oxygen is in use.

3.11  T  F  Legally, no documentation that care was given to a patient means that care was not given.

**Short Answer:** Complete each statement by filling in the correct information in the space(s) provided:

3.12  That form of communication involved in the promotion of health or the prevention of illness best describes _____.

3.13  A patient's pain or depressed level of consciousness is a good example of how _____ noise can affect communication.

3.14  In health communication interactions between a health professional and patient, it is important that each one's expectations be _____.

3.15  In human communication, we express meaning through the use of _____.

3.16  That part of the listening process requiring active discrimination among a message's components best describes _____.

3.17  _____ involves maintaining composure, controlling emotions, and avoiding premature judgments during communication interactions.

3.18  Confirming others' reception of communicated messages requires _____ listening.

3.19  The first step toward effective interaction with others is _____.

3.20  _____ is the primary factor determining the effect of a shock.

**Listing:** Complete each list as directed in its statement.

3.21  List at least three (3) human qualities that may be shared in the process of communication:

1. _____

2. _____

3. _____

3.22  Other than communication skills, list at least three (3) human factors that can affect a communication interaction:

1. _____

2. _____

3. _____

3.23 List two (2) conditions which are needed to start a fire:

1. _____

2. _____

**Matching:**

3.24 Listed below are the major purposes of initiating a health communication dialogue. Below these are several examples of the respiratory care practitioner serving as the *initiator* of a communication interaction. In the space provided next to each purpose, cite (by letter) the example that best represents its intent.

_____ to give instruction

_____ to persuade others

_____ to establish rapport

_____ to relay information

_____ to obtain information

a. In introducing herself to a new patient, a respiratory care practitioner learns that they are both from the same home town. She spends a few minutes discussing the "old haunts" with the patient.

b. A respiratory care practitioner spends time showing the family of a child receiving long–term mechanical ventilatory support in the home what to do in the case of a power failure.

c. In a meeting of the hospital professional union, a respiratory care practitioner stands up and argues against going on strike, citing the potentially disastrous results of a walk–out on the patients' safety and well–being.

d. A respiratory care practitioner calls a patient's attending physician over the phone and describes the results of bedside tests which indicate an improved response to an aerosol drug.

e. In the closing afternoon conference, a clinical instructor asks a respiratory therapy student several technical questions regarding the treatments given that day.

3.25 Listed below are several different types of listening. Below these are several examples of the respiratory care practitioner serving as *listener* in a communication interaction. Match each example to the type of listening that should be applied.

_____ courteous listening

_____ analytical listening

_____ attentive listening

_____ directed listening

_____ exploratory listening

a. A respiratory care practitioner working in the pulmonary function laboratory conducts a patient interview in order to obtain a relevant history.

b. A respiratory care practitioner takes time out to listen to an elderly patient's description of his grandchildren.

c. A respiratory care practitioner asks a patient if he or she has any questions regarding the treatment schedule.

d. A respiratory care practitioner on medical rounds listens to a physician's description of the medical treatment options for one of her patients.

e. A respiratory care practitioner queries a patient regarding her feelings about receiving therapy in the home.

**Multiple Choice:** Circle the letter corresponding to the single best answer from the available choices:

3.26 Failed communication can result in which of the following?
I.   misunderstandings between individuals
II.  personal animosity and mistrust
III. unexpected or adverse patient outcomes

a. I and II          c. I only
b. II and III        d. I, II, and III

3.27 A hospital mounts a campaign to improve the conformance of its employees in maintaining confidentiality in managing AIDS patients. Which types of communication would be appropriate to achieve this end?
I. organizational communication
II. small group communication
III. mass communication
IV. interpersonal health communication

a. I and II
b. II and III
c. I, II, and IV
d. I, II, III, and IV

3.28 You are in a busy emergency room trying to explain a treatment to an extremely anxious patient with chest pain. The patient in the cubicle next to yours is delirious and screaming for her husband. What types of "noise" may be impacting on the effectiveness of communication with your patient?
I. physical noise
II. sensory noise
III. emotional noise

a. I and II
b. II and III
c. I only
d. I, II, and III

3.29 A practitioner who holds strong negative feelings against homosexuals is assigned to treat an AIDS patient. Which of the following types of "noise" is most likely going to impact on their communication?

a. physical noise
b. sensory noise
c. practitioner's emotional noise
d. environmental distractions

3.30 Which of the following represent the primary types of health communication interactions?
I. peer (professional–professional) relationships
II. professional–patient (client) relationships
III. professional–family relationships
IV. patient–family relationships

a. I and II
b. II and III
c. I and III
d. I, II, III, and IV

3.31 In communication interactions, delaying one's responses, taking the other person's point of view, and limiting one's judgment to content (rather than delivery) are all useful in increasing one's:

a. attention
b. understanding
c. concentration
d. tolerance

3.32 Which of the following are components of empathetic listening?
I. attending
II. reflecting feelings
III. requesting clarification
IV. paraphrasing
V. perception checking

a. II, III, IV, and V
b. I, II, III, IV, and V
c. I, II, III, and V
d. III, IV, and V

3.33 The harmful effects of electrical current depend on which of the following?
I. amount of current flowing through the body
II. duration current is applied
III. path the current takes through the body

a. I and II
b. II and III
c. II only
d. I, II, and III

3.34 Each of the following general rules for medical recordkeeping is true *except:*

a. be exact in noting time and results of all treatments
b. record patient complaints and general behavior
c. use standard abbreviations
d. erase documentation notes carefully

## PROBLEMS FOR THOUGHT AND DISCUSSION

3.35 You overhear the following communication between a respiratory care practitioner and a patient:

**Practitioner:** "The desired outcome of this therapeutic regimen is to increase your transpulmonary pressure gradient above that which you are able to generate spontaneously. In order to determine its efficacy, we will conduct pre– and post–intervention assessment of your ventilatory parameters utilizing bedside PFTs. All you have to do is maximize your inspiratory capacity. So let's begin!"
**Patient:** "Well [*long pause*], okay."

a. Identify at least two (2) major errors made by the practitioner in communicating with this patient:

1. _____

_____

_____

2. _____

_____

_____

3.36 Below are several instances of nonverbal communication. For each incident, provide your interpretation by substituting a *verbal* equivalent.

a. A post–op patient who exhibited considerable pain during her last treatment "rolls" her eyes when you walk in to announce your return for additional therapy.

Verbal Equivalent:

_____

_____

_____

_____

b. Your clinical instructor pats you on the shoulder after a difficult cardiac arrest in which you took over responsibility for ventilating the patient.

Verbal Equivalent:

_____

_____

_____

c. A patient's mother turns away after being told by the pediatrician that her child has cystic fibrosis.

Verbal Equivalent:

_____

_____

_____

_____

d. A patient smiles broadly when you enter her room.

Verbal Equivalent:

_____

_____

_____

_____

e. You are assisting a physician with a difficult bronchoscopy. The patient reaches out for your hand.

Verbal Equivalent:

_____

_____

_____

_____

f. While you are interviewing a patient with a diagnosed terminal condition, he consistently stares blankly out the window. You find yourself having to repeat many questions.

Verbal Equivalent:

_____

_____

_____

_____

# 4

# Principles of Infection Control

## CONTENT EXERCISES

**True/False:** For each of the following statements, indicate whether it is mainly true or mainly false by circling the corresponding letter (T=True, F=False):

4.1 T F Among all hospital–acquired infections, nosocomial pulmonary infections are the most frequent cause of death.

4.2 T F Viruses are the most common cause of nosocomial infections in the hospital setting.

4.3 T F Whereas initial classification of bacteria by staining can be done quickly, metabolic tests can require 18 to 48 hours to complete.

4.4 T F The treatment of an infectious disease is usually postponed until final identification of the causative organism.

4.5 T F *Staphylococcus aureus* strains causing in–hospital infections are readily treated with regular penicillin.

4.6 T F The best treatment for pertussis (whooping cough) is prevention by immunization.

4.7 T F Oxygen under pressure (hyperbaric oxygen) helps prevent the spread of gas gangrene.

4.8 T F Spore–forming bacilli are the most difficult microorganisms to kill.

4.9 T F *Shigella dysenteriae* and *Salmonella typhi* are spread mainly via droplet nuclei in the air.

4.10 T F *Legionella pneumophila* (the cause of Legionnaires' disease) is readily communicable between patients.

4.11 T F Viral infections are controlled mainly by antibiotics.

4.12 T F Influenza epidemics are not a major concern in hospital infection control.

4.13 T F Infection of hospital personnel with the human immunodeficiency virus (HIV) occurs at a rate some 10 times greater than in the general population.

4.14 T F It is recommended that all health care personnel at high risk be immunized against hepatitis.

4.15 T F Most health care personnel who have contracted AIDS did so on their jobs.

4.16 T F The great majority of *Rickettsial* infections in the United States are in the form of Rocky Mountain spotted fever.

4.17 T F Opportunistic fungal infections are not a major problem in most hospital settings.

4.18 T F Salmonellosis and hepatitis A infections are transmitted mainly via the vehicle route.

4.19 T F Droplet nuclei do not remain suspended in the air for long periods of time.

4.20 T F Patients who have undergone instrumentation of the respiratory tract are at high risk for aspiration.

4.21 T F The first step in specialized equipment processing is decontamination.

4.22 T F Disinfection always kills spore–forming bacteria.

4.23 T F Soap or detergent residues on equipment can decrease the effectiveness of subsequent sterilization or disinfection procedures.

4.24 T F With heat sterilization, the higher the temperature used, the shorter the sterilization time.

4.25 T F Most of the materials used in respiratory care equipment can be sterilized with a steam autoclave.

4.26 T F Organic coatings on equipment (such as blood or pus) may protect microorganisms and prevent sterilization.

4.27 T F Equipment prepared for steam or ethylene oxide sterilization should be disassembled before processing.

4.28 T F Temperatures used in pasteurization are sufficient to kill all bacterial spores.

4.29 T F The internal machinery of ventilators and breathing machines must be sterilized between patients.

4.30 T F All disposable respiratory care equipment is presterilized by the manufacturer.

4.31 T F Only sterile fluids should be used to fill nebulizers and humidifiers.

4.32 T F Fluid reservoirs of large reservoir nondisposable nebulizers and humidifiers can be safely prefilled and stored for up to three days before use.

4.33 T F Manual resuscitation bags need only be thoroughly cleaned before use on different patients.

4.34 T F As long as they are kept refrigerated, multi–dose medication vials can be used after the expiration date given on the label.

4.35 T F Proper handwashing is the single most important means of preventing the spread of infection in the hospital.

4.36 T F Masks should be used by all persons in situations where airborne transmission of microorganisms is a possibility.

4.37 T F Gowns are necessary for most patient care activities.

4.38 T F Bags used for articles or waste materials that have been contaminated should be clearly labeled or color coded.

4.39 T F Patients requiring intensive care are not at high risk for acquiring serious nosocomial infections.

4.40 T F Immunocompromised patients can be mixed with patients having similar infectious diseases.

4.41 T F Protective isolation for immunocompromised patients is no better in preventing infection than strict adherence to proper handwashing protocols.

4.42 T F It is easy to reliably identify newly admitted patients who are infected with the HIV virus or other blood–borne infectious agents.

4.43 T F The CDC recommends that blood and body fluid precautions be consistently used for all patients.

4.44 T F According to the CDC, gloves and surgical masks are required for all invasive procedures.

4.45 T F The use of chemical indicators is generally sufficient to verify the efficacy of sterilization cycles.

4.46 T F Ventilator circuits with water humidifiers need be changed only every 48 to 72 hours.

**Short Answer:** Complete each statement by filling in the correct information in the space(s) provided:

4.47 The procedure used to broadly categorize bacteria into those that retain an initial stain after alcohol wash and those that do not is called the _____.

4.48 The _____ (also called the Ziehl–Neelsen stain) is used specifically to help identify organisms in the genus *Mycobacterium*.

4.49 _____ causes meningitis but can also cause septicemia, especially in susceptible hosts.

4.50 The highly communicable whooping cough is caused by _____.

4.51 The most important gram–positive non–spore–forming bacilli causing disease in humans is _____ _____.

4.52 A common cause of croup (laryngotracheal bronchitis) in infants is the _____ virus (related to the mumps virus).

4.53 The predominant cause of bronchiolitis in children less than one year old is the _____ virus.

4.54 Besides being the most common cause of blindness in the world, _____ also causes a nongonococcal urethritis and newborn conjunctivitis (by contact with the mother's genital tract).

4.55 Transmission of an infection through the conjunctivae, nose, or mouth of a susceptible host via contact with an infected person or carrier who is coughing or sneezing is an example of _____.

4.56 When a susceptible host is exposed to an infectious agent transmitted through contaminated food or water, the term _____ transmission is used.

4.57 _____ involves the dissemination of an infectious agent in the air, either by aerosol droplets, droplet nuclei, or dust particles.

4.58 The process which renders objects free from all living organisms is called _____.

4.59 The process which destroys only the vegetative form of pathogenic organisms is referred to as _____.

4.60 All heat sterilization methods must be sufficient enough to kill bacterial _____.

4.61 The most efficient sterilization agent is _____ _____.

4.62 That form of infection control designed to eliminate all vegetative bacteria and not just prevent the further growth of microorganisms is termed _____ _____.

4.63 After a large container (bottle) of fluid intended for use in a nebulizer or humidifier has been opened, unused fluid should be discarded within _____ hours.

4.64 Used articles that have been contaminated with infective material should be enclosed in an _____ before removal from the room of a patient on isolation precautions.

4.65 The grouping together of patients with the same infection is called _____.

4.66 The most common source of infection in immuno-compromised patients is _____.

4.67 Most major burn wounds become infected within _____ after the initial incident.

4.68 Health care workers who have _____
_____
should refrain from all direct patient care and from handling patient–care equipment until the condition resolves.

4.69 In order to provide assurance that a sterilization process has worked, one must use a _____ indicator.

4.70 Sampling and culturing in–use equipment helps to establish the frequency with which in–use items should be _____.

**Listing:** Complete each list as directed in its statement.

4.71 List the two (2) clinically significant genera of bacilli capable of spore formation:

1. _____

2. _____

4.72 List at least twelve (12) clinical conditions in which a patient's susceptibility to infection may be increased:

1. _____

2. _____

3. _____

4. _____

5. _____

6. _____

7. _____

8. _____

9. _____

10. _____

11. _____

12. _____

4.73 List several major components of the universal precautions recommended by the Centers for Disease Control (CDC) for health care workers according to the following categories:

a. Regarding Gloves:

_____

_____

_____

b. Regarding Masks and Protective Eyewear:

_____

_____

_____

c. Regarding Gowns or Aprons:

_____

_____

_____

d. Regarding Preventing Needlestick Injuries:

_____

_____

_____

e. Regarding Pregnant Health Care Workers:

_____

_____

_____

**Matching:**

4.74 Match each bacteria listed in the center column to the appropriate category letter label on the left:

| Category | Organism | Answer |
|---|---|---|
| a. Gram⁻ bacillus | *Staphylococcus aureus* | _____ |
| | *Haemophilus influenzae* | _____ |
| b. Spirochete | *Clostridium botulinum* | _____ |
| | *Mycobacterium tuberculosis* | _____ |
| c. Gram⁻ cocco–bacillus | *Leptospirae* | _____ |
| | *Pseudomonas aeruginosa* | _____ |
| d. Gram⁺ coccus | *Clostridium tetani* | _____ |
| | *Bordetella pertussis* | _____ |
| e. Acid–fast bacillus | *Streptococcus pneumoniae* | _____ |
| | *M. avium–intracellulare* | _____ |
| f. Gram⁺ spore–forming bacillus | *Clostridium perfringens* | _____ |
| | *Neisseria meningitidis* | _____ |
| g. Gram⁻ coccus | *Legionella pneumophila* | _____ |
| | *Serratia marcescens* | _____ |
| h. Gram⁺ non–spore–forming bacillus | *Corynebacterium diphtheriae* | _____ |
| | *Escherichia coli* | _____ |
| | *Treponema pallidum* | _____ |
| | *Proteus vulgaris* | _____ |
| | *Klebsiella pneumoniae* | _____ |
| | *Bacillus anthracis* | _____ |
| | *Streptococcus pyogenes* | _____ |

**Multiple Choice:** Circle the letter corresponding to the single best answer from the available choices:

4.75 Approximately what percentage of nosocomial infections are pulmonary in nature?

a. 5–10%
b. 60–70%
c. 40–50%
d. 10–40%

4.76 *Staphylococcus aureus* is implicated in pneumonia and other organ or systemic infections in which of the following groups of patients?
I.   infants and young children
II.  elderly patients
III. those debilitated by other disease processes

a. II and III          c. I and III
b. III only            d. I, II, and III

4.77 The primary cause of pneumococcal pneumonia is:

a. *Staphylococcus aureus*
b. *Streptococcus pyogenes*
c. *Streptococcus pneumoniae*
d. *Haemophilus influenzae*

4.78 The most important gram–negative coccobacillus responsible for respiratory infections in humans is:

a. *Staphylococcus aureus*
b. *Streptococcus pyogenes*
c. *Bordetella pertussis*
d. *Haemophilus influenzae*

4.79 Which of the following disease processes are caused by members of the genus *Clostridium*?
I.   tetanus
II.  gas gangrene
III. botulism
IV.  anthrax

a. I, II, and IV        c. II, III, and IV
b. I, II, and III       d. I, II, III, and IV

4.80 A gram⁻ bacillus which is normally found in the intestinal tract but can cause urinary tract infections and result in pneumonia, neonatal meningitis, and septicemia in debilitated or immunosuppressed patients best describes:

a. *Neisseria meningitidis*
b. *Haemophilus influenzae*
c. *Streptococcus pyogenes*
d. *Escherichia coli*

4.81 A gram⁻ bacillus which is highly resistant to many antibiotics; is often found in hospital sinks, drinking water, food, and respiratory care equipment; and is estimated to be the cause of 10% or more of hospital–acquired infections best describes:

a. *Pseudomonas aeruginosa*
b. *Haemophilus influenzae*
c. *Streptococcus pyogenes*
d. *Escherichia coli*

4.82 An aerobic bacillus that (1) is difficult to culture but appears to be gram⁻; (2) has been found in air conditioning units, shower heads, and respiratory care equipment; (3) is not readily communicable between patients; and (4) can result in high fever, chills, myalgia, nausea, and diarrhea best describes:

a. *Pseudomonas aeruginosa*
b. *Haemophilus influenzae*
c. *Legionella pneumophila*
d. *Klebsiella pneumoniae*

4.83 A formerly rare and highly resistant form of acid–fast bacillus infection now appearing with some frequency among AIDS patients best describes:

a. *Pneumocystis carinii*
b. *Mycobacterium leprae*
c. *Mycobacterium avium–intracellulare*
d. *Mycobacterium tuberculosis*

4.84 Which of the following are true regarding type B hepatitis?
I. it is caused by a DNA virus
II. it is also referred to as infectious hepatitis
III. infection results in a high mortality rate
IV. it is transmitted mainly via contaminated food or water

a. II, III, and IV          c. I and III
b. III and IV               d. I, II, III, and IV

4.85 A virus transmitted mainly by sexual contact or parenteral exposure that directly attacks the T–lymphocytes of the immune system best describes the:

a. herpes simplex virus
b. human immunodeficiency virus
c. varicella–zoster virus
d. Epstein–Barr virus

4.86 Ornithosis, a highly infectious pneumonia transmitted by contact with parrots, parakeets, pigeons, and other birds, is caused by:

a. *Chlamydia psittaci*
b. *Corynebacterium diphtheriae*
c. *Mycoplasma pneumoniae*
d. *Chlamydia trachomatis*

4.87 Which of the following statements regarding the fungi are true?
I. they include both molds and yeasts
II. they may cause primary or opportunistic infections
III. they are more complex and highly organized than bacteria
IV. they have a preference for warm, moist environments

a. II and III               c. I, III, and IV
b. II, III, and IV          d. I, II, III, and IV

4.88 A protozoal–type organism with both intra– and intercellular life stages that causes an acute interstitial pneumonia with high mortality rates, particularly in patients with impaired immune responses, best describes:

a. *Candida albicans*
b. *Rickettsia rickettsii*
c. *Mycoplasma pneumoniae*
d. *Pneumocystis carinii*

4.89 Which of the following are a primary source of infectious agents in the hospital?
I. animals (especially insects)
II. people (patients, personnel, or visitors)
III. contaminated equipment and medications

a. I and II                 c. II and III
b. I and III                d. I, II, and III

4.90 Which of the following factors contribute to the high incidence of nosocomial pneumonias in post–surgical patients?
I. impaired swallowing or respiratory clearance
II. postoperative surgical pain
III. use of narcotics and sedatives
IV. instrumentation of the respiratory tract

a. III and IV               c. I, III, and IV
b. II, III, and IV          d. I, II, III, and IV

4.91 A postoperative patient in ICU develops a *Pseudomonas pneumonia*. What is the most likely source of this infection?

a. indirect contact transmission via contaminated RT equipment
b. direct contact transmission via ICU visitors
c. airborne transmission via dust particles
d. indirect contact transmission via contaminated IV fluid

4.92 When a respiratory care practitioner with unwashed hands spreads an infection to a patient during change of a tracheostomy dressing, what is the route of transmission?

a. direct contact transmission
b. indirect contact transmission
c. vehicle transmission
d. airborne transmission

4.93 Which of the following are examples of infections transmitted via the droplet contact route?
I.   measles
II.  human immunodeficiency virus (HIV)
III. streptococcal pneumonia

a. I and III            c. I only
b. III only             d. I, II, and III

4.94 A patient develops hepatitis A after exposure to contaminated food. This is an example of what route of transmission?

a. direct contact transmission
b. indirect contact transmission
c. vehicle transmission
d. airborne transmission

4.95 Which of the following infections are transmitted mainly via the airborne route?
I.   legionellosis
II.  tuberculosis
III. fungal infections
IV.  AIDS

a. II, III, and IV      c. I, II, and III
b. II and III           d. I, II, III, and IV

4.96 Which of the following are major routes for spread of infectious agents into the lungs?
I.   airborne transmission of infectious agents
II.  blood–borne spread from a distant site
III. aspiration of oropharyngeal secretions

a. II and III           c. III only
b. I and III            d. I, II, and III

4.97 The goal of general sanitation measures is to:

a. kill all microorganisms present in the environment
b. eliminate all environmental sources of infectious agents
c. isolate infectious microorganisms in the environment
d. reduce microorganisms in the environment to a safe level

4.98 Instructions for an electrically powered respirometer clearly specify that it cannot be immersed in water. What procedure would you recommend to decontaminate this piece of equipment before further processing?

a. a quick wash in a fluorocarbon–based liquid
b. microwave heating at low energy for 3 minutes
c. surface disinfection with 70% alcohol
d. immersion in 2% glutaraldehyde for 10 minutes

4.99 Which of the following are correct statements concerning the use of ethylene oxide for sterilization?
I.   the gas is explosive in mixture with air
II.  the gas is toxic to living tissues
III. heat and humidity affect sterilization
IV.  the gas does not damage plastic or rubber

a. I and II             c. I, II, and IV
b. I and III            d. I, II, III, and IV

4.100 As a clinical infection control procedure, the major limitation of pasteurization is:

a. the complexity and cost of processing equipment
b. the potential damage to common respiratory equipment
c. the difficulty in training personnel in its use
d. the difficulty in preventing equipment recontamination

4.101 Which of the following chemical disinfectant solutions would you choose if the objective was to kill both the vegetative and spore forms of bacterial pathogens?

a. a glutaraldehyde solution
b. an alcohol solution (e.g., 70% ethyl alcohol)
c. a phenol solution (e.g., hexachlorophene)
d. a quaternary ammonium compound

4.102 Which of the following types of respiratory care equipment presents the greatest potential for spreading nosocomial infections?

a. small–volume medication nebulizers
b. heated cascade humidifiers
c. large reservoir jet nebulizers
d. unheated oxygen humidifiers

4.103 In order to minimize the likelihood of nebulizers serving as a source for transmission of infectious agents, all of the following procedures should be scrupulously followed *except:*

a. when refilling, discard old fluid remaining in reservoir
b. when checking, drain tubing condensate back into reservoir
c. change and replace with sterile equipment every 24 hours
d. avoid using nebulizers for purposes of room humidification

4.104 Cultures taken from a bedside electronic respirometer that has been used in the intensive care unit to monitor several patients indicate that it is contaminated. The most practical way to prevent cross–contamination would be to:

a. provide a new respirometer for each patient
b. sterilize the respirometer after each use
c. replace the respirometer with a water–sealed spirometer
d. use an extension piece with one–way valving for each patient

4.105 You are making equipment rounds to fill continuous–use nebulizers on a nursing unit. A large bottle of previously sterilized distilled water is dated as opened the prior day. You should:

a. use the water, but only for new equipment set–ups
b. discard the water and obtain an unopened sterile bottle
c. ask the nurse if it is okay to use the water
d. use an unopened IV fluid bottle marked "D5W"

4.106 Your supervisor gives you a multi–dose vial of an expensive medication for aerosol administration to patients on your shift. You note that the expiration date on the label was two days ago. The supervisor says that since the med is kept refrigerated, it is okay to use for another day or so. You should:

a. follow the supervisor's instructions and use the medication
b. check with the pharmacist to see if the med needs refrigeration
c. ask the medical director if it is okay to use the medication
d. discard the medication and obtain a new unexpired vial

4.107 Which of the following conditions conform to the CDC standards set for universal precautions?
I.      extreme care with sharp instruments
II.     gowns for touching blood/body fluids
III.    gloves for touching blood/body fluids
IV.     masks/protective eyewear for procedures involving droplets/splashing of blood or body fluids
V.      immediate skin/handwashing if contamination occurs

a. I and III          c. I, II, and III
b. II, IV, and V      d. I, II, III, IV, and V

4.108 Which of the following conditions conform to the standards set for a patient in tuberculosis (AFB) isolation?
I.      private room with special ventilation
II.     masks only if patient is coughing
III.    gloves required of all persons entering room
IV.     contaminated articles bagged/labeled before removal

a. I and II           c. II, III, and IV
b. II and IV          d. I, II, III, and IV

4.109 You are gathering a sputum specimen from a patient in strict isolation. Which of the following procedures should be followed in gathering, removing, and transporting this specimen?

I. disinfect outside of specimen container if contaminated
II. place specimen in a sturdy container with a secure lid
III. place specimen container in an impervious, labeled bag

a. III only
b. I, II, and III
c. II and III
d. I and III

4.110 During insertion of an arterial line in a patient under blood and body fluid precautions, a substantial amount of blood is spilled on a bedside table. Which of the following is the recommended procedure to deal with this spill?

a. clean the spill immediately with a sodium hypochlorite solution
b. let the spilled blood dry first, then notify housekeeping
c. spray the spill immediately with a phenol solution (e.g., Lysol)
d. wait 10 minutes, then clean the spill with a 70% alcohol solution

4.111 What is the primary purpose of using chemical indicators in equipment sterilization processing?

a. to warn the user about the presence of toxic residues
b. to indicate the remaining safe shelf–life of the equipment
c. to provide visual assurance that the item is truly sterile
d. to show that a package has been through a sterilizing process

4.112 The most critical aspect of equipment processing quality control is:

a. the application of equipment culture sampling methods
b. the existence of well–written policies and procedures
c. the monitoring and evaluation of adherence to procedures
d. the use of specially prepared processing indicators

4.113 Techniques used to monitor the presence of microorganisms on in–use respiratory care equipment include which of the following?

I. aerosol impaction
II. swab sampling
III. use of liquid broths
IV. spore indicator strips

a. I, III, and IV
b. II, III, and IV
c. I, II, and III
d. I, II, III, and IV

4.114 Which of the following is the major disadvantage of using biological indicators in equipment quality control?

a. the cost of the biological indicator systems themselves
b. the equipment down–time necessary to obtain culture results
c. the unreliability of biological indicator systems
d. the hazards of using spore–forming bacteria as indicators

4.115 Your department employs pasteurization to process most of its nondisposable respiratory care equipment. Which of the following techniques would you recommend as best able to evaluate the effectiveness of the pasteurization process?

a. place chemical indicator tape on equipment before immersion
b. culture a biological indicator after immersion in the water bath
c. obtain and culture bacteriologic samples from processed equipment
d. conduct an epidemiological study on all respiratory care patients

# 5

## Legal and Ethical Implications of the Practice

## CONTENT EXERCISES

**True/False:** For each of the following statements, indicate whether it is mainly true or mainly false by circling the corresponding letter (T=True, F=False):

5.1   T   F   Conventional knowledge and technical standards of good practice are always enough to ensure that respiratory care practitioners fulfill their roles competently.

5.2   T   F   The number and complexity of ethical dilemmas in health care have grown dramatically.

5.3   T   F   In the absence of some benchmark of what constitutes morally justifiable behavior, it is possible to argue in favor of almost any position.

5.4   T   F   Most Americans seeking health care want to know the full truth about their problem(s).

5.5   T   F   Confidentiality in health care provider–patient relationships is an absolute obligation in most professional codes of ethics.

5.6   T   F   According to formalist reasoning, an act is considered morally justifiable if and only if it upholds the rules or principles that apply.

5.7   T   F   The principle of utility aims to promote the greatest general good for the greatest number.

5.8   T   F   The most common torts brought against health care professionals fall under the category of malpractice.

5.9   T   F   In regard to the tort of negligence, health care providers are generally held to a higher standard than the average person.

5.10  T   F   Respiratory care practitioners are required by their scope of practice to work under competent medical supervision.

5.11  T   F   The legal scope of practice for respiratory care practitioners is normally defined in hospital policy and procedure manuals.

5.12  T   F   Anyone who willfully solicits, receives, offers, or pays any remuneration in return for Medicare business is guilty of a criminal offense.

5.13  T   F   According to the American Medical Association, the discontinuance of life–prolonging medical treatment is ethical only in the case of clearly terminal illnesses.

**Short Answer:** Complete each statement by filling in the correct information in the space(s) provided:

5.14  Choices and actions that go beyond prevailing technical standards in health care usually involve the areas of _____ or _____.

5.15  When professional _____ are insufficient to address a moral dilemma, one must turn to the concepts and principles of _____.

5.16  Each ethical principle consists of two components: a _____ and a _____.

5.17  The two basic requirements inherent in the principle of autonomy are freedom to _____ and freedom to act _____.

5.18  The tendency among health workers to assume that they know what is best for the patient is called _____.

5.19  Breaching patient confidentiality in order to protect the welfare of the community is based primarily on the ethical viewpoint called _____.

5.20  That type of justice which deals with the allocation of scarce resources and the proper distribution of benefits and burdens in a society is termed _____ _____.

5.21  The ethical viewpoint in which moral principles or rules function apart from the consequences of a particular action is called _____.

5.22  That form of law which seeks to protect individuals from others who might seek to take unfair and unlawful advantage of them is called _____ law.

5.23  When a respiratory care practitioner fails to exercise an adequate degree of care in performing a prescribed therapeutic procedure, she may be guilty of _____.

5.24 The major element of battery is _____ without consent.

5.25 That form of consent which operates when a patient solicits care from a health care practitioner and which allows for ordinary procedures to be performed without formal written consent is called _____ _____.

5.26 The pretrial component of a civil suit during which both parties engage in fact–finding is termed the _____ phase.

5.27 An employer of a respiratory care practitioner may under certain conditions be liable for the actions of the practitioner. This liability is based on the legal principle _____.

5.28 Use of life–prolonging technologies often creates a dilemma between health professionals' obligations to _____ and _____.

5.29 Statutes that protect citizens from civil or criminal liability for acts of omission occurring during attempts to give emergency aid are referred to as _____ _____.

**Listing:** Complete each list as directed in its statement.

5.30 List at least three (3) reasons why the number and complexity of ethical dilemmas in health care are increasing:

1. _____

_____

2. _____

_____

3. _____

_____

5.31 List the two (2) conditions that generally must be met to demonstrate that dereliction occurred in the course of the employer–employee relationship (legal principle of respondeat superior):

1. _____

_____

2. _____

_____

5.32 List at least five (5) key elements normally found in a state practice act:

1. _____

2. _____

3. _____

4. _____

5. _____

5.33 According to the American Hospital Association, a patient has the right to receive from his physician information necessary to give *informed* consent prior to the start of any procedure and/or treatment. List the four (4) major components of informed consent described by the American Hospital Association:

1. _____

_____

2. _____

_____

3. _____

_____

4. _____

_____

**Multiple Choice:** Circle the letter corresponding to the single best answer from the available choices:

5.34 The ethical principle which acknowledges patients' personal liberty and their right to decide upon their own course best describes:

a. nonmaleficence
b. justice
c. veracity
d. autonomy

5.35 The ethical principle which binds the health giver and the patient to tell the truth best describes:

a. nonmaleficence
b. justice
c. veracity
d. beneficence

5.36 The act of "benevolent deception" involves a conflict among which of the following ethical principles?
I.    nonmaleficence
II.   veracity
III.  beneficence

a. I, II, and III      c. I and II
b. II and III          d. II only

5.37 The ethical principle which obligates health care professionals to actively prevent harm to patients best describes:

a. justice
b. veracity
c. beneficence
d. nonmaleficence

5.38 The ethical principle which requires health practitioners to actively contribute to the health and well-being of the patients they serve best describes:

a. justice
b. veracity
c. nonmaleficence
d. beneficence

5.39 The ethical principle which requires that like cases should be treated alike and that different cases be treated differently best describes:

a. justice
b. autonomy
c. veracity
d. nonmaleficence

5.40 A claim of private or civil wrong or injury, other than breach of contract, for which a civil court will provide a remedy in the form of damages is known as a(n):

a. felony
b. misdemeanor
c. tort
d. offense

5.41 Professional negligence represents which type of malpractice?

a. moral malpractice
b. civil malpractice
c. social malpractice
d. ethical malpractice

5.42 Which of the following are examples of criminal malpractice?
I.    negligence
II.   assault and battery
III.  euthanasia

a. I only            c. I and II
b. II and III        d. I, II, and III

5.43 Which of the following are necessary in order to validate a claim of professional negligence?
I.    the health care provider must owe a legal duty to the patient
II.   the duty must have been breached by provision of substandard care
III.  the breach in duty must cause actual harm to the patient

a. III only          c. I and II
b. II and III        d. I, II, and III

5.44 In a civil court, a former patient is suing a respiratory care practitioner for permanent damage to her teeth resulting from an intubation. The plaintiff's lawyer argues that this harm would not have happened if the practitioner had used appropriate care. What legal principle is the plaintiff's lawyer using as a basis for this argument?

a. implied consent
b. respondeat superior
c. res ipsa loquitur
d. strict liability

5.45 A respiratory care practitioner remarks to a post–op patient that her surgeon is a "butcher" and suggests that she not return to him for follow–up care. What act might the respiratory care practitioner be charged with by the surgeon?

a. negligence
b. slander
c. libel
d. assault

5.46 You become aware of a respiratory care staff member accepting gratuities for preferential consideration of a patient. Some time after you express your concerns to this individual and his supervisor, the actions continue. Your next step should be to report these incidents to the:

a. local police force
b. AARC Judicial Committee
c. U.S. Department of Health and Human Services
d. Federal Bureau of Investigation
e. State Hospital Association

**Matching:**

5.47 Below on the left are the key provisions of the AARC Code of Ethics. On the right are listed several incidents representing potential violations of this code. In the space provided next to each incident, cite (by letter) the provision of the code that is being violated.

<u>CODE PROVISION</u>

a. The respiratory care practitioner shall practice medically acceptable methods of treatment and shall not endeavor to extend his practice beyond his competence and the authority vested in him by the physician.

b. The respiratory care practitioner shall continually strive to increase and improve his knowledge and skill and render to each patient the full measure of his ability. All services shall be provided with respect for the dignity of the patient, unrestricted by considerations of social or economic status, personal attributes, or the nature of health problems.

c. The respiratory care practitioner shall be responsible for the competent and efficient performance of his assigned duties and shall expose incompetence and illegal or unethical conduct of members of the profession.

d. The respiratory care practitioner shall hold in strict confidence all privileged information concerning the patient and refer all inquiries to the physician in charge of the patient's medical care.

e. The respiratory care practitioner shall not accept gratuities for preferential consideration of the patient. He shall not solicit patients for personal gain and shall guard against conflicts of interest.

f. The respiratory care practitioner shall uphold the dignity and honor of the profession and abide by its ethical principles. He should be familiar with existing state and federal laws governing the practice of respiratory therapy and comply with those laws.

g. The respiratory care practitioner shall cooperate with other health care professionals and participate in activities to promote community and national efforts to meet the health needs of the public.

<u>INCIDENT</u>

_____ a respiratory care practitioner refuses to cooperate with the nursing staff in planning a community health promotion program

_____ based on her readings of some new animal research studies, a respiratory care practitioner modifies a therapeutic procedure without consulting the ordering physician

_____ a respiratory care practitioner knowingly assigns an individual without formal training to provide bedside care in a state where practice is limited to graduates of accredited respiratory care programs

_____ a respiratory care practitioner refers a patient's family only to her friend's home care equipment company

_____ a respiratory care practitioner refuses to treat a patient who is HIV positive (suspected of having AIDS)

_____ a respiratory care practitioner is overheard discussing a patient's sexual orientation in the elevator, using the patient's name

_____ a respiratory care practitioner observes another staff member on several occasions using an outdated and dangerous therapeutic technique

_____ a respiratory care practitioner who completed an approved therapist program in 1970 does not read the professional literature and has not attended a staff development or continuing education program since graduation

# Terms, Symbols, and Units of Measure

## CONTENT EXERCISES

**Short Answer:** Complete each statement by filling in the correct information in the space(s) provided:

6.1 Use standard root words, combining forms, prefixes, and/or suffixes to derive the appropriate medical term for each of the following:

_____ greater than normal acid in the urine

_____ increased alkalinity in the blood

_____ from the front to the back of the body

_____ an absence of spontaneous breathing

_____ a small artery

_____ without symptoms

_____ the presence of bacteria in the blood

_____ a slow heart rate (less than 60/min)

_____ inflammation of the bronchi

_____ visual examination of the bronchial tree

_____ cancer–causing

_____ enlargement of the heart

_____ of or pertaining to the ribs and diaphragm

_____ difficulty in swallowing

_____ difficult or labored breathing

_____ a tracing of the heart's electrical activity

_____ within the trachea

_____ an increased number of eosinophils in the blood

_____ bleeding from the nose

_____ outside a cell or cell tissue

_____ to withdraw a tube from the body

_____ coughing up of blood from the respiratory tract

_____ the stoppage of bleeding

_____ an accumulation of blood in the thorax

_____ abnormal enlargement of the liver

_____ excess carbon dioxide in the blood

_____ lower than normal glucose in the blood

_____ a condition with decreased muscle tone

_____ a deficiency of oxygen in the blood

_____ within the alveoli

_____ within a blood vessel

_____ a surgical incision into the abdomen

_____ an abnormal decrease in white blood cells

_____ toxic or destructive to a kidney

_____ the presence of air in the thorax

_____ situated behind and to one side or the other

_____ pus–producing

_____ inflammation of the nose

_____ an abnormally rapid rate of breathing

_____ softening of the trachea

_____ the procedure by which an incision is made into the trachea

_____ a narrowing of any blood vessel

6.2   In the space provided, translate each of the following medical terms into plain English:

acidemia _____

anaerobic _____

anemia _____

anesthetic _____

asepsis _____

asystole _____

atelectasis _____

atrophy _____

bacteriocidal _____

bradypnea _____

bronchiectasis _____

bronchiolitis _____

bronchoconstriction _____

bronchopleural fistula _____

capnograph _____

cardiogenic _____

cerebrovascular _____

costochondral _____

cricothyrotomy _____

cyanosis _____

decongestant _____

decontamination _____

diaphoresis _____

diuresis _____

ectopic _____

electromyography _____

embolization _____

empyema _____

endocarditis _____

endogenous _____

epigastric _____

erythema _____

erythrocythemia _____

extrathoracic _____

fungicide _____

genitourinary _____

hematopoiesis _____

hemolysis _____

hyperinflation _____

hyperkalemia _____

hyperoxia _____

hyperplasia _____

hyperpnea _____

hypertrophy _____

hypochloremia _____

hypopnea _____

hypothermia _____

hypoxia _____

infiltrate _____

interstitial _____

intramuscular _____

intrapleural _____

laryngoscopy _____

laryngospasm _____

lobectomy _____

lymphadenopathy _____

midsternal _____

nocturia _____

oliguria _____

orthopnea _____

oximeter _____

pericarditis _____

pleurisy _____

pneumonectomy _____

polycythemia _____

radiolucent _____

sclerosis _____

septicemia _____

tachycardia _____
_____

thoracentesis _____
_____

thoracotomy _____
_____

thrombolysis _____
_____

tracheostomy _____
_____

transbronchial _____
_____

venule _____
_____

6.3   In the space provided, define each of the following medical abbreviations:

ABG _____

a.c. _____

ad lib. _____

ADH _____

AFB _____

AP _____

ARDS _____

ASHD _____

B.I.D., b.i.d. _____

BP _____

$\bar{c}$ _____

CA, Ca _____

CAD _____

CBC _____

CC _____

cc _____

CHF _____

COPD _____

CPR _____

CSF _____

CVA _____

CXR _____

/d _____

Dx _____

ECG, EKG _____

GI _____

Gtt., gtt. _____

GU _____

Gyn _____

HCT, Hct _____

Hg _____

HGB, Hgb, Hb _____

h.s. _____

IM _____

I.V., IV _____

LAT, lat. _____

mcg _____

MI _____

NPO _____

od _____

OR _____

os _____

paren _____

P.C., p.c. _____

PND _____

P.O. _____

p.r.n. _____

q.d. _____

q.h. _____

Q.I.D., q.i.d. _____

qm _____

qn _____

RBC _____

Rx _____

$\overline{s}$ _____

SOB _____

Stat. _____

subcu., SC _____

TB _____

T.I.D, t.i.d. _____

TPR _____

UA _____

URI _____

WBC _____

**Translating Pulmonary Abbreviations:** The following equations make extensive use of selected pulmonary abbreviations. Translate each into one or more sentences which indicate the relationship among the variables:

6.4

$$P_A CO_2 = \frac{\mathring{V}CO_2 \times .863}{V_A}$$

Your Translation:

_____

_____

_____

_____

_____

_____

6.5

$$P_L = P_{alv} - P_{pl}$$

Your Translation:

_____

_____

_____

_____

_____

6.6

$$\mathring{V}_E = f \times V_T$$

Your Translation:

_____

_____

_____

_____

_____

6.7

$$\frac{V_D}{V_T} = \frac{Paco_2 - P\overline{E}co_2}{Paco_2}$$

Your Translation:

_____

_____

_____

_____

_____

6.8

$$\overset{\circ}{Q} = \frac{\overset{\circ}{V}o_2}{C(a - \overline{v})o_2 \times 10}$$

Your Translation:

_____

_____

_____

_____

_____

_____

6.9

$$\frac{\overset{\circ}{Q}s}{\overset{\circ}{Q}_C} = \frac{Cco_2 - Cao_2}{Cco_2 - C\overline{v}o_2}$$

Your Translation:

_____

_____

_____

_____

_____

_____

**Computations:** Compute each conversion as specified, placing your answer in the space provided:

6.10
**Using Prefixes**

a. 35 cm = _____ mm (millimeters)

b. 1 mm = _____ m (micrometers)

c. 250 msec = _____ sec (seconds)

d. 1 dL = _____ L (liters)

e. 2.40 L = _____ ml (milliliters)

f. 4550 ml = _____ L (liters)

g. 2.65 kg = _____ gm (grams)

h. 600 gm = _____ kg (kilograms)

i. .01 gm = _____ mg (milligrams)

j. 35 mg = _____ gm (grams)

k. 2 mg = _____ g (micrograms)

6.11
**Unit Conversions – Length**

a. 6.10 ft = _____ cm (centimeters)

b. 9.50 in = _____ cm (centimeters)

c. 18.50 cm = _____ in (inches)

d. 26.30 cm = _____ m (meters)

e. 2.40 m = _____ cm (centimeters)

f. 1.85 m = _____ ft (feet)

g. .35 m = _____ in (inches)

6.12
## Unit Conversions – Volume

a. 244 ft$^3$ = _____ gallons (US)

b. 22 ft$^3$ = _____ L (liters)

c. 1.50 gallons = _____ L (liters)

d. 6900 L = _____ ft$^3$ (cubic feet)

e. 2.50 L = _____ gallons (US)

f. 6.85 gallons = _____ ft$^3$ (cubic feet)

g. 1.00 dL = _____ cm$^3$ (cubic centimeters; cc)

6.13
## Unit Conversions – Weight

a. 65 kg = _____ lb (pounds)

b. 185 lb = _____ kg (kilograms)

c. 32 g = _____ oz (ounces)

d. 8.50 oz = _____ g (grams; gm)

e. 1500 g = _____ lb (pounds)

f. 5.60 lb = _____ g (grams; gm)

6.14
## Unit Conversions – Pressure

a. 14.70 lb/in$^2$ = _____ Pa (Pascals)

b. 2200 lb/in$^2$ = _____ kPa (kilo/Pascals)

c. 32.50 Pa = _____ dynes/cm$^2$

d. 63 dynes/cm$^2$ = _____ Pa (Pascals)

6.15
## Unit Conversions – Work and Energy

a. 47 BTU = _____ cal (calories)

b. 6500 cal = _____ BTU

c. 50 cal = _____ J (Joule)

d. .0025 J = _____ ergs (dyne–cm)

e. 6845000 ergs = _____ J (Joule)

# 7

# Physical Principles in Respiratory Care

## CONTENT EXERCISES

**True/False:** For each of the following statements, indicate whether it is mainly true or mainly false by circling the corresponding letter (T=True, F=False):

7.1   T   F   Both liquids and gases are considered fluids.

7.2   T   F   Most of the internal energy of a gas is in the form of potential energy.

7.3   T   F   Heat cannot be transferred between two objects unless they are in contact with each other.

7.4   T   F   The energy required to effect the freezing process is the same as that needed to cause melting.

7.5   T   F   The viscosity of a homogenous fluid varies inversely with changes in its temperature.

7.6   T   F   Surface tension forces tend to decrease the pressure within a drop or bubble of liquid.

7.7   T   F   The warmer a gas, the less water vapor it can hold.

7.8   T   F   At a constant temperature and pressure, two gases with the same number of molecules occupy the same volume.

7.9   T   F   With temperature and mass constant, the volume of a gas varies directly with its pressure.

7.10   T   F   If the pressure and mass of a gas are kept constant, its volume will vary directly with changes in its absolute temperature.

7.11   T   F   If the volume and mass of a gas remain fixed, an increase in its temperature will cause the pressure exerted by the gas to rise.

7.12   T   F   No pressure can keep oxygen in its liquid form above a temperature of –118.8°C (–181.1 °F).

7.13   T   F   Under conditions of turbulent flow, driving pressure is linearly proportional to the flow.

7.14   T   F   With a constant driving pressure, if the cross–sectional area of a tube is halved, the velocity of a fluid moving through the tube will double.

**Short Answer:** Complete each statement by filling in the correct information in the space(s) provided:

7.15 The temperature of a substance represents a measure of its _____.

7.16 According to the The First Law of Thermodynamics, the energy gained by a substance in any physical process must be _____ the energy lost by its surroundings.

7.17 When two objects in proximity to each other are at the same temperature, a state of _____ exists.

7.18 The additional heat energy needed to effect the changeover from solid to liquid is referred to as the _____ _____.

7.19 The device used to measure specific gravity in the clinical setting is called the _____.

7.20 In cgs units, the viscosity of a fluid is measured in a unit called a _____.

7.21 The attractive force between like molecules is termed _____.

7.22 The change of state from the liquid to the vapor phase of matter is called _____.

7.23 The temperature at which the vapor pressure of a liquid equals the pressure exerted on the liquid by the surrounding atmosphere is termed the _____ _____.

7.24 The kinetic activity of water vapor molecules in a gas is measured as the _____ _____.

7.25 The actual content or weight of water present in a given volume of air is called the _____ _____.

7.26 The ratio of the actual water vapor present in a gas compared with the capacity of that gas to hold the vapor at a given temperature is called the _____ _____.

7.27 The physical process whereby atoms or molecules tend to move from an area of higher pressure to an area of lower pressure is termed _____.

7.28 The _____ is that combination of temperature and pressure that allows the solid, liquid, and vapor forms of a given substance to exist in equilibrium with one another.

7.29 The highest temperature at which a substance can exist as a liquid is called the _____ _____.

7.30 As a fluid flows through a stricture, its velocity _____ and its lateral pressure _____.

7.31 A venturi tube employs a precise angulation distal to an orifice in order to _____ fluid pressure.

7.32 The major advantages of fluidic devices over comparable mechanical systems is their _____, their _____, and their _____.

7.33 The physical principle underlying most fluidic circuitry is a phenomenon called the _____ effect or the _____ effect.

**Listing:** Complete each list as directed in its statement.

7.34 List two (2) means by which the internal energy of an object may be increased:

1. _____

2. _____

7.35 List three (3) synonyms for the invisible moisture present in the atmosphere:

1. _____

2. _____

3. _____

**Multiple Choice:** Circle the letter corresponding to the single best answer from the available choices:

7.36 Which of the following characteristics correctly describe the gaseous state of matter?
I.   gases exhibit the phenomenon of flow
II.  intermolecular forces of attraction are minimal
III. gases are easily compressible
IV.  gases expand to fill their container

a. I, II, and III      c. II, III, and IV
b. I and II      d. I, II, III, and IV

7.37 The primary means by which heat transfer occurs in fluids, both liquids and gases, is:

a. radiation
b. conduction
c. convection
d. evaporation

7.38 Which of the following will increase the radiant heat loss of an object with a given emissivity (assuming all else remains constant)?
I.   an increase in the surface area of the object
II.  a reduction in the temperature around the object
III. an increase in the object's temperature
IV.  an increase in the temperature around the object

a. I, II, and III      c. II, III, and IV
b. I and II      d. I, II, III, and IV

7.39 According to Pascal's principle, the pressure exerted by a liquid in a container is dependent on which of the following?
I.   the depth of the liquid
II.  the shape of the container
III. the density of the liquid

a. II and III      c. I and III
b. I and II      d. I, II, and III

7.40 The change in state of a substance from its liquid to its gaseous form that occurs below its boiling point best describes:

a. sublimation
b. vaporization
c. evaporation
d. boiling

7.41 An equilibrium condition in which a gas holds all the water vapor molecules it can hold best describes:

a. saturation
b. relative humidity
c. pressure stabilization
d. body humidity

7.42 The molar volume of an ideal gas at STPD is:

a. 6.023 liters
b. 22.4 liters
c. 1034 liters
d. 43.8 liters

7.43 According to Graham's law, which of the following gases would diffuse most quickly (d = density)?

a. d = 1.432 gm/L
b. d = 1.567 gm/L
c. d = 0.834 gm/L
d. d = 0.543 gm/L

7.44 The rate of molecular diffusion of both gases and liquids can be increased by:
I. increasing their temperature
II. mechanically agitating the mixture
III. increasing the ambient pressure

a. I and III          c. II and III
b. I and II           d. I, II, and III

7.45 Which of the following factors determine the pressure exerted by a gas?
I. the frequency of particle collisions
II. the velocity of the particles
III. the number of particles present

a. I and II           c. II and III
b. II only            d. I, II, and III

7.46 Which of the following occurs when water vapor is added to a dry gas at a constant pressure?
I. the volume occupied by the gas mixture will increase
II. the relative humidity of the mixture will decrease
III. the partial pressure of the original gas will be reduced

a. I and II           c. I and III
b. II and III         d. I, II, and III

7.47 Which of the following medical gases can be maintained in the liquid form at room temperature?
I. oxygen
II. carbon dioxide
III. nitrous oxide
IV. helium

a. I and II           c. II and III
b. II, III, and IV    d. I, II, III, and IV

7.48 The temperature necessary to liquefy oxygen at one atmosphere pressure is:

a. −118.8°C
b. −183.0°C
c. −181.1°F
d. −463.3°F

7.49 According to Poiseuille's law, the pressure difference necessary to drive a fluid flowing in a laminar pattern through a tube will increase under which of the following conditions?
I. increased fluid viscosity
II. decreased tube length
III. increased rate of flow
IV. decreased tube radius

a. I and II           c. I, III, and IV
b. II, III, and IV    d. I, II, III, and IV

7.50 Which of the following design components of an air injector would result in entraining the greatest amount of air?
I. a small orifice jet
II. large entrainment ports
III. low velocity gas flow

a. I and II           c. I and III
b. II only            d. I, II, and III

## Computations:

7.51 Fill in the blank temperature values using standard conversion formulae:

| | °K | °C | °F |
|---|---|---|---|
| a. | 347 | _____ | _____ |
| b. | _____ | 20 | _____ |
| c. | _____ | _____ | 104 |
| d. | 330 | _____ | _____ |
| e. | _____ | 10 | _____ |
| f. | _____ | _____ | 93 |

7.52 Compute the pressure in $gm/cm^2$ exerted by the following fluid columns: (Hint: Be sure to first convert all column heights to centimeters.)

| Fluid | Density (gm/cm³) | Column Height | Pressure (gm/cm²) |
|---|---|---|---|
| a. mercury | 13.60 | 740 mm | _____ |
| b. mercury | 13.60 | 76.80 cm | _____ |
| c. water | 1.00 | 99 ft | _____ |
| d. water | 1.00 | 10 in | _____ |

7.53 The following data are known for three liquid bubbles:

| Bubble | Surface Tension (dynes/cm) | Bubble Radius (cm) | Bubble Pressure (dynes/cm²) |
|---|---|---|---|
| a. Bubble 1 | 60 | .01 | _____ |
| b. Bubble 2 | 60 | .005 | _____ |
| c. Bubble 3 | 20 | .005 | _____ |

a. Compute the pressure due to surface tension for each of the three bubbles in $dynes/cm^2$ (right column above).

b. Explain the significance of the difference between bubble 1 and bubble 2 and between bubble 2 and bubble 3.

_____

_____

_____

7.54
a. Using Table 4–5 (Water Vapor Pressures and Contents at Selected Temperatures), compute (1) saturated capacity, (2) percent relative humidity, and (3) the percent body humidity of the following samples of air:

| Air Sample # | Temp °C | H₂O Content (mg/L) | Saturated Capacity (mg/L) | Percent Relative Humidity | Percent Body Humidity |
|---|---|---|---|---|---|
| 1 | 20 | 10.00 | _____ | _____ | _____ |
| 2 | 22 | 12.93 | _____ | _____ | _____ |
| 3 | 33 | 10.50 | _____ | _____ | _____ |
| 4 | 30 | 27.65 | _____ | _____ | _____ |
| 5 | 37 | 30.00 | _____ | _____ | _____ |

b. The American National Standards Institute has set 10 mg/L as the minimum water vapor content needed in medical gases supplied to patients breathing through their intact upper airway. Approximately what % relative and body humidity is this equivalent to at 20°C?

_____ % relative humidity    _____ % body humidity

c. The American National Standards Institute has set 30 mg/L as the minimum water vapor content needed in medical gases supplied to patients whose upper airways have been bypassed. Approximately what % relative and body humidity is this equivalent to at 37°C?

_____ % relative humidity    _____ % body humidity

7.55

a. Compute the densities of the following gas mixtures in gm/L:

| Gas 1 | | | Gas 2 | | | Density of Mixture |
|---|---|---|---|---|---|---|
| Gas | GMW | Percent | Gas | GMW | Percent | |
| oxygen | 32 | 50% + | nitrogen | 28 | 50% | _____ |
| oxygen | 32 | 95% + | carbon dioxide | 44 | 5% | _____ |
| oxygen | 32 | 90% + | carbon dioxide | 44 | 10% | _____ |
| oxygen | 32 | 20% + | helium | 4 | 80% | _____ |
| oxygen | 32 | 30% + | helium | 4 | 70% | _____ |

b. Assuming that the flow pattern is turbulent, which of the above mixtures would result in the least resistance to flow?

_____

c. Assuming that the flow pattern is turbulent, which of the above mixtures would result in the greatest resistance to flow?

_____

7.56 In order to calibrate your blood gas analyzer in the pulmonary function laboratory you must obtain a corrected barometric pressure reading each day of the week. Given the following data, compute the corrected barometric pressure for each day to the nearest 0.1 mm Hg:

| | Temperature (°C) | Uncorrected $P_B$ | Corrected $P_B$ |
|---|---|---|---|
| Monday | 19 | 760 | _____ |
| Tuesday | 21 | 750 | _____ |
| Wednesday | 17 | 740 | _____ |
| Thursday | 20 | 745 | _____ |
| Friday | 23 | 755 | _____ |

7.57 Complete the following table using standard pressure unit conversion factors:

| | cm $H_2O$ | kPa | mm Hg |
|---|---|---|---|
| a. | 40.00 | _____ | _____ |
| b. | _____ | 6.00 | _____ |
| c. | _____ | _____ | 120.00 |
| d. | 8.00 | _____ | _____ |
| e. | _____ | 3.50 | _____ |
| f. | _____ | _____ | 80.00 |

7.58

a. Assuming a corrected barometric pressure of 755 mm Hg, compute the partial pressures of the following gases in air to the nearest hundredth (.01). Check your computations by summing the partial pressures (TOTAL).

| Gas in Air | Percent (as decimal) | Partial Pressure |
|---|---|---|
| nitrogen | .7808 | _____ mm Hg |
| oxygen | .2095 | _____ mm Hg |
| argon | .0093 | _____ mm Hg |
| carbon dioxide | .0003 | _____ mm Hg |
| | TOTAL | _____ mm Hg |

b. Explain why the total pressure you computed does not exactly equal the barometric pressure.

_____

_____

7.59  The following oxygen/nitrogen mixtures are fully saturated with water vapor at 37°C ($PH_2O$ = 47 mm Hg). Compute the corrected partial pressure of oxygen in each mixture:

| Percent Oxygen | Corrected $P_B$ | Partial Pressure of Oxygen ($Po_2$) |
| --- | --- | --- |
| 21% | 758 | _____ |
| 40% | 765 | _____ |
| 70% | 749 | _____ |
| 100% | 760 | _____ |

7.60  The following represent the partial pressures of the key gases in the lungs breathing room air at a barometric pressure of 760 mm Hg. Compute the percentage of each gas in the lungs. Then check your computations by totaling both the partial pressures and percentages.

| Gas in Lungs | Partial Pressure | Percent of Total |
| --- | --- | --- |
| nitrogen | 573 | _____ |
| oxygen | 100 | _____ |
| carbon dioxide | 40 | _____ |
| water vapor | 47 | _____ |
| TOTALS | _____ | _____ |

# Computer Applications in Respiratory Care

## CONTENT EXERCISES

**True/False:** For each of the following statements, indicate whether it is mainly true or mainly false by circling the corresponding letter (T=True, F=False):

8.1   T   F   Computers are capable only of quickly performing mathematical computations.

8.2   T   F   There are few things that people can do better than computers.

8.3   T   F   A computer can decide if the answers it provides make sense.

8.4   T   F   Computers can simulate some intellectual processes that resemble human thought.

8.5   T   F   Data stored in a computer's random access memory (RAM) are lost when the power is shut off.

8.6   T   F   All keyboard function keys do the same thing in all application programs.

8.7   T   F   Analog data can be directly analyzed by a digital computer.

8.8   T   F   A computer monitor is the most common output device.

8.9   T   F   Most conventional computer programs are based on a logical structure called an algorithm.

8.10  T   F   A computer can "acquire" knowledge from human experts.

8.11  T   F   Most artificial intelligence software uses traditional algorithmic processes.

8.12  T   F   Digital computers have been used in respiratory care for less than a decade.

8.13  T   F   Simple algorithmic processes are satisfactory for computer–based diagnosis of diseases.

8.14  T   F   Interpretation of arterial blood gas test results by health professionals remains highly unreliable.

8.15  T   F   Computer–based patient data systems in most hospitals are well integrated.

**Short Answer:** Complete each statement by filling in the correct information in the space(s) provided:

8.16  Computer data and instructions are stored in the form of binary digits called _____.

8.17  Problems which cannot be reduced to objective numeric or logical equations are termed _____ problems.

8.18  An _____ is a small silicon–base semiconductor "chip" consisting of thousands of miniaturized transistors.

8.19  The capability of a computer to rapidly "juggle" two or more activities using separate time allocations is called _____.

8.20  _____ is a method used to speed computations by dividing a single large task into many smaller tasks, each performed by a separate microprocessor.

8.21  Electronic "space" where data or instructions are stored best describes a computer's _____.

8.22  Eight binary digits (bits) combine to form a _____.

8.23  Permanent preprogrammed instructions are stored in a computer's _____.

8.24  Semiconductor chips that temporarily store binary data or instructions for use by a computer's CPU best describes _____.

8.25  The storage capacity of tape and disk media varies according to the _____ of the magnetized material on its surface.

8.26  The most common way for a user to enter data into a computer is through a _____.

8.27  In graphic–intensive applications, cursor control may be separately provided by an additional input device such as a _____.

8.28  _____ is a standardized input code designed to make various types of data processing and communications machines compatible.

8.29  An _____ is a device which scans visual information, translates it into digital form, and inputs it into a computer.

8.30  A tiny dot of light that can be turned on or off on the monitor screen display best describes a _____ _____.

8.31  In scientific applications, most computer input data is in _____ format.

8.32  In order to convert computer output into hard copy, you need a _____.

8.33  A human operator instructs a computer what to do and how to do it using _____ _____.

8.34  An _____ is a clearly defined, step–by–step procedure for solving a specific problem.

8.35  A series of operating system commands designed to function in sequence is called a _____ _____.

8.36  A common multipurpose application program designed specifically for numeric manipulation is the _____.

8.37  Application software used to manipulate numeric data use mathematical algorithms called _____ to handle computations.

8.38  A database is simply a collection of _____.

8.39  The process by which a remote computer accesses and receives data stored on a host system is called _____.

8.40  Most communication protocols provide an _____ mechanism to help identify errors occurring during data transmission.

**Multiple Choice:** Circle the letter corresponding to the single best answer from the available choices:

8.41  A computer's ability to take charge of or operate external devices best describes which of the following functions?

a. retrieve function
b. sort function
c. control function
d. translate function

8.42  A computer which is observing external events and is programmed to take action if certain conditions are met is performing which of the following functions?

a. retrieve function
b. monitor function
c. control function
d. translate function

8.43  When a computer examines data and puts it in a particular order or format, it is:

a. storing
b. retrieving
c. calculating
d. sorting

8.44  A computer can do all of the following *except*:

a. perform mathematical operations
b. reason about input or output values
c. reach conclusions based on certain conditions
d. control and operate external devices

8.45  Major software advances likely to occur throughout the 1990s include which of the following?
I.    expert systems/artificial intelligence
II.   Computer–Aided Software Engineering
III.  automated programming
IV.   natural language processing

a. II and IV            c. I and III
b. I, II, and III       d. I, II, III, and IV

8.46  The binary number 01101110 equals what base 10 value?

a. 640
b. 512
c. 356
d. 110

8.47  In computer programming, groups of letters (such as those forming words) are called:

a. bits
b. strings
c. bytes
d. integers

8.48 A modern digital computer consists of which of the following key hardware components?

I. an arithmetic logic unit
II. a memory to store data
III. an input mechanism
IV. a central control unit
V. an output mechanism

a. II, III, IV, and V
b. I, III, and IV
c. I, II, IV, and V
d. I, II, III, IV, and V

8.49 A friend accidentally trips over and disconnects the electrical cord powering your computer while you are editing a term paper. Which of the following will occur?

a. the computer will automatically restart with no data loss
b. any changes made since you last saved data will be lost
c. the CPU will save any new information to read only memory
d. any changes made since you last saved data will be saved

8.50 For a computer to interact with its user, which of the following conditions are necessary?

I. there must be a means to pass results back to users (output)
II. a means must exist to provide data to the computer (input)
III. the user must be able to communicate in machine language

a. I and II
b. II and III
c. II only
d. I, II, and III

8.51 Common devices used to input data or instructions to a computer include which of the following?

I. mouse/light pen
II. ADC converters
III. keyboards
IV. X–Y plotters
V. optical scanners

a. I, III, and IV
b. II, III, IV, and V
c. I, II, III, and V
d. I, II, III, IV, and V

8.52 A specialized input device designed to convert the freehand movements of a pen or mouse on a flat surface into a digital image best describes a:

a. trackball
b. ADC converter
c. X–Y plotter
d. digitizing pad

8.53 Computer output may take which of the following forms?

I. control signals
II. graphics
III. words
IV. numbers

a. II and IV
b. I, II, and III
c. I and III
d. I, II, III, and IV

8.54 A complete set of computer instructions, designed to accomplish a specific task, is called a(n):

a. loop
b. algorithm
c. branch
d. program

8.55 Which of the following are common to all conventional computer programming algorithms?

I. conditional branching
II. simple sequence
III. conditional looping
IV. search/pattern matching

a. II and IV
b. I, II, and III
c. I and III
d. I, II, III, and IV

8.56 When a computer program performs a sequence of operations over and over again until some condition is satisfied, it is:

a. looping
b. storing
c. branching
d. sequencing

8.57 Which of the following are true regarding true programming languages?

I. they consist of a set of English–like instructions
II. each command translates into many machine level statements
III. commands are directly dependent on processor/CPU design
IV. they can be used on many different types of computers

a. II and IV
b. I, II, and IV
c. I and III
d. I, II, III, and IV

8.58 Which of the following functions are provided by a typical computer operating system?
I.  applications interface
II.  command and program execution
III.  multitasking
IV.  memory management
V.  input/output (I/O) control

a. II, III, IV, and V    c. I, II, IV, and V
b. I, III, and IV        d. I, II, III, IV, and V

8.59 As director of a new respiratory care department, you need to create and store a text–based procedure manual. You will also need to retrieve and edit portions of the document over time. Which of the following application programs would best meet your needs?

a. database
b. expert system
c. graphic
d. word processor

8.60 As shift supervisor for a respiratory care department, you need to generate weekly productivity reports using weighted numerical time units. Which of the following application programs would best meet your needs?

a. spreadsheet
b. database
c. word processor
d. graphic

8.61 A system for organizing text and numeric data in such a way that it can be easily stored, retrieved, and manipulated is called a:

a. telecommunications system
b. artificial intelligence system
c. statistical analysis system
d. database management system

8.62 A database management system consists of which of the following components?
I.  a program that provides the storage and retrieval functions
II.  a knowledge base consisting of numerous production rules
III.  one or more collections of categorical data (databases)

a. I and III    c. II only
b. II and III   d. I, II, and III

8.63 Each "piece" of categorical information within a database record is called a:

a. byte
b. field
c. string
d. file

8.64 A collection of categorical data describing a single object, person, or event best describes a:

a. list
b. database
c. record
d. field

8.65 In order to share data between databases, which of the following is needed?

a. a production rule
b. a common link field
c. a numeric formula
d. a hard disk system

8.66 Computer programs used to assess the result of blood gas analysis are examples of what type of expert system application?

a. prediction
b. instruction
c. interpretation
d. planning

8.67 Monitoring and control expert systems are useful under which of the following conditions?
I.  when a human cannot analyze data fast enough to make a response
II.  when experts are not always available to provide consultation
III.  when round–the–clock monitoring of a system is necessary

a. I and II     c. I and III
b. II and III   d. I, II, and III

8.68 When a monitoring and control computer system automatically takes action based on sensor–provided input data (without the need for operator input), it is said to be operating as a:

a. prediction system
b. open loop system
c. host–remote system
d. closed loop system

8.69 The capacity of a computer program to use current data to determine what may happen if conditions change is termed:

a. monitoring
b. interpreting
c. modeling
d. controlling

8.70 In electronic data communication, which of the following is the correct order of steps needed to share data between computers?

a. sending, encoding, decoding
b. encoding, decoding, sending
c. decoding, sending, encoding
d. encoding, sending, decoding

8.71 Which of the following are necessary for a host and remote computers to "talk" to each other over the telephone?
I.   binary data must be sent over the telephone lines
II.  the same communications protocol must be used
III. the computers must be linked by coaxial cables

a. I and II
b. II and III
c. II only
d. I, II, and III

8.72 A device used to convert a computer's digital data to and from the acoustic analog format used by telephone lines is:

a. router
b. multiplexer
c. modem
d. network

8.73 In the absence of a hospital–wide patient information system, a respiratory care computer system is commonly used for which of the following?
I.   log and track physician orders
II.  create billing/procedural summaries
III. record patient treatments

a. II and III
b. I and II
c. III only
d. I, II, and III

8.74 The most common application of computers encountered in respiratory care is their use in:

a. computer–aided bedside monitoring
b. computerized patient diagnosis
c. closed–loop control of mechanical ventilation
d. computerized departmental management

8.75 A common example of a closed–loop control system used in respiratory care is the:

a. automated blood gas analyzer
b. servo–controlled heated humidifier
c. computerized pulmonary function system
d. departmental scheduling program

8.76 The only true application of closed–loop computer control of mechanical ventilation to have reached the bedside is:

a. positive end–expiratory pressure (PEEP)
b. pressure support ventilation (PSV)
c. continuous mandatory ventilation (CMV)
d. mandatory minute ventilation (MMV)

**Introduction to Computer Programming:**

8.77 Below is a simple computer program designed to convert a temperature in degrees Fahrenheit to degrees Celsius. The program was written in the GW–BASIC programming language (Microsoft) and will run under most IBM–PC compatible versions of BASIC.

```
10 CLS
20 PRINT
30 PRINT "This program converts degrees Fahrenheit
to Celsius"
40 PRINT
50 INPUT "First enter the number of conversions you
want to compute:",X
60 FOR S=1 TO X
70 PRINT
80 PRINT "Conversion#"S
90 INPUT "Enter the temperature in degrees
Fahrenheit:",F$
100 IF VAL(F$)=0 THEN 170
110 C=(5*((VAL(F$)–32)/9))
120 PRINT F$ "degrees Fahrenheit equals" C "degrees
Celsius"
130 PRINT
140 NEXT
150 PRINT "Thank you for your input"
160 END
170 PRINT
180 PRINT F$ "is not a number. Hit return key to try
again"
190 INPUT "",Z
200 GOTO 80
```

Access any IBM–PC compatible having a BASIC interpreter and enter the lines of the program exactly as written above (the numbers at the left margin are line numbers and are required in most versions of BASIC). After entering all 20 lines, SAVE your program and then enter the RUN command (if you receive a message that there is a syntax error, use the BASIC editor to correct any errors). Once the program begins, respond to the prompts for input while carefully observing how the program functions.

After running the program and observing its function, take a careful look at the program code. Then answer the following questions:

First, identify the INPUT used by the program. (Hint: Look for INPUT statements.) What input is used? Who supplies the input? What is done with the input?

Second, identify the program's OUTPUT. (Hint: The PRINT statement directs output to the computer monitor.) What is the primary output of the program?

All computer programs use *variables*. Variables can be thought of as "places" which store numeric values or strings (groups of letters). Try to identify all the variables used by the program. (Hint: In this program, all variables are designated by a single letter.) What are the variables used for? Do the variables change? Why?

Next, identify where the program performs the following common algorithmic functions:

1. **Simple sequencing,** i.e., when each step is performed in sequence, one after another. (Hint: Look at lines 10–50.)

2. **Looping,** i.e., when an operation or sequence of operations is done over and over again until some condition is satisfied. (Hint: Look at lines 60–140, the FOR...NEXT structure.)

3. **Conditional branching,** i.e., when the program branches to other portions of the algorithm based on the value of a conditional statement. (Hint: Look at line 100.)

Last, although computers cannot reason about input or output values, they can be programmed to catch input errors, for example, entering a letter instead of a number. Examine the program carefully and try to identify whether it is programmed to catch an input error. If you are not sure about the program code itself, rerun the program and enter a letter when it asks for a Fahrenheit temperature. What happens? Why? What do you think would happen if there were no mechanism to catch input errors?

# 9

## Functional Anatomy of the Respiratory System

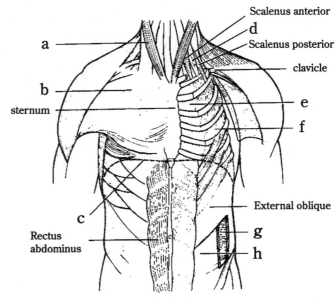

**Figure 9–2** Muscles of ventilation

### CONTENT EXERCISES

**Labeling:** Match the structures listed on the right to the letter labels in each of the following figures:

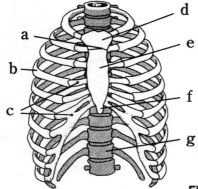

**Figure 9–1** Chest cage

9.1

a. _____ manubrium

b. _____ thoracic vertebrae

c. _____ angle of Louis

d. _____ xiphoid process

e. _____ ribs

f. _____ costal cartilages

g. _____ body of sternum

9.2

a. _____ internal oblique

b. _____ transverse abdominus

c. _____ internal intercostal

d. _____ sternomastoid

e. _____ diaphragm

f. _____ pectoralis major

g. _____ scalenus medius

h. _____ external intercostal

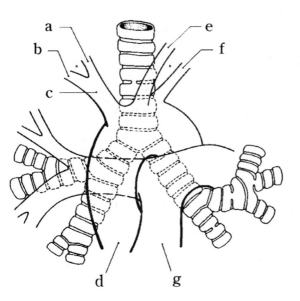

**Figure 9–3** Great vessels of the thorax

9.3
a. _____ innominate artery

b. _____ left carotid artery

c. _____ pulmonary artery

d. _____ left subclavian artery

e. _____ right carotid artery

f. _____ right subclavian
artery

g. _____ aorta

9.4
a. _____ hard palate

b. _____ eustachian tube

c. _____ epiglottis

d. _____ palatine tonsil

e. _____ middle concha

f. _____ cricothyroid
membrane

g. _____ thyroid cartilage

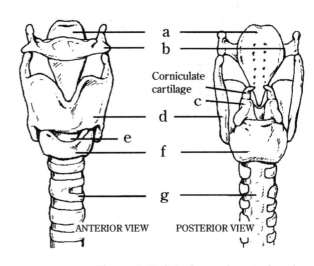

**Figure 9–5** Anterior and posterior view
of larynx and trachea

9.5
a. _____ cricothyroid ligament

b. _____ thyroid cartilage

c. _____ hyoid bone

d. _____ epiglottis

e. _____ trachea

f. _____ arytenoid cartilage

g. _____ cricoid cartilage

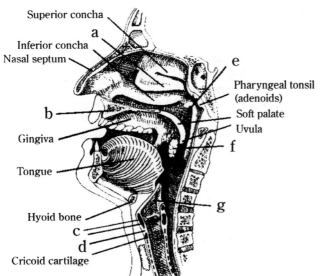

**Figure 9–4** Structures of upper airway and oral cavity

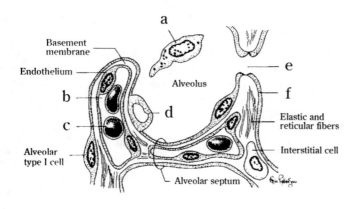

**Figure 9–6** High power view of alveolus

9.6
a. _____ alveolar type I cell

b. _____ pore of Kohn

c. _____ alveolar type II cell

d. _____ red blood cell

e. _____ capillary

f. _____ alveolar macrophage

9.7
a. For each numbered lung segment in Figure 9–7, specify the segment name and lung lobe:

| Right Lung | Left Lung |
|---|---|
| 1. _____ | 1. _____ |
| 2. _____ | 2. _____ |
| 3. _____ | 3. _____ |
| 4. _____ | 4. _____ |
| 5. _____ | 5. _____ |
| 6. _____ | 6. _____ |
| 7. _____ | 7. _____ |
| 8. _____ | 8. _____ |
| 9. _____ | 9. _____ |
| 10. _____ | 10. _____ |

b. Which left lung segment(s) correspond to those constituting the middle lobe of the right lung?

_____

_____

**Multiple Choice:** Circle the letter corresponding to the single best answer from the available choices:

9.8   Which of the following events occur between 4 and 5 weeks' gestation?
I.     development of the bronchial buds
II.    development of the palate
III.   development of the diaphragm
IV.   development of surfactant–producing cells

a. I and II              c. II, III, and IV
b. I, II, and III        d. I, II, III, and IV

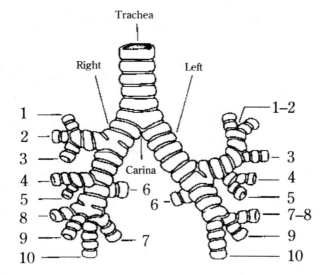

**Figure 9–7** Bronchopulmonary segments

9.9   By the end of the pseudoglandular stage (after 15 weeks' gestation), which of the following are true?
I.    all upper airway structures are recognizable
II.   cartilaginous support structures are developing
III.  the mediastinum has been formed
IV.   the pleural cavities and diaphragm have been formed
V.    the respiratory tract mucosal cells have begun differentiation

a. I, III, and IV          c. I, II, and V
b. II, III, IV, and V      d. I, II, III, IV, and V

9.10  The development of a stable pathway for production of surfactant (the phosphocoline transferase system) and the appearance of type II alveolar cells occurs at approximately how many weeks' gestation?

a. 16 weeks
b. 26 weeks
c. 35 weeks
d. 42 weeks

9.11  Which of the following statements regarding lung development during the first eight to ten years of life are true?
I.    growth is mainly hypertrophic (increase in size)
II.   growth is mainly hyperplastic (increase in number)
III.  alveolar development is intense
IV.   the surface area increases 10– to 15–fold

a. I only                  c. II, III, and IV
b. II and III              d. I, II, III, and IV

9.12  The middle compartment of the mediastinum contains which structures?
I.    pericardium and heart
II.   great vessels (aortic arch and vena cava)
III.  esophagus
IV.   trachea and mainstem bronchi
V.    thymus gland

a. I only                  c. I, II, and IV
b. II and IV               d. I, II, III, IV, and V

9.13  The thin mesothelial layer covering the outer surface of the lungs and extending onto the hilar bronchi and vessels and into the major fissures is called the:

a. parietal pleura
b. mesothelioma
c. cupula
d. visceral pleura

9.14  Which of the following are true regarding the normal pleural cavity?
I.    it is a potential space (not really a cavity)
II.   it is normally occupied by small amounts of serous fluid
III.  introduction of air or blood can separate the pleural surfaces, turning the potential into a real space

a. II and III              c. II only
b. I and III               d. I, II, and III

9.15  What functions do the bones of the thorax serve?
I.    they protect the thoracic viscera
II.   they are origin and insertion points for the respiratory muscles
III.  with the respiratory muscles, they provide the mechanism for ventilation (cyclical gas flow)

a. I and III               c. III only
b. II and III              d. I, II, and III

9.16  The angle of Louis, or sternal angle, serves as a landmark for which of the following?
I.    the point of sternal articulation with the second ribs
II.   the point of articulation between corpus sterni and manubrium
III.  the top of the heart and pericardium
IV.   the point at which the trachea divides into left and right mainstem bronchi

a. III and IV              c. I, III, and IV
b. II, III, and IV         d. I, II, III, and IV

9.17  In contrast to the first rib, during inspiration ribs 2 through 7 move simultaneously about the axis of the rib neck and the axis between the angle of the rib and its sternal junction. These movements result in:
I.    an increase in the anteroposterior (AP) diameter of the chest
II.   a decrease in the anteroposterior (AP) diameter of the chest
III.  an increase in the lateral (side–to–side) dimensions of the chest

a. II and III              c. I and III
b. I only                  d. I, II, and III

9.18 Which of the following muscles are considered secondary or accessory muscles of ventilation?
I.   diaphragm
II.  scalene group
III. sternomastoid
IV.  abdominals
V.   intercostals

a. I, III, IV, and V
b. I and V
c. II, III, and IV
d. I, II, III, IV, and V

9.19 Which of the following statements regarding the action of the diaphragm are true?
I.   it takes no active part in exhalation
II.  during forced exhalation it is pushed upward by increased abdominal pressure
III. contraction draws the central tendon down, increasing thoracic volume
IV.  rigidity of the abdominal wall interferes with its descent during inspiration
V.   contraction of its costal fibers raises and everts the lateral costal margins

a. I, III, and IV
b. II, IV, and V
c. I, III, IV, and V
d. I, II, III, IV, and V

9.20 As ventilatory muscles, the sternomastoids pull from their skull insertions and elevate the sternum during inspiration, thereby:

a. elevating the sternum and increasing the AP diameter of the chest
b. lowering the sternum and increasing the AP diameter of the chest
c. elevating the ribs and decreasing the AP diameter of the chest
d. fixing the ribs against abdominal contraction

9.21 The primary sources of motor innervation to the larynx are the:

a. phrenic nerves
b. recurrent laryngeal nerves
c. superior laryngeal nerves
d. intercostal nerves

9.22 Autonomic motor fibers influence:
I.   the caliber of the conducting airways
II.  the activity of the bronchial glands
III. the tone of the pulmonary blood vessels

a. I only
b. II and III
c. I and III
d. I, II, and III

9.23 Which of the following are true regarding the Hering–Breuer reflex (inflation reflex)?
I.   it is based on receptors located in bronchial smooth muscle
II.  its activation increases nerve impulse discharge during inflation
III. it is weak or absent during normal quiet breathing in adults
IV.  it probably influences the length of the pause between breaths

a. III and IV
b. II, III, and IV
c. I and III
d. I, II, III, and IV

9.24 Stimulation of the irritant receptors in the lung can result in:
I.   bronchoconstriction
II.  reflex closure of the glottis
III. reflex slowing of the heart (bradycardia)

a. I only
b. II and III
c. I and III
d. I, II, and III

9.25 The pulmonary venous circulation:
I.   empties into the left atrium
II.  empties into the pulmonary artery
III. delivers unoxygenated blood to the lungs
IV.  delivers oxygenated blood back to the heart

a. I and IV
b. II and IV
c. III only
d. I, II, III, and IV

9.26 Which of the following statements are true regarding the pulmonary lymphatic system?
I.   it consists of two sets of vessels: superficial and deep
II.  vessels begin as dead–end lymphatic channels in lung tissue
III. together with phagocytes, it defends against foreign material
IV.  it drains into the right lymphatic or thoracic duct

a. I, III, and IV
b. II and III
c. I and III
d. I, II, III, and IV

9.27 The functions of the upper airway include all the following *except:*

a. conducting gases
b. heat exchange
c. humidification
d. gas exchange

9.28 The smallest cross-sectional area in the upper respiratory tract of the adult occurs at the:

a. anterior nares
b. cricoid cartilage
c. hypopharynx (laryngopharynx)
d. oropharynx

9.29 The defense function of the nose involves which of the following?
I.      gross filtration by the large hairs of the nasal vestibule
II.     impaction of particulate foreign matter on the nasal mucosa
III.    the antibacterial properties of nasal secretions
IV.     clearance of foreign matter by ciliary action

a. II, III, and IV          c. III and IV
b. I, II, and IV            d. I, II, III, and IV

9.30 Three folds of tissue at the posterior base of the tongue that attach to the epiglottis form a small space between these two structures that is a key landmark in oral intubation. This space is called the:

a. vestibule
b. false vocal cords
c. vallecula
d. palatine fold

9.31 For which of the following purposes might the cricothyroid ligament be punctured or opened?
I.      to open the airway in an emergency (cricothyrotomy)
II.     to remove secretions (transtracheal aspiration)
III.    to provide supplementary oxygen (transtracheal oxygenation)
IV.     to ventilate the patient (high frequency jet ventilation)

a. I, III, and IV           c. I and IV
b. II, III, and IV          d. I, II, III, and IV

9.32 The adult trachea is approximately how long?

a. 5 cm
b. 12 cm
c. 18 cm
d. 20 cm

9.33 According to the Jackson–Huber classification, which of the following statements regarding segmental anatomy of the lungs is true?

a. the left lung has 8 segments, the right has 10
b. the right lung has 8 segments, the left has 10
c. the right lung has 2 lobes, the left has 3
d. both lungs have an equal number of lobes

9.34 The primary cell type constituting the mucosa of the larger airways is a:

a. pseudostratified ciliated columnar epithelium
b. pseudostratified ciliated cuboidal epithelium
c. stratified unciliated squamous epithelium
d. stratified unciliated serous endothelium

9.35 Which of the following can impair or inhibit ciliary activity?
I.      drying of the respiratory tract mucosa
II.     parasympatholytic drugs (e.g., atropine)
III.    excessive production of mucus

a. I only                   c. II and III
b. II only                  d. I, II, and III

9.36 The major source of respiratory tract secretions in the normal lung are the:

a. goblet cells
b. mast cells
c. Clara cells
d. bronchial glands

9.37 Release of histamine and other chemical mediators from the mast cells in the submucosa of the airways can cause:
I.      vasodilation
II.     vasoconstriction
III.    bronchoconstriction

a. I only                   c. I and III
b. II only                  d. I, II, and III

9.38 The patency of airways less than 1 to 2 mm in size is maintained by which of the following mechanisms?
I.      cartilaginous support
II.     transmural pressure gradients
III.    the traction of surrounding elastic tissue

a. I only                   c. II and III
b. II only                  d. I, II, and III

9.39 Which of the following are true regarding the terminal respiratory unit of the lung (also called the primary lobule or acinus)?

I.    it begins at a point about 17 generations beyond the trachea
II.   it consists of all structures distal to a terminal bronchiole
III.  it consists of 2 to 5 orders of respiratory bronchioles
IV.   it is the site of pulmonary gas exchange

a. I and II
b. I, II, and III
c. II and III
d. I, II, III, and IV

9.40 Pulmonary surfactant is most likely secreted by:

a. type I cells (squamous pneumocytes)
b. type II pneumocytes (granular pneumocytes)
c. type II cells (alveolar macrophages)
d. ciliary cells of the mucosa

9.41 Which of the following layers must gases pass through in order to transverse the alveolar–capillary septum or membrane?

I.    alveolar lining fluid
II.   alveolar epithelium
III.  basement membrane(s)
IV.   interstitial space
V.    capillary endothelium

a. II, III, IV, and V
b. I, III, IV, and V
c. III, IV, and V
d. I, II, III, IV, and V

9.42 Intercommunicating channels that permit collateral ventilation between adjacent alveoli and primary lobules include which of the following?

I.    interalveolar channels (pores of Kohn)
II.   bronchiole–alveolar channels (canals of Lambert)
III.  interbronchiolar channels

a. I and II
b. I and III
c. II and III
d. I, II, and III

# CHAPTER 10

# The Cardiovascular System

## CONTENT EXERCISES

**Labeling:** Match the structures listed on the right to the letter labels in each of the following figures:

10.1

| | | |
|---|---|---|
| a. | ____________ | right ventricle |
| b. | ____________ | left ventricle |
| c. | ____________ | orifices of coronary arteries |
| d. | ____________ | papillary muscles |
| e. | ____________ | left atrium |
| f. | ____________ | interventricular septum |
| g. | ____________ | tricuspid valve |
| h. | ____________ | pulmonary veins |
| i. | ____________ | pulmonary artery |
| j. | ____________ | aorta |
| k. | ____________ | superior vena cava |

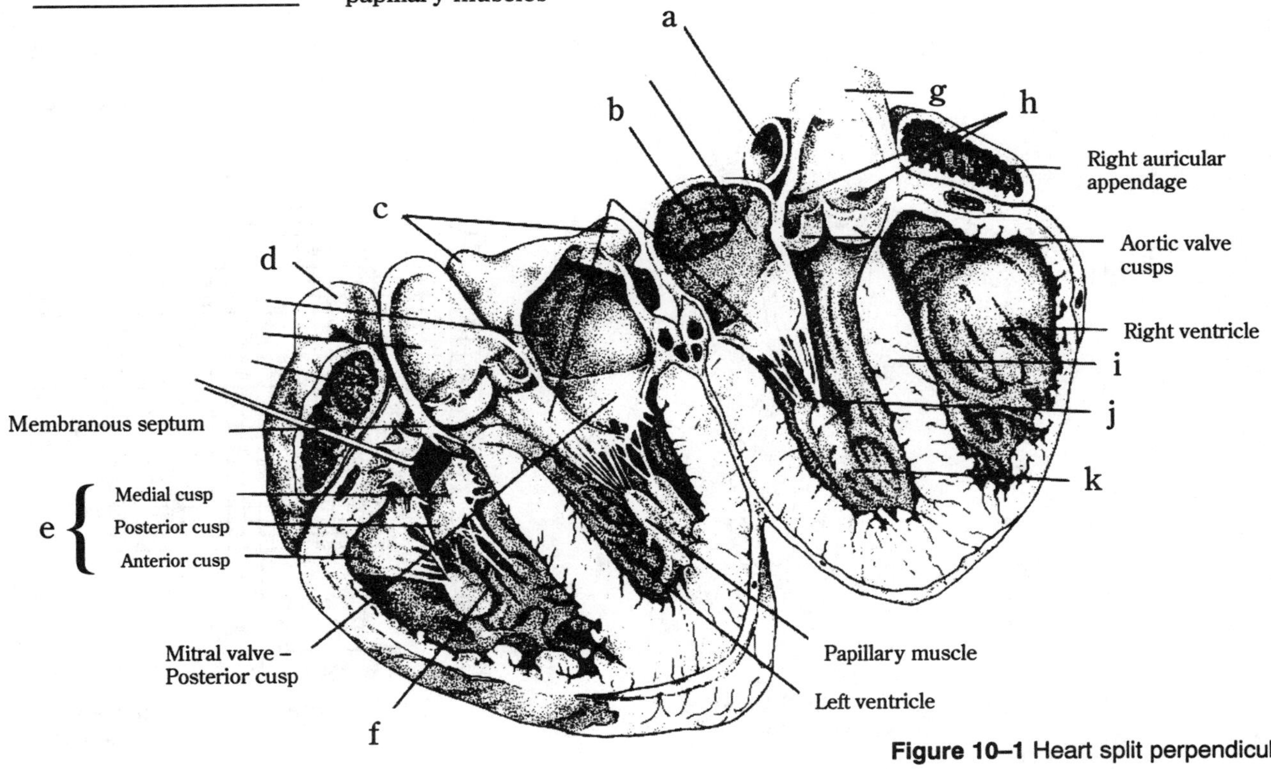


**Figure 10–1** Heart split perpendicular

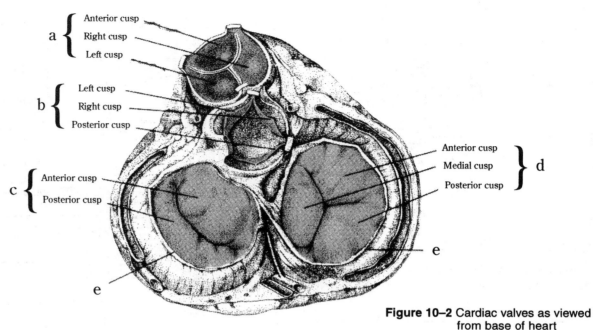

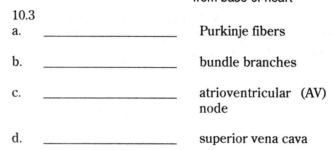

Figure 10–2 Cardiac valves as viewed from base of heart

10.2

a. _____ tricuspid valve

b. _____ pulmonic valve

c. _____ anulus fibrosus

d. _____ aortic valve

e. _____ mitral (bicuspid) valve

10.3

a. _____ Purkinje fibers

b. _____ bundle branches

c. _____ atrioventricular (AV) node

d. _____ superior vena cava

e. _____ sinoatrial (SA) node

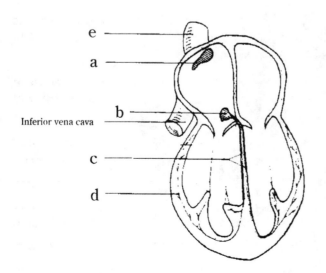

Figure 10–3 The electrical conducting system of the heart

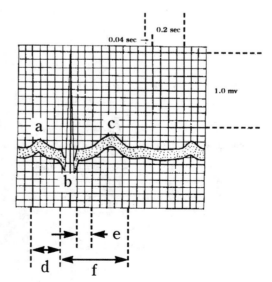

Figure 10–4 Normal electrocardiographic pattern

10.4

a. _____ T wave

b. _____ P–R interval

c. _____ P wave

d. _____ Q–T segment

e. _____ QRS complex

f. _____ S–T segment

g. Which of the above ECG components represent ventricular repolarization?

_____

h. Which of the above ECG components represent atrial depolarization?

_____

i. The time interval between atrial depolarization and ventricular depolarization is depicted by which of the above ECG components?

_____

j. "Electrical systole" corresponds to which of the above ECG components?

_____

k. Which of the above time intervals corresponds to the heart's refractory period?

_____

**Short Answer:**

10.5   Answer the following questions by referring to Figure 10–5:

a. The _____, indicating atrial contraction, immediately follow the P wave of the electrocardiogram.

b. The upward bulge of the AV valves during ventricular contraction is recorded as the _____, representing a slight rise in pressure in the atria.

c. The AV valves open when the pressure in the atria _____ the pressure in the ventricles.

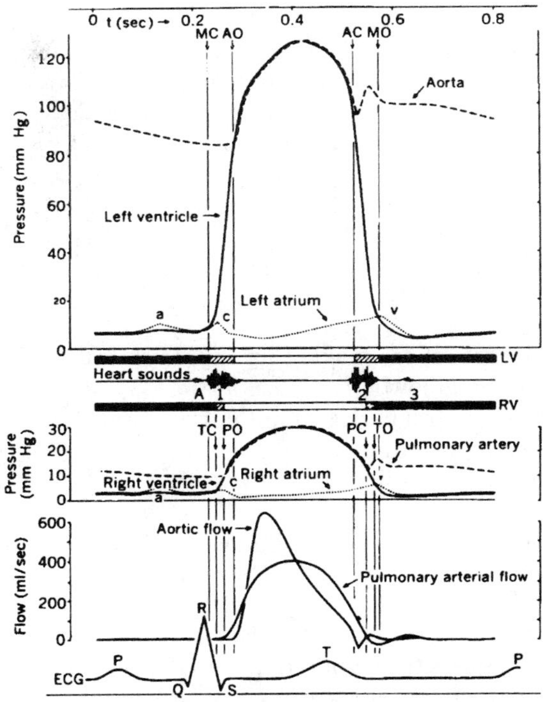

**Figure 10–5** Events of the cardiac cycle

d. The semilunar valves close when the pressure in the ventricles _____ the pressure in the outflow arteries.

e. Throughout the period of ventricular systole, atrial pressures exhibit a steady _____.

f. The second part of the first heart sound (if heard) is associated with opening of the _____ and _____ valves.

g. The dicrotic notch in the aorta occurs between closure of the _____ valve and opening of the _____ valve.

h. The rapid drop in atrial pressures toward the end of ventricular systole (indicated by the v wave) corresponds to opening of the _____.

i. Commencing with the T wave on the electrocardiogram, ventricular pressures begin to drop rapidly, indicating _____.

j. The central venous pressure is recorded as the _____ in the right atrium.

**Multiple Choice:** Circle the letter corresponding to the single best answer from the available choices:

10.6   The pointed end or apex of the heart is formed by the tip of the left ventricle and lies just above the diaphragm at a level corresponding to which intercostal space?

a. the 3rd right intercostal space
b. the 3rd left intercostal space
c. the 5th left intercostal space
d. the 5th right intercostal space

10.7   Tissue layers making up the heart wall include which of the following?
I.     the visceral pericardium (epicardium)
II.    the myocardium
III.   the endocardium

a. II and III           c. III only
b. I and III            d. I, II, and III

10.8   The mitral (bicuspid) valve:
I.     separates the right atrium and the right ventricle
II.    prevents atrial backflow during ventricular contraction
III.   separates the left atrium and the left ventricle
IV.    separates the right ventricle and the pulmonary artery

a. II only              c. II and III
b. I only               d. I, II, III, and IV

10.9   The first arteries branching off the aorta are the:

a. subclavian arteries
b. brachiocephalic arteries
c. carotid arteries
d. coronary arteries

10.10 The branches of the right coronary artery normally supply which areas of the heart?
I.     most of the interventricular septum
II.    most of the right ventricular myocardium
III.   most of the right atrial myocardium
IV.    the sinoatrial (SA) node

a. III and IV           c. I, and III
b. II, III, and IV      d. I, II, III, and IV

10.11 Which of the following properties of cardiac muscle are unique to this tissue type?

a. excitability
b. contractility
c. conductivity
d. inherent rhythmicity

10.12 Myocardial responsiveness to stimulation caused by electrical, chemical, or mechanical factors in the cell or in its surrounding environment is called:

a. excitability
b. contractility
c. conductivity
d. automaticity

10.13 It is thought that shortening of the sarcomere, and thus the myofibrils and cardiac muscle fiber as a whole, occurs when the reversible cross–bridges formed by actin and myosin cause these filaments to slide over one another. This model of myocardial contraction is called the:

a. cross–bridge concept
b. thoracic pump theory
c. sliding filament theory
d. Frank–Starling relationship

10.14 Oxygenated blood returns to the left atrium through the:

a. pulmonary veins
b. pulmonary arteries
c. superior vena cava
d. coronary arteries

10.15 Which of the following best describes the role of arterioles?

a. as variable resistors, they control blood flow into the capillaries
b. they maintain the head of perfusion pressure generated by the heart
c. they transport and exchange gases and nutrients with the tissues
d. they serve as a volume reservoir for the systemic circulation

10.16 The vessels of the venous system, particularly the small venules and veins, are termed capacitance vessels because:

a. they transmit and maintain the head of perfusion pressure
b. they determine the afterload on the left ventricle
c. they maintain a constant internal environment for the body's cells
d. they can alter their capacity to maintain perfusion pressures

10.17 Which of the following mechanisms facilitate venous return to the heart?
I.    the thoracic pump mechanism
II.   sympathetic venomotor tone
III.  cardiac suction
IV.   skeletal muscle contraction

a. I and II              c. II and IV
b. II, III, and IV       d. I, II, III, and IV

10.18 During blood loss due to hemorrhage, perfusing pressures can be kept near normal until the volume loss overwhelms the system. This is because:

a. venules constrict, decreasing vascular capacity
b. arterioles dilate, decreasing vascular capacity
c. arterioles constrict, increasing vascular resistance
d. muscle vessels dilate, increasing vascular capacity

10.19 The underlying goal of the body's cardiovascular control mechanisms is to ensure that:

a. all tissues receive perfusion according to their metabolic needs
b. all tissues receive equivalent amounts of blood flow
c. all tissues receive perfusion according to their size
d. all tissues receive perfusion according to their mass

10.20 The cardiovascular system regulates perfusion mainly by altering:

a. the rate of cardiac contractions
b. the volume of cardiac contractions
c. the strength of cardiac contractions
d. the capacity and resistance of blood vessels

10.21 Autoregulation of blood flow in the tissues in response to changing levels of oxygen, carbon dioxide, pH, and lactic acid is called:

a. myogenic control
b. humoral control
c. central control
d. metabolic control

10.22 Smooth muscle relaxation and vessel dilation in the arterioles and veins are caused mainly by:
I.    parasympathetic/cholinergic stimulation (via acetylcholine)
II.   the selective action of specialized adrenergic receptors
III.  the action of local metabolites

a. II and III            c. I and III
b. I and II              d. I, II, and III

10.23 Cardiac output per minute is equal to:

a. rate (f) times stroke volume (SV)
b. stroke volume (SV) divided by rate (f)
c. blood pressure (BP) times stroke volume (SV)
d. blood pressure (BP) divided by stroke volume (SV)

10.24 Significant loss of blood volume causes which of the following?
I.    an increase in vascular tone
II.   increased secretion of ADH (antidiuretic hormone)
III.  an increase in heart rate

a. II and III            c. I and III
b. I and II              d. I, II, and III

10.25 Alteration of the resting potential of cardiac tissue by electrical stimulation results in:
I.    rapid diffusion of sodium ions into the cell
II.   release of calcium ions into the myofibrils
III.  electrical depolarization (reversal of charge)
IV.   activation of the myocardial contractile process

a. II, III, and IV       c. I, II, and III
b. II and III            d. I, II, III, and IV

10.26 During most of the depolarization stage of the cardiac action potential, muscle fibers cannot respond to further electrical stimulation. This period is called the:

a. isovolume contract period
b. isovolume relaxation period
c. refractory period
d. repolarization period

10.27 Under which of the following conditions can latent pacemakers or ectopic foci develop in cardiac tissues?
I.      when their excitability is increased
II.     when normal nodal tissues are depressed
III.    when conducting pathways are blocked

a. II and III          c. III only
b. I and III           d. I, II, and III

10.28 The dominant pacemaker in the normal heart is the:

a. AV node
b. bundle of His
c. Purkinje system
d. sinus (SA) node

10.29 Strong vagal (parasympathetic) stimulation of the heart causes:

a. a decrease in heart rate
b. an increase in heart rate
c. greater contractility
d. faster electrical conduction

10.30 Should the sinus node fail to function because of disease:

a. the heart will always completely cease beating (asystole)
b. the atria will not depolarize, but the ventricles will
c. the AV node will normally take over at a slower rate
d. the bundle branches will normally take over at a faster rate

10.31 The length of time taken by the atrial impulse to transverse the AV node and reach the ventricles is measured on the EKG as the:

a. S–T segment
b. QRS width
c. R–R interval
d. P–R interval

10.32 The first heart sound is associated with what mechanical event of the cardiac cycle?

a. AV valve opening
b. AV valve closure
c. semilunar valve closure
d. semilunar valve opening

10.33 Central venous pressures (the CVP) correspond to those measured in the:

a. right ventricle
b. right atrium
c. left ventricle
d. left atrium

10.34 A balloon–directed Swan–Ganz catheter measures pressures in the:

a. right ventricle
b. right atrium
c. left ventricle
d. pulmonary artery

# Ventilation

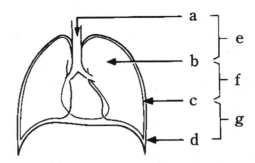

**Figure 11–2** Pressures involved in ventilation

## CONTENT EXERCISES

**Labeling:** Match the components listed on the right to the letter labels in each of the following figures:

11.1

a. _____ expiratory reserve volume

b. _____ residual volume

c. _____ vital capacity

d. _____ total lung capacity

e. _____ inspiratory capacity

f. _____ resting tidal volume

g. _____ functional residual capacity

h. _____ inspiratory reserve volume

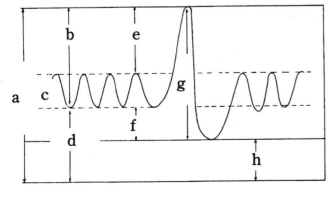

**Figure 11–1** Lung volumes and capacities

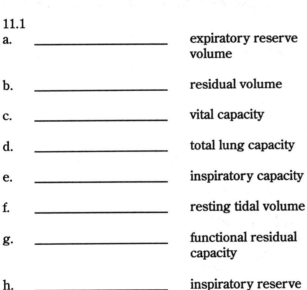

11.2

a. _____ transpulmonary gradient ($P_L$)

b. _____ pleural pressure ($P_{pl}$)

c. _____ body surface pressure ($P_{bs}$)

d. _____ transthoracic gradient ($P_W$)

e. _____ mouth pressure ($P_{ao}$)

f. _____ alveolar pressure ($P_{alv}$)

g. _____ transrespiratory gradient ($P_{rs}$)

h. Which of the above pressures or pressure gradients vary throughout the normal breathing cycle?

_____

i. Which of the above pressures normally remains negative (relative to atmospheric pressure) throughout the breathing cycle?

_____

j. Which of the above pressure gradients is directly responsible for the normal flow of gases into and out of the alveoli?

_____

k. Which of the above pressure gradients is directly responsible for the inflation volume of the alveoli?

_____

**Multiple Choice:** Circle the letter corresponding to the single best answer from the available choices:

11.3 Which of the following is equal to total lung capacity (TLC)?

a. IC + TV + ERV
b. VC + ERV
c. $V_T$ + ERV + IRV + RV
d. FRC + IRV

11.4 After the most strenuous expiratory effort, air still remains in the lungs and cannot be removed voluntarily. This volume is known as the:

a. expiratory reserve volume (ERV)
b. functional residual capacity (FRC)
c. vital capacity (VC)
d. residual volume (RV)

11.5 Which of the following is being measured if a respiratory care practitioner instructs a patient to take a maximum deep breath and then exhale completely?

a. inspiratory force
b. vital capacity (VC)
c. total lung capacity (TLC)
d. residual volume (RV)

11.6 Which of the following statements regarding alveolar pressure ($P_{alv}$) during normal quiet breathing is true?

a. it is positive during inspiration, negative during expiration
b. it is the same as intrapleural pressure ($P_{pl}$)
c. it always remains less than atmospheric pressure
d. it is negative during inspiration, positive during expiration

11.7 Which of the following pressure measurements normally remains negative (relative to atmospheric pressure) during quiet breathing?

a. alveolar pressure ($P_{alv}$)
b. mouth pressure ($P_{ao}$)
c. pleural pressure ($P_{pl}$)
d. body surface pressure ($P_{bs}$)

11.8 Which of the following pressure gradients is responsible for the actual flow of gas into and out of the alveoli during breathing?

a. the transrespiratory pressure gradient ($P_{alv} - P_{ao}$)
b. the transpulmonary pressure gradient ($P_{alv} - P_{pl}$)
c. the transthoracic pressure gradient ($P_{pl} - P_{bs}$)
d. the transcanadian pressure gradient ($P_{ca} - P_{ks}$)

11.9 Which of the following pressure gradients is responsible for maintaining alveolar inflation?

a. the transthoracic pressure gradient ($P_{pl} - P_{bs}$)
b. the transcanadian pressure gradient ($P_{ca} - P_{ks}$)
c. the transpulmonary pressure gradient ($P_{alv} - P_{pl}$)
d. the transrespiratory pressure gradient ($P_{alv} - P_{ao}$)

11.10 During normal inspiration:
I. the transthoracic pressure gradient becomes more negative
II. the pleural pressure decreases further below atmospheric
III. the transpulmonary pressure gradient widens
IV. alveolar pressure drops below that at the airway opening
V. air moves from the airway opening to the alveoli

a. I, II, III, and IV        c. III, IV, and V
b. II, III, IV, and V        d. I, II, III, IV, and V

11.11 During normal tidal ventilation, the transpulmonary pressure gradient ($P_{alv} - P_{pl}$) reaches its maximum value at what point in the cycle?

a. early inspiration
b. mid–inspiration
c. end–inspiration
d. end–expiration

11.12 Forces which must be overcome to move air into the respiratory system include which of the following?
I. tissue viscous resistance
II. elastic forces of lung tissue
III. airway resistance
IV. surface tension forces

a. II and III        c. II, III, and IV
b. III only          d. I, II, III, and IV

11.13 Normal (unforced) expiration:
I.    is accomplished passively (without muscular effort)
II.   uses energy stored during inspiration to expel gases
III.  requires large active energy expenditures

a. I and II                    c. III only
b. II only                     d. I, II, and III

11.14 The presence of surfactant in the alveoli tends to:

a. increase elastance
b. decrease compliance
c. increase resistance during gas flow
d. increase compliance

11.15 Compliance of the human lung:
I.    equals the volume change per unit pressure change
II.   averages about 0.2 liters per cm $H_2O$
III.  is the reciprocal (inverse) of elastance

a. I only                      c. III only
b. I and II                    d. I, II, and III

11.16 A lung which loses elastic fibers (as in emphysema) would exhibit which of the following characteristics?

a. decreased compliance
b. increased resistance
c. increased compliance
d. decreased time constant

11.17 Exhalation below the resting level requires active muscular effort in order to:

a. overcome the tendency of the chest wall to contract
b. overcome the tendency of the lungs to expand
c. overcome the tendency of the airways to expand
d. overcome the tendency of the chest wall to expand

11.18 Normal airway resistance ($R_{aw}$) is approximately:

a. 0.1–0.2 cm $H_2O$/liter/sec
b. 0.5–2.5 cm $H_2O$/liter/sec
c. 10–15 cm $H_2O$/liter/sec
d. 15–20 cm $H_2O$/liter/sec

11.19 Which of the following factors affect airway resistance?
I.    the pattern of gas flow, e.g., laminar, turbulent, etc.
II.   the density and viscosity of gas breathed
III.  the size, shape, and caliber of the airways

a. I and II                    c. II and III
b. I only                      d. I, II, and III

11.20 Most of the drop in pressure due to frictional resistance to gas flow occurs in what region?

a. the respiratory bronchioles
b. the terminal respiratory unit
c. the terminal bronchioles
d. the nose, mouth, and large airways

11.21 Which of the following statements regarding airway resistance is true?

a. as lung volume decreases toward RV, airway resistance drops
b. as lung volume increases toward TLC, airway resistance rises
c. the greater the lung volume, the less the airway resistance
d. the greater the lung volume, the greater the airway resistance

11.22 Which of the following statements regarding the equal pressure point (EPP) is *false*?

a. the EPP is the point at which the pressure inside an airway equals the pleural pressure
b. beyond the EPP (toward the airway opening) pleural pressure exceeds the pressure inside the airway, encouraging airway collapse
c. once the EPP is reached, greater expiratory effort will only further increase pleural pressure and further restrict flow
d. in healthy subjects, the dynamic compression occurs at lung volumes just above the resting expiratory level

11.23 Which of the following statements are true regarding the work of breathing?

I. even during tidal breathing, the respiratory muscles do work
II. in inspiration, both elastic and frictional forces must be overcome
III. during tidal breathing, expiratory work is recovered from the potential energy stored in the expanded lung–thorax
IV. forced exhalation requires additional work by the expiratory muscles

a. I, II, and III
b. II, III, and IV
c. II and IV
d. I, II, III, and IV

11.24 Which of the following formulae is used to compute the mechanical work of breathing?

a. $\Delta P$/flow
b. $\Delta P / \Delta V$
c. $\Delta V / \Delta P$
d. $\Delta P \times \Delta V$

11.25 In health, about what proportion of the total work of breathing is attributable to elastic forces opposing ventilation?

a. 1/2
b. 2/3
c. 3/4
d. 1/3

11.26 On inspecting a volume–pressure curve for a patient with restrictive lung disease, which of the following abnormalities would you expect to find?

I. an increase in the area of the volume–pressure curve
II. a decrease in the slope of the volume–pressure curve
III. a positive intrapleural pressure during exhalation

a. I and II
b. I and III
c. II and III
d. I, II, and III

11.27 Compared with a normal individual, when a patient with a severe obstructive impairment such as emphysema increases ventilation, which of the following occurs?

a. oxygen consumption increases at a faster rate than normal
b. oxygen consumption decreases compared with normal
c. oxygen consumption rises faster than carbon dioxide production
d. the anaerobic threshold is reached later than normal

11.28 Which of the following statements regarding the distribution of ventilation throughout the normal lung are true?

I. the distribution of ventilation is not uniform
II. uneven distribution results in imperfect gas exchange
III. regional and local factors contribute to uneven distribution

a. I and II
b. II and III
c. II only
d. I, II, and III

11.29 Compared with the apices, the bases of the normal upright lung:

a. receive about the same amount of ventilation
b. receive about four times less ventilation
c. receive about twice as much ventilation
d. receive about four times as much ventilation

11.30 Which of the following statements are true regarding a lung unit with higher resistance than normal?

I. it will fill and empty slower than normal
II. there will be less volume change for a given pressure change
III. a given volume change will require a greater pressure change

a. I and III
b. I and II
c. II and III
d. I, II, and III

11.31 Which of the following lung units would empty and fill most quickly?

a. a unit with low resistance and high compliance
b. a unit with high resistance and high compliance
c. a unit with high resistance and low compliance
d. a unit with low resistance and low compliance

11.32 In patients with small airways disease breathing at higher than normal frequencies:

I.    dynamic compliance drops
II.   the work of breathing increases
III.  oxygen consumption increases
IV.  the distribution of ventilation worsens

a. I, II, and III       c. I and III
b. I and IV          d. I, II, III, and IV

11.33 Anatomical deadspace plus alveolar deadspace is called:

a. mechanical deadspace
b. partial deadspace
c. total lung capacity
d. physiological deadspace

11.34 If the frequency of breathing increases without any change in total minute ventilation ($\dot{V}_E$ constant):

a  the alveolar ventilation per minute will increase
b. the alveolar ventilation per minute will decrease
c. the deadspace ventilation per minute will decrease
d. the alveolar ventilation per minute will remain constant

11.35 Blockage of the pulmonary arterial circulation to a portion of the lung would cause which of the following?

a. an increase in anatomic deadspace
b. a decrease in physiologic deadspace
c. an increase in alveolar deadspace
d. a decrease in anatomic deadspace

11.36 The single best indicator of the adequacy or effectiveness of alveolar ventilation is the:

a. $Pao_2$
b. $Paco_2$
c. $Pao_2$
d. $Sao_2$

11.37 In normal individuals, approximately what fraction of the tidal volume is considered wasted ventilation, in that it does not participate in gaseous exchange?

a. 1/2
b. 1/3
c. 1/4
d. 2/3

11.38 A patient has a $Pco_2$ of 22 mm Hg. Based on this information you may rightly conclude that:

a. the patient's $CO_2$ production is higher than normal
b. the patient is hypoventilating
c. the patient is hyperventilating
d. the patient's tidal volume is less than normal

**Computations:**

11.39
Lung Compliance

a. Listed below are data obtained on six patients. Compute each patient's lung compliance ($C_L$) in L/cm $H_2O$:

| Patient # | $\Delta V$ (liters) | $\Delta P$ ($P_{pl}$) (cm $H_2O$) | $C_L$ (L/cm $H_2O$) |
|---|---|---|---|
| 1 | .500 | 3.50 | _____ |
| 2 | 1.250 | 5.80 | _____ |
| 3 | .800 | 7.20 | _____ |
| 4 | .675 | 7.20 | _____ |
| 5 | 1.650 | 2.95 | _____ |
| 6 | .450 | 8.25 | _____ |

b. Which of the above patients' lung compliance ($C_L$) is within the normal range?

_____

c. Which of the above patients' lung compliance ($C_L$) indicates greater than normal elastance?

_____

d. Which of the above patients' lung compliance ($C_L$) indicates greater than normal distensibility?

_____

## 11.40
### Lung, Thorax, and Total Compliance

a. Listed below are compliance data obtained on eight patients. Compute the missing compliance values for each patient in L/cm $H_2O$:

| Patient # | $C_L$ | $C_T$ | $C_{LT}$ |
|---|---|---|---|
| 1 | .20 | .10 | _____ |
| 2 | .05 | .20 | _____ |
| 3 | .15 | .03 | _____ |
| 4 | _____ | .08 | .030 |
| 5 | _____ | .25 | .080 |
| 6 | _____ | .15 | .100 |
| 7 | .25 | _____ | .140 |
| 8 | .01 | _____ | .005 |

b. Assuming that a normal total compliance for the lungs and thorax together ($C_{LT}$) is between 0.05 and 0.15 L/cm $H_2O$, which of the above patients exhibit an abnormally low total compliance?

_____

c. Of those patients exhibiting an abnormally low total compliance, for which is this finding due mainly to a decrease in lung compliance ($C_L$)?

_____

d. Of those patients exhibiting an abnormally low total compliance, for which is this finding due mainly to a decrease in thoracic or chest wall compliance ($C_T$)?

_____

e. Of those patients exhibiting an abnormally low total compliance, for which is this finding due to a decrease in both lung and thoracic compliance?

_____

## 11.41
### Airway Resistance

a. Given the following data, compute (1) the change in pressure due to flow (P) between the airway opening and alveoli and (2) the resulting airway resistance in cm $H_2O$/L/sec (be sure to convert the flow from L/min to L/sec):

| $P_{ao}$ (cm $H_2O$) | $P_{alv}$ (cm $H_2O$) | $\Delta P$ (cm $H_2O$) | V (L/min) | $R_{aw}$ (cm $H_2O$/L/sec) |
|---|---|---|---|---|
| 0 | −5.00 | _____ | 35 | _____ |
| 0 | −8.50 | _____ | 120 | _____ |
| 0 | −3.80 | _____ | 80 | _____ |
| 40 | 20 | _____ | 45 | _____ |
| 50 | 35 | _____ | 75 | _____ |
| 60 | 50 | _____ | 55 | _____ |

b. Based on these data, are we measuring inspiratory or expiratory airway resistance? How do you know?

_____

_____

_____

c. In the first three examples, pressure at the airway opening is 0, while the alveolar pressure is negative. In the next three cases, both $P_{ao}$ and $P_{alv}$ are positive. Why?

_____

_____

_____

## 11.42
### Time Constants Versus Filling and Emptying of Lung Units

a. Below are compliance and resistance values for various lung units. Compute the time constant for each unit.

| Example # | Compliance (L/cm H$_2$O) | Resistance (cm H$_2$O/L/sec) | Time Constant (seconds) |
|---|---|---|---|
| 1 | .20 | 2.00 | _____ |
| 2 | .01 | 2.00 | _____ |
| 3 | .18 | 40.00 | _____ |
| 4 | .80 | 2.20 | _____ |
| 5 | .15 | .30 | _____ |
| 6 | .90 | 25.00 | _____ |
| 7 | .06 | .25 | _____ |
| 8 | .04 | 10.00 | _____ |
| 9 | .05 | .20 | _____ |

b. Under what conditions will filling and emptying of a lung unit be more rapid than normal (low time constant)? Which of the above examples demonstrate this effect?

_____

_____

_____

c. Under what conditions will filling and emptying of a lung unit be slower than normal (high time constant)? Which of the above examples demonstrate this effect?

_____

_____

_____

d. Does a normal time constant mean that the lung unit has normal compliance and resistance? Which of the above examples demonstrate this effect?

_____

_____

_____

## 11.43
### Minute Ventilation, Frequency of Breathing, Deadspace and Alveolar Ventilation

a. Given the following data on six patients, compute the missing values for each (all volumes should be expressed in milliliters):

| Case # | f | $\overset{\circ}{V}_T$ | $\overset{\circ}{V}_E$ | V$_D$ | $\overset{\circ}{V}_A$ |
|---|---|---|---|---|---|
| 1 | 12 | 500 | _____ | 150 | _____ |
| 2 | 24 | 250 | _____ | 150 | _____ |
| 3 | 6 | _____ | 6000 | 150 | _____ |
| 4 | 12 | _____ | 6000 | 300 | _____ |
| 5 | _____ | 650 | 7800 | 300 | _____ |
| 6 | 40 | _____ | 6000 | 150 | _____ |

b. Assuming that the minute ventilation remains constant, what effect does increasing the frequency of breathing have on the alveolar ventilation per minute? Why? (Hint: Compare Case #1 with Case #2.)

_____

_____

_____

c. Assuming that the minute ventilation remains constant, what effect does decreasing the frequency of breathing have on the alveolar ventilation per minute? (Hint: Compare Case #3 with Case #1.)

_____

_____

_____

d. Assuming that the frequency of breathing and minute ventilation remain constant, what effect does increasing the physiologic deadspace per breath have on the alveolar ventilation? (Hint: Compare Case #4 with Case #1.)

_____

_____

_____

e. How can a patient maintain a normal alveolar ventilation when his or her physiologic deadspace increases? (Hint: Compare Case #5 with Case #4.)

_____

_____

_____

f. What effect does rapid shallow breathing have on alveolar ventilation? (Hint: Compare Case #6 with Case #1.)

_____

_____

_____

g. Is the minute ventilation always a good indicator of the amount of alveolar ventilation (cite examples from the above table)?

_____

_____

_____

11.44

Physiologic Deadspace and the Bohr Equation

Given the following data on five patients, compute the missing values for each. (Hint: First compute the $V_T$, then use the Bohr equation to compute the $V_{Dphys}$, then compute the $V_D/V_T$.) All volumes should be expressed in milliliters.

| f | $\mathring{V}_E$ | $V_T$ | $Pa_{CO_2}$ | $P\bar{E}_{CO_2}$ | $V_D/V_T$ | $V_{Dphys}$ |
|---|---|---|---|---|---|---|
| 24 | 8400 | _____ | 32 | 22 | _____ | _____ |
| 15 | 7200 | _____ | 46 | 25 | _____ | _____ |
| 10 | 9600 | _____ | 30 | 15 | _____ | _____ |
| 32 | 16000 | _____ | 34 | 16 | _____ | _____ |
| 8 | 8800 | _____ | 65 | 25 | _____ | _____ |

# Gas Exchange and Transport

## CONTENT EXERCISES

**Multiple Choice:** Circle the letter corresponding to the single best answer from the available choices:

12.1 The movement of gases between lungs and the body tissues depends mainly on:

a. active transport
b. osmosis
c. gaseous diffusion
d. dialysis

12.2 The highest $P_{O_2}$ levels are found in:

a. the trachea and upper airways
b. the arterial blood
c. atmospheric air
d. the cells

12.3 The lowest $P_{CO_2}$ would normally be found in what location?

a. the trachea and upper airways
b. the arterial blood
c. room air
d. within the cells

12.4 The normal whole body carbon dioxide production per minute ($\dot{V}_{CO_2}$) for a 70–kg man is about:

a. 250 ml/min
b. 200 ml/min
c. 4,200 ml/min
d. 6,000 ml/min

12.5 Under what conditions will the alveolar partial pressure of carbon dioxide fall below normal?

I. if $CO_2$ production decreases relative to alveolar ventilation
II. if alveolar ventilation increases relative to $CO_2$ production
III. if the metabolic rate increases (as during exercise)

a. II and III
b. I and II
c. III only
d. I, II, and III

12.6 The partial pressure of oxygen in the alveoli depends on which of the following factors?
I. Fractional concentration of oxygen inspired ($F_{IO_2}$)
II. the level of alveolar ventilation ($\dot{V}_A$)
III. the whole body carbon dioxide production ($\dot{V}_{CO_2}$)
IV. the atmospheric pressure ($P_B$)

a. I, III, and IV
b. I and II
c. III and IV
d. I, II, III, and IV

12.7 Which of the following best represent the partial pressures of all gases in the normally ventilated and perfused alveolus when breathing room air at sea level?

a. $P_{O_2}$ = 40 mm Hg; $P_{CO_2}$ = 100 mm Hg; $P_{N_2}$ = 573 mm Hg; $P_{H_2O}$ = 47 mm Hg
b. $P_{O_2}$ = 100 mm Hg; $P_{CO_2}$ = 40 mm Hg; $P_{N_2}$ =713 mm Hg; $P_{H_2O}$ = 47 mm Hg
c. $P_{O_2}$ =149 mm Hg; $P_{CO_2}$ = 40 mm Hg; $P_{N_2}$ = 573 mm Hg; $P_{H_2O}$ = 47 mm Hg
d. $P_{O_2}$ =100 mm Hg; $P_{CO_2}$ = 40 mm Hg; $P_{N_2}$ = 573 mm Hg; $P_{H_2O}$ = 47 mm Hg

12.8 Assuming a constant $F_{IO_2}$ and $CO_2$ production, which of the following statements are true?
I. $P_{A}O_2$ varies inversely with the $P_{A}CO_2$
II. increases in $\dot{V}_A$ decrease the $P_{A}CO_2$ and increase the $P_{A}O_2$
III. decreases in $\dot{V}_A$ increase the $P_{A}CO_2$ and decrease the $P_{A}O_2$

a. II and III
b. I and II
c. II only
d. I, II, and III

12.9 What is the highest $P_{A}O_2$ one could expect to observe in an individual breathing room air at sea level?

a. 120–130 mm Hg
b. 640–670 mm Hg
c. 90–100 mm Hg
d. 710–760 mm Hg

12.10 The physical process whereby gas molecules move from an area of high partial pressure to an area of low partial pressure is called:

a. ventilation
b. diffusion
c. active transport
d. membrane exchange

12.11 The rate of gaseous diffusion across a biologic membrane is decreased when:
I. the gas diffusion constant is low
II. the surface area is low
III. the diffusion distance is large
IV. the partial pressure gradient is high

a. I and IV          c. I and II
b. I, II, and III     d. I, II, III, and IV

12.12 Which of the following values correspond most closely to the normal partial pressures of oxygen and carbon dioxide in the mixed venous blood returning to the lungs from the right heart?

a. $Po_2 = 40$ mm Hg; $Pco_2 = 100$ mm Hg
b. $Po_2 = 100$ mm Hg; $Pco_2 = 40$ mm Hg
c. $Po_2 = 100$ mm Hg; $Pco_2 = 46$ mm Hg
d. $Po_2 = 40$ mm Hg; $Pco_2 = 46$ mm Hg

12.13 Due mainly to its high solubility coefficient, carbon dioxide diffuses across the alveolar–capillary membrane at a rate how many times greater than oxygen?

a. 2 times greater
b. 20 times greater
c. 200 times greater
d. 50 times greater

12.14 The time available for diffusion in the lung is mainly a function of the:

a. level of alveolar ventilation
b. functional residual capacity
c. inspired oxygen concentration
d. rate of pulmonary blood flow

12.15 In order to assess the events occurring at the tissue level, especially tissue oxygenation, you would sample and measure:

a. left heart blood parameters
b. pulmonary venous blood parameters
c. systemic arterial blood parameters
d. systemic venous blood parameters

12.16 Even in healthy young subjects, the alveolar partial pressure of oxygen is somewhat higher than the arterial level. This normal alveolar–arterial oxygen tension gradient, or $P(A - a)O_2$, is due to:
I. anatomic shunts in the pulmonary and cardiac circulations
II. regional differences in pulmonary ventilation and blood flow
III. normal limitations to oxygen diffusion in the lung

a. II and III         c. III only
b. I and II           d. I, II, and III

12.17 Which of the following would you expect to occur if perfusion ($\dot{Q}_c$) to an area of the lung remained constant, but alveolar ventilation ($\dot{V}_A$) to this same area decreased?
I. the alveolar $Pco_2$ should rise
II. the ventilation–perfusion ratio should rise
III. the alveolar $Po_2$ should fall

a. II and III         c. III only
b. I and III          d. I, II, and III

12.18 Which of the following would you expect to occur if ventilation ($\dot{V}_A$) to an area of the lung remained constant, but perfusion ($\dot{Q}_c$) to this same area decreased?
I. the alveolar $Pco_2$ should fall
II. the ventilation–perfusion ratio should drop
III. the alveolar $Po_2$ should fall

a. II and III         c. I only
b. I and II           d. I, II, and III

12.19 An area of the lung has no ventilation but is normally perfused by the pulmonary circulation. Which of the following statements are true regarding this area?
I. the $\dot{V}_A/\dot{Q}_c$ ratio is zero
II. the alveolar gas is like venous blood ($Po_2 = 40$, $Pco_2 = 46$)
III. the area represents an alveolar shunt

a. II and III         c. III only
b. I and III          d. I, II, and III

12.20 At the bases of the upright lung:
I. the $\dot{V}_A/\dot{Q}_c$ ratio is low
II. the respiratory exchange ratio is low
III. the alveolar $Po_2$ is low

a. II and III         c. III only
b. I and II           d. I, II, and III

12.21 In what forms is oxygen transported in the blood?
I.     in simple physical solution
II.    chemically combined with hemoglobin
III.   chemically combined with plasma proteins

a. II and III                 c. III only
b. I and II                   d. I, II, and III

12.22 The amount of oxygen which dissolves in the plasma is:
I.     directly proportional to its solubility coefficient
II.    directly proportional to its partial pressure
III.   inversely proportional to the temperature

a. II and III                 c. III only
b. I and II                   d. I, II, and III

12.23 Each hemoglobin molecule is capable of binding how many oxygen molecules?

a. one
b. two
c. three
d. four

12.24 At a normal arterial blood $Pao_2$ of 100 mm Hg, what is the approximate percent saturation of hemoglobin with oxygen?

a. 82%
b. 87%
c. 94%
d. 97%

12.25 At a normal venous blood $Po_2$ of 40 mm Hg, what is the approximate percent saturation of hemoglobin with oxygen?

a. 40%
b. 87%
c. 73%
d. 66%

12.26 Compared with normal, a shift in the oxyhemoglobin curve to the left has which of the following effects?
I.     the hemoglobin saturation for a given $Po_2$ falls
II.    the hemoglobin saturation for a given $Po_2$ rises
III.   the affinity of hemoglobin for $O_2$ increases

a. II and III                 c. III only
b. I and II                   d. I, II, and III

12.27 According to the Bohr effect, normal changes in blood pH:
I.     aid oxygen loading in the pulmonary capillaries
II.    impede oxygen unloading in the tissue capillaries
III.   aid oxygen unloading in the tissue capillaries

a. II and III                 c. III only
b. I and III                  d. I, II, and III

12.28 When the temperature of the blood rises:
I.     the hemoglobin saturation for a given $Po_2$ falls
II.    the oxyhemoglobin dissociation curve shifts to the right
III.   the affinity of hemoglobin for $O_2$ decreases

a. II and III                 c. III only
b. I and III                  d. I, II, and III

12.29 When the erythrocyte concentration of 2,3 DPG increases:
I.     the hemoglobin saturation for a given $Po_2$ falls
II.    the oxyhemoglobin dissociation curve shifts to the right
III.   the affinity of hemoglobin for $O_2$ increases

a. II and III                 c. I and II
b. I and III                  d. I, II, and III

12.30 In which of the following conditions will erythrocyte concentration of 2,3 DPG be decreased?

a. high pH
b. anemia
c. hypoxemia
d. banked blood

12.31 The oxidation of the hemoglobin molecule's iron ions to the ferric state (Fe+++) results in:
I.     the formation of methemoglobin (metHb)
II.    the inability of hemoglobin to bind with oxygen
III.   a form of anemia called methemoglobinemia

a. II and III                 c. I and II
b. I and III                  d. I, II, and III

12.32 The affinity of carbon monoxide for hemoglobin is approximately how many times greater than that for oxygen?

a. 2–3 times greater
b. 20–30 times greater
c. 200–300 times greater
d. 50–60 times greater

12.33 A patient has a P50 value of 22 mm Hg. This would indicate:

a. a decreased affinity of hemoglobin for $O_2$
b. a shift in the oxyhemoglobin curve to the right
c. improved delivery of oxygen to the tissues
d. an increased affinity of hemoglobin for $O_2$

12.34 The total amount of $CO_2$ transported in the blood is about:

a. 75–97 ml/dL
b. 15–20 ml/dL
c. 50–60 ml/dL
d. 90–100 ml/dL

12.35 In which of the following forms is $CO_2$ transported by the blood?
I. in simple physical solution
II. ionized as bicarbonate ($HCO_3$)
III. chemically combined with proteins

a. III only
b. II and III
c. I and III
d. I, II, and III

12.36 When hemoglobin saturation with oxygen is high, less carbon dioxide is carried in the blood. This relationship is called the:

a. Bohr effect
b. Haldane effect
c. chloride shift
d. dissociation constant

12.37 The conversion of oxyhemoglobin to reduced hemoglobin:
I. helps buffer $H^+$ ions
II. enhances $CO_2$ loading on Hb
III. decreases blood $CO_2$ content

a. II and III
b. I and II
c. III only
d. I, II, and III

12.38 In the red blood cell, the rate of the hydrolysis of $CO_2$ is increased by:

a. carboxyhemoglobin
b. carbonic anhydrase
c. cholinesterase
d. 2,3 DPG

12.39 Which of the following are true regarding the relationship between the $CO_2$ combined as bicarbonate (basic salt) to that physically dissolved in the plasma (acid)?
I. they normally exist in a constant 20:1 ratio
II. their relative concentrations determine the blood's pH
III. together they form the primary body buffer system

a. II and III
b. I and II
c. II only
d. I, II, and III

**Computations:**

12.40
a. Using the data provided for the following six patients, compute the alveolar partial pressure of carbon dioxide ($P_ACO_2$) for each:

| Case # | $\dot{V}_{CO_2}$ ml/min | $\dot{V}_A$ L/min | $P_ACO_2$ mm Hg |
|---|---|---|---|
| 1 | 200 | 4.20 | _____ |
| 2 | 300 | 4.20 | _____ |
| 3 | 300 | 6.50 | _____ |
| 4 | 200 | 2.40 | _____ |
| 5 | 200 | 7.10 | _____ |
| 6 | 800 | 16.85 | _____ |

b. Which of the above cases represent normal values for a healthy 70–kg adult male? _____

_____

_____

c. Assuming the alveolar ventilation remains constant, what effect does an increase in carbon dioxide production have on the alveolar partial pressure of carbon dioxide ($P_ACO_2$)? (Hint: Compare Case #2 with Case #1.)

_____

_____

_____

d. When faced with an increase in metabolic rate (resulting in an increase in carbon dioxide production), how does the body maintain normal levels of alveolar carbon dioxide ($P_{A}CO_2$)? (Hint: Look at Cases #2 and #6.)

_____

_____

_____

e. Assuming the carbon dioxide production remains constant, what effect does a decrease in alveolar ventilation have on the alveolar partial pressure of carbon dioxide ($P_{A}CO_2$)? (Hint: Compare Case #4 with Case #1.)

_____

_____

_____

f. Assuming the carbon dioxide production remains constant, what effect does an increase in alveolar ventilation have on the alveolar partial pressure of carbon dioxide ($P_{A}CO_2$)? (Hint: Compare Case #5 with Case #1.)

_____

_____

_____

g. In which of the above cases are the patients exhibiting alveolar hypoventilation? On what evidence do you base your conclusions?

_____

_____

_____

h. In which of the above cases are the patients exhibiting alveolar hyperventilation? On what evidence do you base your conclusions?

_____

_____

_____

12.41

a. Using the alveolar air equation and the data provided for the following 10 patients, compute the alveolar partial pressure of oxygen ($P_{A}O_2$) for each. (Hint: If the $F_{IO_2}$ is greater than .60, use the simplified form of the equation.)

| Case # | $P_B$ mm Hg | $F_{IO_2}$ (%/100) | $P_aCO_2$ mm Hg | $P_{A}O_2$ mm Hg |
|--------|-------------|---------------------|------------------|-------------------|
| 1 | 760 | .21 | 40 | _____ |
| 2 | 760 | .21 | 75 | _____ |
| 3 | 760 | .21 | 22 | _____ |
| 4 | 630 | .21 | 40 | _____ |
| 5 | 2280 | .21 | 40 | _____ |
| 6 | 752 | .28 | 43 | _____ |
| 7 | 763 | .40 | 38 | _____ |
| 8 | 755 | .70 | 36 | _____ |
| 9 | 760 | 1.00 | 45 | _____ |
| 10 | 250 | 1.00 | 45 | _____ |

b. Which of the above cases represent normal values for a healthy young adult?

_____

_____

_____

c. Assuming a constant $P_B$ and $F_{IO_2}$, what effect do changes in alveolar ventilation (as manifested by changes in the $P_aCO_2$) have on the alveolar partial pressure of oxygen ($P_{A}O_2$). Which of the above cases demonstrate this effect?

_____

_____

_____

d. Assuming a constant $FIO_2$ and alveolar ventilation, what effect do changes in the barometric pressure have on the alveolar partial pressure of oxygen ($P_AO_2$)? Which of the above cases demonstrate this effect?

_____

_____

_____

e. If our desire was to increase the partial pressure of oxygen in the lungs and blood without increasing the $FIO_2$ above that available in room air, how might this be accomplished? Which of the above cases demonstrate this effect?

_____

_____

_____

f. In healthy individuals, what effect does increasing the $FIO_2$ have on the alveolar partial pressure of oxygen ($P_AO_2$)? Which of the above cases demonstrate this effect?

_____

_____

_____

g. Exposure of the lung to partial pressures of oxygen above 250 to 300 mm Hg for prolonged periods is known to result in a variety of tissue and cellular injuries, yet our astronauts breathe 100% oxygen ($FIO_2$ = 1.0) for days or weeks when in space without suffering harm. How is this possible? (Hint: Look at Case #10.)

_____

_____

_____

| Case # | Po$_2$ mm Hg | Dis O$_2$ ml/dL | Hb Sat % | Hb gm/dL | HbO$_2$ ml/dL | TOT O$_2$ ml/dL |
|--------|--------------|-----------------|----------|----------|---------------|-----------------|
| 1 | 100 | _____ | 97% | 15.0 | _____ | _____ |
| 2 | 40 | _____ | 73% | 15.0 | _____ | _____ |
| 3 | 625 | _____ | 100% | 15.0 | _____ | _____ |
| 4 | 100 | _____ | 97% | 7.5 | _____ | _____ |
| 5 | 200 | _____ | 97% | 7.5 | _____ | _____ |
| 6 | 50 | _____ | 82% | 18.6 | _____ | _____ |
| 7 | 100 | _____ | 10% | 15.0 | _____ | _____ |
| 8 | 3040 | _____ | 100% | 5.6 | _____ | _____ |

12.42

a. Using the data provided for the above eight patients, compute the dissolved O$_2$ content, chemically combined O$_2$ content (HbO$_2$), and total O$_2$ content of their blood in ml/dL. Use 1.34 ml/gm as the factor for computing HbO$_2$. _____

_____

_____

b. Which of the above cases represent normal values for a healthy young adult?

_____

c. Assuming a normal concentration of hemoglobin, what effect does a lower than normal blood Po$_2$ have on the total oxygen content of the blood? What is the main cause of this effect? Which of the above cases demonstrate this effect?

_____

_____

d. Assuming a normal concentration of hemoglobin, what effect does a higher than normal blood Po$_2$ have on the total oxygen content of the blood? Which of the above cases demonstrate this effect?

_____

_____

_____

_____

e. Comparing your answers to c and d above, which effect has the greater impact on total oxygen contents, i.e., a low or high blood Po$_2$? Why?

_____

_____

_____

f. What effect does a decrease in hemoglobin concentration have on the total oxygen content of the blood? Which of the above cases demonstrate this effect?

_____

_____

_____

g. With normal atmospheric pressures, if the blood hemoglobin concentration is below normal, does increasing the blood Po$_2$ significantly increase the total oxygen contents? Why/why not? Which of the above cases demonstrate this effect?

_____

_____

h. Look carefully at Case #7. Why is the total oxygen content of the blood so low? Name two clinical conditions that might explain this problem.

_____

_____

_____

i. Look carefully at Case #8. The hemoglobin concentration is dangerously low, yet the patient has an acceptable total oxygen content. How is this possible?

_____

_____

_____

12.43

a. Using the data provided for the following five patients, first compute each patient's arterial–venous oxygen content difference. Then apply the Fick principle to calculate their cardiac outputs.

| Case # | $\dot{V}_{O_2}$ ml/min | $Ca_{O_2}$ ml/dL | $C\bar{v}_{O_2}$ ml/dL | $C(a-\bar{v})_{O_2}$ | $\dot{Q}_T$ L/min |
|--------|------|-------|-------|------|------|
| 1 | 265 | 19.40 | 14.60 | _____ | _____ |
| 2 | 265 | 19.40 | 12.30 | _____ | _____ |
| 3 | 265 | 19.40 | 16.70 | _____ | _____ |
| 4 | 740 | 19.40 | 14.60 | _____ | _____ |
| 5 | 150 | 19.40 | 14.60 | _____ | _____ |

b. Assuming that Case #1 represents a normal patient and that the oxygen consumption ($\dot{V}_{O_2}$) and total arterial oxygen contents ($Ca_{O_2}$) remain constant, what effect do changes in cardiac output have on the mixed venous oxygen content? On the arterial–venous oxygen content difference? Which of the above cases demonstrate this effect? _____

_____

_____

_____

c. During moderate exercise in normal individuals, the oxygen consumption increases markedly, but the mixed venous oxygen content and arterial–venous oxygen content difference remain near normal. How is this possible? Which of the above cases demonstrate this effect?

_____

_____

_____

d. Whole–body hypothermia reduces total oxygen consumption. What impact would hypothermia have on the demands placed on the heart? Which of the above cases demonstrate this effect?

_____

_____

_____

# Solutions, Body Fluids, and Electrolytes

## CONTENT EXERCISES

**True/False:** For each of the following statements, indicate whether it is mainly true or mainly false by circling the corresponding letter (T=True, F=False):

13.1 T F In general, the solubility of most solid solutes increases with temperature; the solubility of gases, however, varies inversely with temperature.

13.2 T F A 4% solution will exert twice the osmotic pressure of a 2% solution.

13.3 T F The larger the concentration of ions made available by a solute, the stronger the electrolyte is.

13.4 T F Any solution having a hydrogen ion concentration less than $1.0 \times 10^{-7}$ moles per liter is acid in its reactions.

13.5 T F Most body water is normally found within the cells.

13.6 T F The extracellular fluid compartment of the infant is approximately twice as large as that of the adult.

13.7 T F The composition of solutes in the intracellular and extracellular fluid compartments are just about the same.

13.8 T F A loss of chloride by the body is equivalent to a gain in bicarbonate.

13.9 T F The serum $K^+$ level is a direct indicator of the total body potassium.

13.10 T F As the pH of body fluids rises, $K^+$ moves out of the cells.

13.11 T F Unlike many electrolytes, the kidney does not have the capability to conserve potassium.

**Short Answer:** Complete each statement by filling in the correct information in the space(s) provided:

13.12 _____ is a stable mixture of two substances, with one evenly dispersed throughout the other.

13.13 A _____ solution is one with the maximum amount of solute that can be held by a given volume of a solvent at a constant temperature, in the presence of an excess of solute.

13.14 _____ is the process by which the ions of an electrovalent substance are freed from their mutual bonds and distribute themselves uniformly throughout a solvent.

13.15 Any solution with a $[H^+]$ greater than _____ nM/L is considered acidic.

13.16 A 1–unit change in pH is equivalent to a _____ change in $[H^+]$.

13.17 As the pH value of a solution decreases below 7, the $[H^+]$ _____, and the solution becomes more _____.

13.18 The total body water of the average adult male is about _____ % of his body weight, whereas that of the average adult female is about _____ %.

13.19 The average urine output in the normal adult ranges between _____ and _____ ml per day.

13.20 The _____ is the difference between the humidity content of the inspired air and the normal BTPS conditions in the lung.

13.21 A patient with an artificial airway who is not provided adequate airway humidification may lose as much as _____ ml of additional water per day.

13.22 Mean pressures in the pulmonary circulation are about _____ those in the systemic circulation.

13.23 _____ hormone levels largely govern sodium reabsorption in the kidneys.

13.24 _____ is the most prominent anion in the body.

13.25 The concentration of _____ in the extracellular compartment is inversely proportionate to that of chloride.

13.26 Chloride is usually excreted by the kidney with
_____.

13.27 A precise ratio of _____ is the normal ratio of bicarbonate to carbonic acid, resulting in a normal pH of 7.4.

13.28 Calcium is an important mediator of _____ and cellular enzyme processes.

**Listing:** Complete each list as directed in its statement.

13.29 List the two (2) mechanisms by which the kidneys maintain the volume and composition of body fluids relatively constantly:

1. _____

_____

2. _____

_____

13.30 List at least five (5) clinical examples of conditions causing abnormal additive fluid losses:

1. _____

2. _____

3. _____

4. _____

5. _____

13.31 List the normal serum (intravascular) ranges for the following electrolytes:

| | Electrolyte | Normal Range (mEq/L) |
|---|---|---|
| 1. | sodium ($Na^+$) | _____ |
| 2. | chloride ($Cl^-$) | _____ |
| 3. | bicarbonate ($HCO_3^-$) | _____ |
| 4. | potassium ($K^+$) | _____ |
| 5. | calcium ($Ca^{++}$) | _____ |
| 6. | phosphorus ($HPO_4^-$) | _____ |

13.32 List the three (3) forms of calcium present in the blood:

1. _____

2. _____

3. _____

**Multiple Choice:** Circle the letter corresponding to the single best answer from the available choices:

13.33 Which of the following effects are observed when a solute is added to a solvent to create a solution?
I.   the vapor pressure of the solution is decreased
II.  the boiling point of the solution is lowered
III. the freezing point of the solution is lowered
IV.  the osmotic pressure of the solution increases

a. I and II                 c. I, III, and IV
b. I, II, and III           d. I, II, III, and IV

13.34 The primary intracellular cation is:

a. sodium ($Na^+$)
b. potassium ($K^+$)
c. calcium ($Ca^{++}$)
d. magnesium ($Mg^{++}$)

13.35 The primary intravascular cation is:

a. sodium ($Na^+$)
b. potassium ($K^+$)
c. calcium ($Ca^{++}$)
d. magnesium ($Mg^{++}$)

13.36 Compared with the interstitial compartment, the higher osmotic pressure of the plasma is due primarily to its high concentration of:

a. plasma proteins, mainly albumin
b. sodium chloride (NaCl)
c. organic acids
d. sodium hydrogen phosphate

13.37 Sensible water loss includes which of the following categories?
I.   urinary excretion
II.  intestinal losses
III. loss due to sweating
IV.  evaporation via skin/lungs

a. I and II                 c. II, III, and IV
b. I, II, and III           d. I, II, III, and IV

13.38 The primary mechanism responsible for the exchange of fluids between the systemic capillaries and the interstitial fluid is:

a. active transport
b. osmosis
c. filtration
d. passive diffusion

13.39 According to the Starling equilibrium equation, which of the following factors would increase fluid movement into the interstitial space?
I.   increased capillary hydrostatic pressure
II.  decreased capillary osmotic pressure
III. increased capillary permeability

a. I and II            c. III only
b. II and III          d. I, II, and III

13.40 Factors aiding reabsorption of tissue fluid in areas with high hydrostatic pressures (such as in the feet) include which of the following?
I.   proportionately higher interstitial pressures
II.  lower venous pressures (due to the pumping action of skeletal muscle)
III. lower lymph pressures (due to the pumping action of skeletal muscle)

a. III only            c. II and III
b. I and II            d. I, II, and III

13.41 The alveolar–capillary region is kept relatively free of excess interstitial water because:

a. hydrostatic pressures are lower than in the systemic circulation
b. capillary osmotic pressures are high in the pulmonary circulation
c. alveolar capillary permeability is less than in the tissue capillaries
d. alveolar capillary permeability is greater than in the tissue capillaries
e. lymphatic pressures are higher in the lung than in the tissues

13.42 The ability of some cells to maintain significant differences in the concentrations of electrolytes (such as potassium) across their cell walls is due mainly to which of the following phenomena?

a. active transport
b. osmosis
c. filtration
d. passive diffusion

13.43 Which of the following are common causes of hyponatremia?
I.   gastrointestinal losses
II.  excessive sweat or fever
III. prolonged use of certain diuretics
IV.  Addison's disease

a. I, II, and III      c. II and III
b. II, III, and IV     d. I, II, III, and IV

13.44 Hypochloremia is usually associated with which of the following acid–base abnormalities?

a. respiratory acidosis
b. respiratory alkalosis
c. metabolic alkalosis
d. metabolic acidosis

13.45 Hypokalemia can result in:
I.   muscle weakness
II.  paralysis
III. cardiac arrest
IV.  ileus

a. II and III          c. II and IV
b. II, III, and IV     d. I, II, III, and IV

13.46 Clinical manifestations of hypocalcemia include which of the following?
I.   a shortened Q–T interval on the EKG
II.  abdominal cramps
III. muscular twitching and spasm
IV.  hyperactive tendon reflexes

a. II and III          c. II and IV
b. II, III, and IV     d. I, II, III, and IV

13.47 Clinical manifestations of hypercalcemia include which of the following?
I.   fatigue
II.  muscle weakness
III. nausea and vomiting
IV.  hyperactive tendon reflexes

a. I, II, and III      c. II and IV
b. II, III, and IV     d. I, II, III, and IV

## Computations:

13.48 For each of the following W/V solutions, compute (1) the total grams of solute in the given volume of the solution and (2) the number of milligrams of solute in each milliliter of the solution (mg/ml):

| Solution Volume in ml | Concentration of Solution (W/V) | Total Solute Content in grams | Solute Content in mg/ml |
|---|---|---|---|
| a.  10 | 1.00% | _____ | _____ |
| b.  2 | 3.00% | _____ | _____ |
| c.  50 | 20.00% | _____ | _____ |
| d.  1000 | 10.00% | _____ | _____ |

13.49 For each hydrogen ion concentration listed below, (1) compute the pH of the solution and (2) calculate the nanomolar hydrogen ion concentration:

| $[H^+]$ M/L | pH | nanomole/L (nM/L) |
|---|---|---|
| a.  $4.80 \times 10^{-8}$ | _____ | _____ |
| b.  $8.50 \times 10^{-8}$ | _____ | _____ |
| c.  $1.20 \times 10^{-7}$ | _____ | _____ |
| d.  $6.10 \times 10^{-7}$ | _____ | _____ |
| e.  $2.40 \times 10^{-6}$ | _____ | _____ |

# Acid–Base Balance and the Regulation of Respiration

## CONTENT EXERCISES

**True/False:** For each of the following statements, indicate whether it is mainly true or mainly false by circling the corresponding letter (T=True, F=False):

14.1　T　F　Carbonic acid is considered a nonvolatile or fixed acid.

14.2　T　F　Fixed acids are produced primarily from the catabolism of proteins.

14.3　T　F　$CO_2$ excretion is inversely proportional to the level of alveolar ventilation.

14.4　T　F　In regard to overall body acid–base homeostasis, the retention of base has the same effect as the excretion of acid.

14.5　T　F　Most bicarbonate reabsorption occurs in the distal tubules of the kidney.

14.6　T　F　For each hydrogen ion excreted by the kidney, one bicarbonate ion is returned to the blood.

14.7　T　F　According to the Henderson–Hasselbalch equation, if either the buffer capacity or $CO_2$ decreases, the pH will fall.

14.8　T　F　Compensatory responses in acid–base imbalances require that the unaffected system be functioning normally.

14.9　T　F　Correction of compensated acid–base abnormalities should be accomplished as quickly as possible.

14.10　T　F　In compensation for acute respiratory acidosis, bicarbonate reabsorption and urine acidification by the kidneys may not reach maximum efficiency for 3 or 4 days.

14.11　T　F　In acute or uncompensated respiratory acidosis, the base excess range is +/– 2 mEq/L.

14.12　T　F　Metabolic acidosis due to either a loss of $HCO_3$ or a gain of $Cl^-$ generally does not increase the anion gap.

14.13　T　F　Compensation for metabolic acidosis occurs via increased ventilation by the lungs.

14.14　T　F　Hypokalemia can be both a cause and effect of metabolic alkalosis.

14.15　T　F　The expected compensatory response to metabolic alkalosis (hypoventilation) is generally not observed.

14.16　T　F　The major factor responsible for changes in ventilation is neural input to the medullary centers through the chemoreceptors.

14.17　T　F　The blood–brain barrier is freely permeable to hydrogen and bicarbonate ions.

14.18　T　F　Compared with the central chemoreceptors, the carotid and aortic bodies are not very sensitive to $CO_2$ changes.

14.19　T　F　Stimulation of breathing due to hypoxia is solely through the peripheral chemoreceptor mechanism.

14.20　T　F　Hypercapnea and hypoxemia together exert an additive effect on increasing ventilation.

14.21　T　F　In patients with chronic hypercapnea, oxygen administration can depress ventilation.

**Short Answer:** Complete each statement by filling in the correct information in the space(s) provided:

14.22 Normal aerobic metabolism of carbohydrates and fats results in the production of _____.

14.23 About _____ mM of $CO_2$ are eliminated from the body daily via normal ventilation.

14.24 _____ is a fixed acid produced by the incomplete oxidative metabolism of carbohydrates and fats.

14.25 The average amount of fixed acid produced by the body per day is about _____ mEq per kilogram of body weight.

14.26 The body reclaims about _____ mEq of bicarbonate from the blood per day.

14.27 Renal tubular cells produce ammonia by the deamidization of _____.

14.28 In health, the body maintains the arterial blood pH within a narrow normal range of _____.

14.29 According to the Henderson–Hasselbalch equation, the pH of the blood will rise if either the buffer capacity _____ or $CO_2$ content _____.

14.30 The difference in mEq/L between the normal buffer base (NBB) and the actual buffer base (BB) in a whole blood sample is called the _____.

14.31 The difference in concentration between the two primary anions ($Cl^-$ and $HCO_3$ ) and two primary cations ($Na^+$ and $K^+$ ) is called the _____ _____.

14.32 A _____ represents a group of nerve cells that sense and respond to changes in the chemical composition of their fluid environment.

14.33 In addition to the input from the chemoreceptors, the brainstem receives and processes sensory information from a variety of "mechanical" sensors called _____.

**Multiple Choice:** Circle the letter corresponding to the single best answer from the available choices:

14.34 Normally, the kidneys excrete about how much fixed acid?

a. 200–300 mM/day
b. 20,000–24,000 mM/day
c. 50–70 mM/day
d. 5–10 mM/day

14.35 Which of the following are components of the body's nonbicarbonate buffer system?
I.    hemoglobin
II.   the plasma proteins
III.  organic phosphates
IV.  inorganic phosphates

a. II, III, and IV          c. II and IV
b. I, III, and IV          d. I, II, III, and IV

14.36 Under normal physiologic conditions, the negative log of the equilibrium constant of the acid component of the bicarbonate buffer system (abbreviated as pK) is:

a. 7.4
b. 6.1
c. 40
d. 24

14.37 A patient has a bicarbonate concentration of 36 mEq and a $Pco_2$ of 60 mm Hg. What is her approximate pH?

a. 7.4
b. 7.3
c. 7.2
d. 7.5

14.38 If the blood $Pco_2$ is 80 mm Hg, what is the $CO_2$ content in millimoles per liter mM/L?

a. 1.2 mM/L
b. .03 mM/L
c. 80 mM/L
d. 2.4 mM/L

14.39 Which of the following are true regarding the renal reabsorption of bicarbonate?
I.     $HCO_3$ occurs via active transport mechanisms
II.    $HCO_3$ is selectively reabsorbed with sodium ions
III.   its transport is facilitated by conversion to $CO_2$

a. II and III          c. I and III
b. II only             d. I, II, and III

14.40 If the maintenance of acid–base homeostasis demands increased excretion of $HCO_3$, the kidneys will:

a. preferentially retain chloride ions
b. preferentially excrete chloride ions
c. excrete greater numbers of hydrogen ions
d. increase bicarbonate reabsorption

14.41 Most of the body's nonvolatile acids are excreted via which of the following mechanisms?

a. the reabsorption and generation of $HCO_3$
b. the acidification of hydrogen phosphate
c. the production of ammonium ions
d. the selective reabsorption of chloride

14.42 During both the reabsorption of $HCO_3$ and the elimination of fixed acids by the kidneys:
I.     sodium ions (and water) are retained
II.    $HCO_3$ is reabsorbed in proportion to the $H^+$ excreted
III.   bicarbonate buffer capacity is restored

a. II and III          c. I and III
b. II only             d. I, II, and III

14.43 According to the Henderson–Hasselbalch equation, which of the following events can cause alkalemia?
I.   an increase in $HCO_3$
II.  a decrease in $CO_2$
III. a decrease in buffer base

a. II and III
b. I and III
c. I and II
d. I, II, and III

14.44 Correction of acute respiratory acidosis is accomplished by:

a. increasing $HCO_3$ reabsorption
b. increasing alveolar ventilation
c. decreasing $HCO_3$ reabsorption
d. decreasing alveolar ventilation

14.45 Which of the following potential causes of respiratory acidosis are associated with abnormal lungs?

a. neuromuscular disorders
b. spinal cord trauma
c. anesthesia
d. acute airway obstruction

14.46 Renal compensation for respiratory acidosis involves which of the following mechanisms?
I.   preferential reabsorption of $HCO_3^-$ over $Cl^-$
II.  increased acidification of the urine
III. preferential reabsorption of $Na^+$ over $H^+$

a. I and III
b. II and III
c. I and II
d. I, II, and III

14.47 Which of the following would be common findings in "chronic" or compensated respiratory acidosis?
I.   an elevated $HCO_3$
II.  a pH well below 7.35
III. a low serum chloride
IV.  a low urine pH

a. I, III, and IV
b. II and III
c. I, II, and III
d. I, II, III, and IV

14.48 In chronic respiratory acidosis, for each 10 mm Hg rise in $P_{CO_2}$ the plasma $HCO_3$ can be expected to increase by about:

a. 4 mEq/L
b. 1 mEq/L
c. 10 mEq/L
d. 40 mEq/L

14.49 Which of the following are potential causes of respiratory alkalosis?
I.   anxiety
II.  fever
III. hypoxemia
IV.  CNS depression
V.   pain

a. I and III
b. II, III, IV, and V
c. I, II, III, and V
d. I, II, III, IV, and V

14.50 The most common cause of iatrogenic respiratory alkalosis is:

a. CNS stimulation
b. severe hypoxemia
c. mechanical hyperventilation
d. vagal stimulation

14.51 Which of the following are potential manifestations or effects of acute respiratory alkalosis?
I.   paresthesia
II.  impaired cerebral circulation
III. hyperactive neural reflexes
IV.  tetanic muscle contractions
V.   cardiac arrhythmias

a. II, III, IV, and V
b. I, III, and IV
c. II, IV, and V
d. I, II, III, IV, and V

14.52 In patients with chronic or compensated respiratory alkalosis, for every 10 mm Hg decrease in $P_{CO_2}$, the plasma $HCO_3$ can be expected to drop by about:

a. 10 mEq/L
b. 5 mEq/L
c. 1 mEq/L
d. 20 mEq/L

14.53 A patient has an anion gap of 21 mEq/L. Based on this information, you may conclude that:
I.   there is an abnormal excess of anions in the plasma
II.  the patient probably has metabolic acidosis
III. the concentration of organic acids is increased

a. I only
b. I and II
c. II and III
d. I, II, and III

14.54 A patient has an anion gap of 15 mEq/L, a $P_{CO_2}$ of 38 mm Hg, and a pH of 7.29. Based on this information, you may conclude that:

I. the patient has a metabolic acidosis
II. the plasma $HCO_3$ is probably low
III. the plasma $Cl^-$ is probably high

a. I only
b. I and II
c. II only
d. I, II, and III

14.55 Which of the following represent potential causes of metabolic acidosis with an increased anion gap (gain of fixed acid)?

I. renal tubular acidosis
II. parenteral nutrition
III. diabetic ketoacidosis
IV. diarrhea
V. lactic acidosis

a. II and III
b. II, III, IV, and V
c. III and IV
d. I, II, III, IV, and V

14.56 Which of the following are potential causes of hyperchloremic metabolic acidosis?

I. hyperalimentation
II. pancreatic fistula
III. diarrhea
IV. $NH_4Cl$ administration
V. renal tubular acidosis

a. II and III
b. II, III, IV, and V
c. I, III, IV, and V
d. I, II, III, IV, and V

14.57 Which of the following is not a drug– or chemical–induced cause of metabolic acidosis?

a. salicylate intoxication
b. carbenicillin therapy
c. starvation
d. methanol ingestion

14.58 Primary metabolic or nonrespiratory alkalosis is associated with which of the following?

I. a gain in fixed (nonvolatile) acids
II. a loss in blood carbonic acid ($CO_2$)
III. an excessive gain of buffer base

a. I only
b. I and II
c. III only
d. I, II, and III

14.59 Augmented renal excretion of $H^+$, $K^+$, or $Cl^-$ can be caused by:

I. administration of certain diuretic agents
II. administration of certain corticosteroids
III. clinical entities such as Cushing's syndrome

a. I and II
b. I only
c. III only
d. I, II, and III

14.60 The medulla contains which of the following areas?

I. inspiratory/expiratory "centers"
II. chemoreceptor cells
III. pneumotaxic center
IV. apneustic center

a. I only
b. I and II
c. I, II, and III
d. I, II, III, and IV

14.61 The apneustic center:

I. is located in the pons
II. helps terminate normal inspiration
III. receives afferent vagal input

a. I and II
b. I only
c. III only
d. I, II, and III

14.62 Peripheral chemoreceptors are located:

I. on the ventrolateral surfaces of the medulla
II. in the bifurcations of carotid arteries
III. in the arch of the aorta

a. I and II
b. I only
c. II and III
d. I, II, and III

14.63 Which of the following are true regarding the effect of breathing carbon dioxide?

I. breathing carbon dioxide stimulates the central chemoreceptors
II. concentrations below 20% increase ventilation
III. concentrations above 20% have an anesthetic effect

a. I only
b. I and II
c. III only
d. I, II, and III

14.64 Anemia and carbon monoxide poisoning both can cause severe hypoxia. Yet, neither condition results in a major stimulation of breathing. This is because:

a. the peripheral chemoreceptors are responsive mainly to a decreased $Pa_{O_2}$, not a decreased $Ca_{O_2}$
b. anemia and carbon monoxide poisoning depress the peripheral chemoreceptors
c. anemia and carbon monoxide poisoning depress the central chemoreceptors
d. anemia and carbon monoxide cause stagnant hypoxia, not hypoxemia

14.65 Which of the following are true regarding the Hering–Breuer inflation reflex?
I. its receptors are located mostly in the bronchi and bronchioles
II. its impulses travel via the vagus nerve to the apneustic center
III. it is weak or absent during quiet breathing in healthy adults
IV. it mainly affects the length of the expiratory pause between breaths

a. I only
b. I and II
c. I, II, and III
d. I, II, III, and IV

14.66 Which of the following can cause stimulation of the pulmonary irritant receptors?
I. physical manipulation
II. inhalation of noxious gases
III. asphyxia
IV. pulmonary microembolization

a. I and II
b. I only
c. I, II, and III
d. I, II, III, and IV

14.67 Otherwise normal individuals with chronic hypoxemia tend to hyperventilate. If a chronic hypoxic stimulus to breathe is removed, this hyperventilation tends to continue for some time, albeit at a lesser magnitude. This response is due to the fact that:

a. chronic hypoxemia causes the CSF pH to remain alkalotic (high pH)
b. chronic hypoxemia resets the central chemoreceptors to a lower $P_{CO_2}$
c. chronic hypoxemia decreases central sensitivity to carbon dioxide
d. chronic hypoxemia increases peripheral sensitivity to carbon dioxide

14.68 A patient with renal tubular acidosis has the following arterial blood gas values: pH = 7.34; $P_{CO_2}$ = 27 mm Hg; $HCO_3$ = 14 mEq/L. After treatment by dialysis, the following ABGs are obtained: pH = 7.62; $P_{CO_2}$ = 22 mm Hg; $HCO_3$ = 22 mEq/L. Why does her hyperventilation persist despite correction of the metabolic acidosis?

a. in chronic metabolic acidosis the CSF pH remains acid (low pH)
b. in chronic metabolic acidosis the central chemoreceptors become less sensitive to $CO_2$ changes
c. in chronic metabolic acidosis the central chemoreceptors become more sensitive to $CO_2$ changes
d. in chronic metabolic acidosis the CSF pH remains alkaline (high pH)

**Computations and Analysis:**

14.69
a. For each of the five patients listed below, apply the Henderson–Hasselbalch equation to compute their blood pH (a log table will be required):

| Case # | $P_{CO_2}$ mm Hg | $HCO_3$ mEq/L | Blood pH |
|---|---|---|---|
| 1 | 40 | 24 | _____ |
| 2 | 65 | 26 | _____ |
| 3 | 22 | 22 | _____ |
| 4 | 72 | 38 | _____ |
| 5 | 18 | 12 | _____ |

14.70 Given the following data on the twenty patients, provide a correct interpretation of their acid–base status in the space provided. Where evidence of compensation exists, but the pH has not been restored to the normal range, use the term "partially compensated."

| | pH | $P_{CO_2}$ mm Hg | $HCO_3$ mEq/L | Acid–Base Interpretation |
|---|---|---|---|---|
| a. | 7.24 | 47 | 19.5 | _____ |
| b. | 7.43 | 39 | 25.1 | _____ |
| c. | 7.62 | 41 | 40.9 | _____ |
| d. | 7.42 | 20 | 12.6 | _____ |
| e. | 6.89 | 24 | 4.7 | _____ |
| f. | 7.45 | 48 | 29.6 | _____ |
| g. | 7.08 | 39 | 11.8 | _____ |
| h. | 7.79 | 23 | 33.9 | _____ |
| i. | 7.29 | 51 | 25.8 | _____ |
| j. | 7.56 | 51 | 44.3 | _____ |
| k. | 7.09 | 86 | 28.2 | _____ |
| l. | 7.35 | 21 | 11.7 | _____ |
| m. | 7.81 | 12 | 21.2 | _____ |
| n. | 7.35 | 68 | 34.3 | _____ |
| o. | 7.61 | 25 | 21.2 | _____ |
| p. | 7.68 | 14 | 16.3 | _____ |
| q. | 7.36 | 52 | 29.2 | _____ |
| r. | 7.31 | 77 | 39.6 | _____ |
| s. | 7.45 | 28 | 18.9 | _____ |
| t. | 7.36 | 44 | 23.5 | _____ |

# Patterns of Cardiopulmonary Dysfunction

## CONTENT EXERCISES

**True/False:** For each of the following statements, indicate whether it is mainly true or mainly false by circling the corresponding letter (T=True, F=False):

15.1  T   F   A decrease in tissue perfusion can cause hypoxia.

15.2  T   F   An increase in alveolar ventilation relative to metabolic need will result in hypercapnia, or an elevated arterial $P_{CO_2}$.

15.3  T   F   The partial pressure of oxygen in the alveoli varies inversely with the $P_{A}CO_2$.

15.4  T   F   A pure diffusion limitation is a common cause of hypoxemia at rest.

15.5  T   F   Normal individuals do not have anatomic shunts.

15.6  T   F   The arterial $P_{O_2}$ is less than the alveolar $P_{O_2}$.

15.7  T   F   Low V/Q ratios are a more common cause of hypoxemia than are true physiologic shunts.

15.8  T   F   A normal $Pa_{O_2}$ guarantees adequate arterial oxygen content and delivery.

15.9  T   F   Hypoxia can occur in the presence of a normal arterial oxygen content.

15.10  T   F   Cyanosis is a reliable indicator of hypoxemia and hypoxia.

15.11  T   F   An increase in the viscosity of the blood decreases cardiac work load.

15.12  T   F   In hypoxemia caused by physiologic shunting, high $O_2$ concentrations are usually effective to achieve a satisfactory arterial oxygen content.

15.13  T   F   Ventilation–perfusion imbalance is a common physiologic cause for a reduced $Pa_{O_2}$.

15.14  T   F   An increase in $P_{O_2}$ levels above 100 mm Hg contributes little to increasing the oxygen content of the blood.

15.15  T   F   A drop in $P_{O_2}$ from low V/Q units can be compensated for by a rise in the $P_{O_2}$ in high V/Q units.

15.16  T   F   High viscosity respiratory tract secretions can usually be cleared by coughing.

15.17  T   F   Pursed–lip breathing can increase the efficiency of ventilation.

15.18  T   F   All obstructive disorders are characterized by impedance to the flow of air.

**Short Answer:** Complete each statement by filling in the correct information in the space(s) provided:

15.19 A condition in which oxygen delivery to the tissues is inadequate to meet cellular needs best defines _____.

15.20 Unlike healthy individuals, those with respiratory disease may exhibit an _____ in $P_{CO_2}$ during exercise.

15.21 When blood bypasses the lungs by flowing from the venous to the arterial side of the circulation, a _____ shunt exists.

15.22 A physiologic shunt exists when a portion of the pulmonary blood perfuses _____ alveoli.

15.23 The term used to describe a reduction in the blood hemoglobin level below normal is _____ _____.

15.24 In order for cyanosis to be detected, the capillaries generally must contain at least _____ reduced hemoglobin.

15.25 With right–to–left shunting, administration of a higher $FI_{O_2}$ typically _____ the $P(A - a)_{O_2}$.

15.26 A blood gas change indicating that hypoxemia is due to reduced blood flow is a reduction in the _____.

15.27 _____ secretions are the result of invasion of the respiratory tract by pathogenic bacteria and the effect of such infection on the sputum.

**Listing:** Complete each list as directed in its statement.

15.28 List the three (3) primary physiologic causes of tissue hypoxia:

1. _____

   _____

2. _____

   _____

3. _____

   _____

15.29 List at least four (4) pathologic causes of acute hypoxia:

1. _____

   _____

2. _____

   _____

3. _____

   _____

4. _____

   _____

**Multiple Choice:** Circle the letter corresponding to the single best answer from the available choices:

15.30 General causes of cardiopulmonary dysfunction include which of the following?
I.   impaired oxygen delivery
II.  impaired carbon dioxide removal
III. prohibitively excessive energy costs

a. II and III          c. I and II
b. I and III           d. I, II, and III

15.31 The alveolar partial pressure of carbon dioxide, or $P_{A}CO_2$, is:
I.   directly proportional to whole body carbon dioxide production
II.  inversely proportional to the level of alveolar ventilation
III. normally maintained at about 38–42 mm Hg

a. I and II            c. III only
b. II and III          d. I, II, and III

15.32 Which of the following equations best describes oxygen delivery *to* the tissues?

a. arterial oxygen content/cardiac output
b. cardiac output/arterial oxygen content
c. cardiac output x vascular resistance
d. arterial oxygen content x cardiac output

15.33 Which of the following factors limit the increase in workload that patients with cardiovascular disease can sustain?
I.   dyspnea (subjective difficulty in breathing)
II.  an inadequate heart rate
III. an inadequate stroke volume

a. I and III           c. II only
b. II and III          d. I, II, and III

15.34 Since an elevated $Paco_2$ increases ventilatory drive in normal subjects, the presence of hypercapnia clinically suggests which of the following?
I.   a failure of the breathing stimulus to get through to the respiratory muscles
II.  a failure to respond normally to the elevated $Pco_2$
III. pulmonary restriction or muscular fatigue

a. II and III          c. II only
b. I and III           d. I, II, and III

15.35 Mild to moderate hypoxia in normal subjects usually manifests itself in which of the following signs or symptoms?
I.   hyperventilation and tachypnea
II.  restlessness and disorientation
III. tachycardia and mild hypertension

a. I and III           c. II only
b. II and III          d. I, II, and III

15.36 The most critical target organ of hypoxia is the:

a. liver
b. kidney
c. lung
d. brain

15.37 Simple oxygen therapy techniques (those capable of providing $FIO_2$s between 0.21 and 0.50) are generally effective in treating which of the following types of hypoxemia?
I.    hypoxemia due to a low alveolar $PO_2$
II.   hypoxemia due to a left–to–right shunt
III.  hypoxemia due to a moderately low V/Q imbalance

a. III only
b. I and III
c. I only
d. I, II, and III

15.38 The primary therapeutic goal in the treatment of hypoxia is to provide sufficient oxygen to the cells to preserve their normal function. Specific clinical objectives under this goal include which of the following?
I.    the restoration of arterial oxygen content
II.   the assurance of tissue perfusion
III.  the avoidance of toxic $PO_2$s

a. I and II
b. I and III
c. II only
d. I, II, and III

15.39 Which of the following statements regarding *peripheral* cyanosis is true?

a. it is caused by poor tissue perfusion or blood stasis
b. it is an indicator of central hypoxemia
c. it is observed in the lips and gums
d. it is rare when the arterial oxygen content is normal

15.40 Assuming normal conditions, the appearance of central cyanosis in adults *first* manifests itself when the arterial hemoglobin saturation drops below:

a. 95%
b. 90%
c. 85%
d. 80%

15.41 A patient with a normal $PaO_2$, $P(A - a)O_2$, Hb content, and cardiac output is exhibiting signs and symptoms of tissue hypoxia. What is the most likely cause of her hypoxia?

a. hypoventilation (decreased $\dot{V}_A$)
b. a right–to–left physiologic shunt
c. impaired lung diffusion
d. a hemoglobin saturation abnormality

15.42 Which of the following are common to the normal aging process?
I.    a predictable decrease in the $PO_2$ over time
II.   a predictable increase in the $P(A - a)O_2$ over time
III.  a loss of lung tissue elastic recoil over time
IV.   a worsening of the V/Q balance over time

a. I, II, and IV
b. II, III, and IV
c. I, II, and III
d. I, II, III, and IV

15.43 Which of the following are good examples of conditions in which ischemia results in *localized* hypoxia and tissue death?
I.    myocardial infarction
II.   cardiogenic shock
III.  stroke (cerebral vascular accident)

a. I and III
b. II and III
c. II only
d. I, II, and III

15.44 Regarding ventilation ($\dot{V}_A$) and pulmonary blood flow ($\dot{Q}_c$) in the upright lung, which of the following statements are true?
I.    $\dot{Q}_c$ decreases from the bases to the apices
II.   $\dot{V}_A$ decreases from the bases to the apices
III.  up the lung, $\dot{Q}_c$ decreases more than $\dot{V}_A$
IV.   at the bottom of the lung there is more $\dot{Q}_c$ than $\dot{V}_A$
V.    toward the apices of the lung the $\dot{V}_A/\dot{Q}_c$ is high

a. I, II, and III
b. II, III, IV, and V
c. II, IV, and V
d. I, II, III, IV, and V

15.45 An area of the lung has no ventilation but is normally perfused by the pulmonary circulation. Which of the following statements are true regarding this area?
I.    the ventilation–perfusion ratio is zero
II.   the alveolar gas is like venous blood ($PO_2$ = 40, $PCO_2$ = 46)
III.  the area represents an alveolar shunt

a. I and III
b. I and II
c. III only
d. I, II, and III

15.46 The oxygen content of the blood leaving lung units with higher than normal V/Q ratios is not much greater than that leaving units with normal V/Q ratios. This is because:

a. less blood flows through areas with higher than normal V/Q ratios
b. more blood flows through areas with normal V/Q ratios
c. hemoglobin is already almost fully saturated at a $P_{O_2}$ of 100 mm Hg
d. areas with higher than normal V/Q ratios have lower $P_{O_2}$s

15.47 The most common physiologic cause for a reduced $Pa_{O_2}$ (arterial hypoxemia) is:

a. low inspired $P_{O_2}$
b. diffusion abnormalities
c. anatomic shunts
d. ventilation–perfusion (V/Q) imbalances

15.48 All of the following statements are true regarding a left–to–right anatomic shunt except:

a. blood flows from the arterial to the venous side of the circulation
b. it lowers the oxygen content of the arterial blood
c. it can increase the work load imposed on the heart
d. it can lead to failure of the heart

15.49 What can you assume about a patient who has a V/Q imbalance and exhibits hypercapnea ($P_{CO_2}$ 45 mm Hg)?

a. he is compensating for an acute metabolic alkalosis
b. he is compensating for a chronic metabolic acidosis
c. he cannot sustain the higher $\dot{V}_E$ to overcome the increased $V_D$
d. his CNS is not responding to the increased $P_{CO_2}$

15.50 Chronically recurring bronchial spasm can result in:

a. edema of the respiratory tract mucosa
b. loss of elastic tissue support
c. induration of the respiratory tract mucosa
d. hypertrophy of the bronchial smooth muscle

15.51 The most common cause of increased bronchial secretions is:

a. airway trauma
b. mechanical irritation
c. infection
d. chemical irritation

15.52 Which of the following components may be found in bronchial secretions?
I.     water
II.    DNA and RNA
III.   plasma fluid
IV.    mucopolysaccharides
V.     plasma proteins

a. I, II, and III            c. I, IV, and V
b. II, III, IV, and V        d. I, II, III, IV, and V

15.53 All of the following statements are true regarding an asthmatic attack except:

a. it is associated with diffuse bronchial spasm
b. the FRC may be markedly increased
c. the diaphragm may be lower than normal
d. the pulmonary distention is irreversible

15.54 On which of the following pulmonary function tests will a patient with pulmonary distention exhibit an abnormally increased value?
I.     functional residual capacity
II.    helium equilibration time
III.   inspiratory capacity
IV.    nitrogen washout time

a. II, III, and IV           c. I and III
b. I, II, and IV             d. I, II, III, and IV

15.55 Contraction of a diaphragm that is abnormally low and flat will result in which of the following?
I.     a greater drop in pleural pressure during inspiration
II.    a greater expansion of the lateral costal margins
III.   a narrowing of the lateral costal margins during inspiration
IV.    diminished vertical excursion (less change in thoracic volume)

a. III and IV                c. III only
b. II, III, and IV           d. I, II, III, and IV

15.56 An abnormal increase in the amount of interstitial fluid surrounding the body cells is termed:

a. transudation
b. edema
c. desiccation
d. bronchorrhea

15.57 Which of the following are considered extrapulmonary causes of pulmonary restriction?
I.     pleurisy
II.    pleural effusion
III.   pleural empyema
IV.    pneumothorax
V.     hemothorax

a. II, IV, and V          c. III, IV, and V
b. I, III, IV, and V      d. I, II, III, IV, and V

15.58 The common denominator in all disorders categorized under the general term "pulmonary restriction" is:

a. an increase in lung volumes
b. a decrease in expiratory flows
c. an increase in inspiratory flows
d. a decrease in lung volumes

## Laboratory Assessment of Hypoxia:

15.59
a. The following table provides relevant laboratory data used to assess the cause of hypoxia for several patients. Based on this information, specify in the blanks below this table the most likely cause of hypoxia for each case.

$N$ = a normal value
$D$ = a decrease in the value below normal
$I$ = an increase in the value above normal

| Case # | $P(A-a)O_2$ $Pao_2$ | Air | $O_2$ | $Cao_2$ | $C\bar{v}o_2$ |
|--------|---------|-----|-----|------|------|
| 1 | N | N | N | N | D |
| 2 | N or D | N | N | D | D |
| 3 | N | N | N | N | I |
| 4 | D | I | I | D | N |
| 5 | D | N | N | D | N |
| 6 | D | I | I | D | N |
| 7 | D | I | N | D | N |

Cause of Hypoxia:

1. _____          5. _____

2. _____          6. _____

3. _____          7. _____

4. _____

b. Hypoxemia due to a diffusion defect, right–to–left shunt, and V/Q imbalance all manifest themselves in a reduced $P(A-a)O_2$ breathing room air. How could you differentiate among these causes of hypoxemia? Cite case examples from the above table to support your conclusion.

_____

_____

_____

_____

c. In the presence of arterial hypoxemia (reduced $Ca_{O_2}$), the oxygen content of the mixed venous blood ($C\bar{v}_{O_2}$) can remain normal. Using case examples from the above table, explain how this is possible.

_____

_____

_____

_____

d. In some clinical conditions, the $Pa_{O_2}$, $P(A - a)_{O_2}$, and $Ca_{O_2}$ may all be normal, but the patient may still suffer the effects of tissue hypoxia. How is this possible? Cite case examples from the above table to support your conclusion.

_____

_____

_____

_____

e. It is often stated that the "best" laboratory indicator of the presence or absence of tissue hypoxia is the $C\bar{v}_{O_2}$. Is this always true? Cite case examples from the above table to support your conclusion.

_____

_____

_____

_____

# Bedside Assessment of the Patient

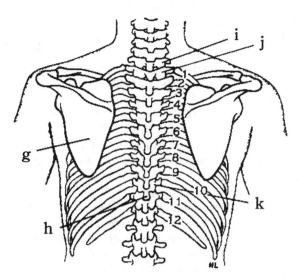

Figure 16–2 Thoracic cage landmarks on posterior chest

## CONTENT EXERCISES

**Labeling:** Match the diagram components listed on the right to the letter labels in the following figures:

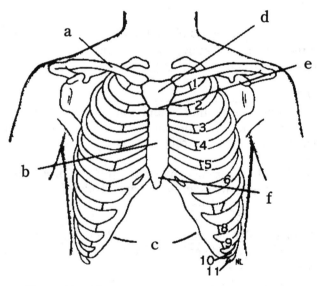

Figure 16–1 Thoracic cage landmarks on anterior chest

16.1

a. _____ spinous process of T10

b. _____ xiphoid

c. _____ manubrium of sternum

d. _____ scapula

e. _____ clavicle

f. _____ T10

g. _____ manubriosternal junction

h. _____ T1

i. _____ body of sternum

j. _____ C7

k. _____ costal angle

**True/False:** For each of the following statements, indicate whether it is mainly true or mainly false by circling the corresponding letter (T=True, F=False):

16.2  T  F  Before conducting a physical exam, the practitioner should review the patient's history of present illness and past medical history.

16.3  T  F  Adequate cerebral oxygenation must be present for the patient to be conscious, alert, and well oriented.

16.4  T  F  With elevated venous pressure, the neck veins of a patient sitting upright may be distended as high as the angle of the jaw.

16.5  T  F  The level of jugular venous distention may vary with breathing.

16.6  T  F  When the peripheral pulses are difficult to identify, one should determine the heart rate by auscultation over the precordium.

16.7  T  F  The left hemidiaphragm is usually a little higher anatomically than the right hemidiaphragm.

16.8 T F In patients with emphysema the lungs lose their elastic recoil and become hyperinflated.

16.9 T F The normal chest wall expands symmetrically during inhalation.

16.10 T F During percussion of the chest wall, movement of the hand striking the chest should be generated at the elbow or shoulder.

16.11 T F Low–pitched sounds, such as those produced by the heart, are best heard with the diaphragm of the stethoscope.

16.12 T F The diaphragm piece of the stethoscope is used most often in auscultation of the lungs.

16.13 T F Normal lung tissue preferentially passes high–frequency sounds.

16.14 T F Hyperinflated lung tissue inhibits normal transmission of sounds through the lungs.

16.15 T F Expiratory flow rates in patients with chronic airflow obstruction who wheeze are not likely to improve after bronchodilator administration.

16.16 T F Crackles occur only in patients with excessive respiratory secretions.

16.17 T F Percussion is an essential component in the examination of the precordium.

16.18 T F The presence of a third heart sound (S3) is considered normal in adults.

16.19 T F Digital clubbing is often associated with a chronic decrease in oxygen supply to the body tissues.

16.20 T F Cyanosis is a reliable indicator of hypoxemia and hypoxia.

16.21 T F When cardiac output is reduced and digital perfusion is poor, capillary refill is slow.

**Short Answer:** Complete each statement by filling in the correct information in the space(s) provided:

16.22 Nasal flaring observed in neonates with respiratory distress indicates an increase in the _____ _____.

16.23 Jugular venous pressure (JVP) reflects the volume and pressure of the venous blood in the _____.

16.24 With a patient sitting up at a 45–degree angle, abnormal venous distention is indicated if the jugular venous blood level rises more than _____ centimeters above the sternal angle.

16.25 With a patient's arm raised above the head, the inferior border of the scapula approximately overlies the lung's _____ fissures.

16.26 At end–expiration, the lower borders of the lungs on the anterior chest extend to about the _____ rib at the midclavicular line and to the _____ rib on the lateral chest wall.

16.27 During palpation of a patient, normal posterior thoracic expansion would be indicated during a full, deep breath if each of the practitioner's thumbs moved equally approximately _____ cm.

16.28 As assessed by the percussion method, the normal diaphragm excursion during a deep breath is about _____ centimeters.

16.29 When attempting to auscultate low–frequency sounds, the bell piece of the stethoscope should be pressed _____ against the chest.

16.30 High–pitched, loud sounds with an expiratory component as long or longer than inspiration best describes _____ breath sounds.

16.31 Short–duration adventitious lung sounds that are intermittent, crackling, or bubbling in nature are referred to as _____.

16.32 A _____ is a creaking or grating sound that occurs when the pleural surfaces become inflamed and the roughened edges rub together during breathing.

16.33 Right ventricular hypertrophy often produces a systolic thrust that can be felt and visualized near the _____ border.

16.34 In order for cyanosis to be detected, the capillaries generally must contain at least _____ gm/dL reduced hemoglobin.

16.35 When the heart does not circulate the blood at a sufficient rate, compensatory _____ occurs in the extremities.

16.36 Right ventricular hypertrophy or failure associated with chronic hypoxemia of pulmonary origin is called _____.

**Listing:** Complete each list as directed in its statement.

16.37 List the four (4) basic components of the physical examination:

1. _____

2. _____

3. _____

4. _____

16.38 List three (3) disorders commonly associated with digital clubbing:

1. _____

2. _____

3. _____

16.39 List at least five (5) clinical signs of acute hypoxemia:

1. _____

2. _____

3. _____

4. _____

5. _____

**Multiple Choice:** Circle the letter corresponding to the single best answer from the available choices:

16.40 Which of the following represents the most effective way for a respiratory care practitioner to initially determine a patient's alertness?

a. determine the patient's pupillary reactivity to light
b. query the family regarding the patient's alertness
c. check the medical record for a history of confusion
d. ask the patient who and where they are and the date/time

16.41 Which of the following are possible causes for an abnormal patient sensorium?
I.   chronic degenerative brain disorders
II.  side effect of certain medications
III. cerebral hypoxia
IV.  overdose of certain drugs
V.   inadequate cerebral perfusion

a. I, III, and IV          c. I, II, IV, and V
b. II, III, IV, and V      d. I, II, III, IV, and V

16.42 In examining the neck of a patient, you note that the trachea is shifted away from the midline. Which of the following conditions could this finding indicate?
I.   lobar collapse
II.  pneumothorax
III. pleural effusion
IV.  lung tumor

a. I, II, and III          c. III and IV
b. II and IV               d. I, II, III, and IV

16.43 On the anterior chest wall, one may localize the upper lobe of the right lung as being:

a. below the 4th rib
b. above the 4th rib
c. between the 4th and 6th ribs
d. between the 5th and 7th ribs

16.44 At end–expiration, the lower border of the lungs on the *anterior* chest wall is at what level?

a. 4th rib
b. 10th rib
c. 8th rib
d. 6th rib

16.45 Upon visually inspecting the thorax of a 73–year–old male, you notice that his chest appears to be overinflated, with the ribs held in a horizontal position. Upon further inspection you observe that the transverse chest diameter is almost equal to its AP diameter. Which of the following terms best describes this thoracic configuration?

a. kyphoscoliosis
b. bucket–handle movement
c. pectus excavatum
d. barrel chest

16.46 Activity of the accessory muscles of ventilation at rest suggests:

a. normal ventilation
b. increased pulmonary compliance
c. increased work of breathing
d. increased physiologic deadspace

16.47 In observing a patient, you note a repeating cycle of gradual increases and decreases in the depth of breathing, followed by a period of apnea. Which of the following terms would you use in charting this observation?

a. Biot's breathing
b. Cheyne–Stokes breathing
c. Kussmaul's breathing
d. paradoxic breathing

16.48 While palpating a patient's chest while she repeats the word "ninety–nine," you note an area of increased tactile fremitus over the left lower lobe. Which of the following could explain this finding?
I.      pneumothorax
II.     pneumonia
III.    emphysema
IV.     atelectasis

a. II, III, and IV          c. II and IV
b. I and III                d. I, II, III, and IV

16.49 During posterior thoracic palpation of an adult, you note little or no right movement during a full, deep breath. Which of the following conditions could explain this finding?
I.      right–sided pleural effusion
II.     atelectasis of the right lower lobe
III.    right lobar consolidation
IV.     bilateral phrenic nerve paralysis

a. I, II, and III           c. III and IV
b. II and III               d. I, II, III, and IV

16.50 On palpation of the neck region of a patient on a mechanical ventilator, you note a crackling sound and sensation. What is the most likely cause of this observation?

a. decreased intrapleural pressure
b. upper bronchial obstruction
c. subcutaneous emphysema
d. pneumonia of the upper lobes

16.51 While percussing a patient's chest wall, you encounter an area which produces a dull or flat percussion note. Which of the following are potential causes of this finding?
I.      pleural effusion
II.     pneumonia
III.    atelectasis
IV.     pneumothorax

a. II and III               c. I, II, and III
b. II and IV                d. I, II, III, and IV

16.52 While percussing an adult patient's posterior chest wall to estimate her diaphragmatic excursion during a deep breath, you note a total movement of about 3 to 4 cm. Which of the following clinical conditions would be most consistent with this finding?
I.      pulmonary hyperinflation
II.     a neuromuscular disorder
III.    hyperventilation syndrome

a. I and II                 c. II only
b. II and III               d. I, II, and III

16.53 While auscultating a patient's posterior lung bases, you hear high–pitched, harsh breath sounds with an expiratory component equal to or slightly longer than inspiration. What conditions might explain this finding?
I.      increased secretions in the lower lobe airways
II.     consolidation or atelectasis in the lower lobes
III.    obstruction of the airways leading to the lower lobes

a. I and II                 c. II only
b. II and III               d. I, II, and III

16.54 During auscultation of a patient's chest, you hear low–pitched continuous sounds to either side of the sternum. Which of the following chart entries best describes this finding?

a. "bilateral bronchial sounds heard"
b. "continuous wheezes heard bilaterally"
c. "rhonchi heard bilaterally throughout cycle"
d. "inspiratory crackles (rales) heard"

16.55 Which of the following are common causes of stridor?
I.      laryngotracheobronchitis (croup)
II.     inflammation of the epiglottis
III.    pulmonary emphysema
IV.     postextubation edema

a. II and IV
b. I, II, and IV

c. III and IV
d. I, II, III, and IV

16.56 In which of the following conditions would you expect breath sounds to be diminished?
I. air or fluid in the pleural space
II. hyperinflation of lung tissue
III. obstruction of the airways
IV. shallow or slow breathing

a. I, II, and III
b. II and IV

c. II and III
d. I, II, III, and IV

16.57 While auscultating a patient's chest, you hear a high–pitched sound that continues throughout expiration. Which of the following conditions could cause this type of adventitious sound?
I. asthma
II. fibrosis
III. congestive heart failure
IV. bronchitis

a. I, II, and III
b. III and IV

c. I, III, and IV
d. I, II, III, and IV

16.58 Which of the following are true regarding early inspiratory crackles?
I. they most often occur in patients with COPD
II. they generally indicate severe airway obstruction
III. they are not affected by coughing or positional change
IV. they are usually scanty (few in number)

a. I, II, and III
b. II and IV

c. II, III, and IV
d. I, II, III, and IV

16.59 During auscultation of a patient's chest, you hear course crackling sounds throughout both inspiration and expiration. These sounds clear when the patient coughs. Which of the following is the most likely cause of these adventitious sounds?

a. the opening of closed smaller airways or alveoli
b. the opening of collapsed large, proximal airways
c. the movement of excessive secretions in the airways
d. a variable obstruction to flow in the upper airway

16.60 In conducting chest auscultation, you have a patient whisper the words "one, two, three." While listening over the lung periphery, you clearly hear these spoken words as high–pitched sounds. Which of the following conditions best explains this finding?

a. obstruction of air flow to a bronchus
b. consolidation of lung tissue (e.g., pneumonia)
c. fluid in the pleural space (pleural effusion)
d. hyperinflation of the lung parenchyma

16.61 The normal apical impulse (PMI) usually is identified where?

a. 3rd right intercostal space
b. 3rd left intercostal space
c. 5th right intercostal space
d. 5th left intercostal space

16.62 In which of the following patient categories would the intensity of the apical impulse (PMI) most likely be reduced?

a. mitral (bicuspid) stenosis
b. aortic valvular insufficiency
c. left ventricular hypertrophy
d. chronic pulmonary hyperinflation (emphysema)

16.63 In order to better detect abnormalities associated with the pulmonary valve, which area would you choose for auscultation?

a. 5th left intercostal space, midclavicular line
b. 2nd left intercostal space, sternal border
c. 2nd right intercostal space, midclavicular line
d. 5th right intercostal space, midclavicular line

16.64 The first heart sound (S1) is created primarily by:

a. closure of the semilunar valves
b. closure of the atrioventricular valves
c. opening of the semilunar valves
d. opening of the atrioventricular valves

16.65 In auscultating the precordium of a patient with chronic hypoxemia, you note a marked increase in the intensity of the second heart sound (S2) and no splitting during inhalation. This finding is most consistent with which of the following?

a. mitral insufficiency
b. pulmonary hypertension
c. left ventricular hypertrophy
d. tricuspid valve stenosis

16.66 In auscultating the precordium of a patient, you hear a high-pitched "whooshing" noise occurring simultaneously with S1. This finding is most consistent with which of the following?

a. a stenotic semilunar valve
b. an incompetent semilunar valve
c. an incompetent atrioventricular valve
d. a stenotic atrioventricular valve

16.67 Which of the following may result from abdominal distention or pain?
I.    impaired movement of the diaphragm
II.   inhibition of proper coughing
III.  failure to breathe deeply

a. II and III          c. I and III
b. I and II            d. I, II, and III

16.68 Which of the following pulmonary disorders is most likely to result in hepatomegaly?

a. pulmonary edema due to left ventricular failure
b. acute viral pulmonary infections
c. chronic pulmonary hemosiderosis
d. chronic right heart failure secondary to COPD

16.69 In patients with chronic respiratory disease, pedal edema is a sign of:

a. impaired pulmonary diffusion
b. hypercapnia (impaired $CO_2$ removal)
c. right ventricular hypertrophy
d. systemic hypertension

16.70 On physical assessment of a patient who does not appear acutely ill, you note the following: prolonged expiratory time; increased AP chest diameter; inspiratory intercostal retractions with accessory muscle usage; and a bilateral decrease in fremitus, breath sounds, and chest expansion. These findings suggest:

a. chronic airways obstruction
b. acute upper airway obstruction
c. bronchial obstruction with atelectasis
d. diffuse interstitial fibrosis

16.71 Upon physical exam of an acutely ill patient, you note the following: fever; tachypnea; cyanosis; and increased tactile/vocal fremitus, bronchial breath sounds and inspiratory crackles, bronchophony, and a dull percussion note—all localized to the right lower lobe. These findings suggest:

a. right lobar obstruction/atelectasis
b. right-sided tension pneumothorax
c. right lower lobe consolidation
d. right-sided pleural effusion

16.72 Upon physical exam of an acutely dyspneic and hypotensive patient, you note the following (all limited to the left hemithorax): reduced chest expansion, a hyperresonant percussion note, absence of breath sounds and tactile fremitus, and a tracheal shift to the right. These findings suggest:

a. acute upper airway obstruction
b. left-sided pleural effusion
c. left-sided consolidation
d. left-sided pneumothorax

16.73 On physical assessment of a patient in no apparent respiratory distress, you note the following (all in the region of the right lower lobe): decreased expansion, a dull percussion note, and the absence of breath sounds/tactile fremitus. The trachea is shifted to the left. These findings suggest:

a. diffuse interstitial fibrosis
b. right-sided pneumothorax
c. right-sided consolidation
d. right-sided pleural effusion

16.74 On physical assessment of an acutely ill patient, you note the following (all in the region of the left lower lobe): decreased expansion, a dull percussion note, and the absence of breath sounds/tactile fremitus. You also observe a shift in the trachea toward the left, more prominent during inspiration. These findings suggest:

a. diffuse interstitial fibrosis
b. left-sided obstruction/atelectasis
c. left-sided consolidation
d. left-sided pleural effusion

# 17

# Analysis of Gas Exchange

## CONTENT EXERCISES

**True/False:** For each of the following statements, indicate whether it is mainly true or mainly false by circling the corresponding letter (T=True, F=False):

17.1 T F Arterial blood sampling is more difficult and has greater risk than venous sampling.

17.2 T F Of all ABG samples, 99% are taken from the brachial artery, which is the vessel of choice in the adult.

17.3 T F The $Pao_2$ and $Paco_2$ are measured in millimeters of mercury (mm Hg).

17.4 T F Because of the sample size and electrode function, lithium heparin is now used in most ABG kits.

17.5 T F A blood sample from any patient should be treated with full precautions, as if it were known to be contaminated.

17.6 T F Femoral punctures should be held for three minutes because of the appreciably higher pressure in the artery.

17.7 T F Two syringes are needed to obtain a sample from an arterial line.

17.8 T F An optode is a sensor that operates on optical detection and quantification rather than electrochemical properties.

17.9 T F Transcutaneous monitoring of oxygen started in the adult intensive care units of the 1970s.

17.10 T F Patient age and cardiac output have very little effect on the accuracy of transcutaneous oxygen measurements.

17.11 T F The pulse oximeter is the most common tool used in the modern ICU to assess gas exchange status of oxygen.

17.12 T F False–positive alarms caused by pulse oximeters are uncommon.

17.13 T F A capnometer is a device that displays a graphical display of the patient's exhaled breath.

17.14 T F End–tidal carbon dioxide values should not equal carbon dioxide values in arterial blood.

**Short Answer:** Complete each statement by filling in the correct information in the space(s) provided:

17.15 Before an arterial puncture in the radial artery is performed, the respiratory care practitioner (RCP) must determine the presence of adequate _____ _____.

17.16 The _____ is the most common technique used to determine the adequacy of ulnar circulation.

17.17 Of the three most common sites for arterial puncture, the _____ is the least desirable.

17.18 The recommended international system of units (SI) used for measurement of blood gases is _____.

17.19 The RCP should be aware that the _____ and _____ of arterial puncture causes changes in ventilation that affect results.

17.20 _____ should always be worn when acquiring an ABG sample.

17.21 Virtually all transcutaneous monitoring systems now incorporate _____ and _____ electrodes combined in the same skin proble.

17.22 _____ is the technique of measuring the amount of light absorbed by a substance.

17.23 _____ uses light to measure arterial pressure waveforms generated by the pulse in the capillaries.

17.24 In healthy subjects with normal lungs and pulmonary blood flow, the $PETCO_2$ value is _____ less than the $Paco_2$.

**Multiple Choice:** Circle the letter corresponding to the single best answer from the available choices:

17.25 Which of the following laboratory tests is most frequently ordered in the critical care patient area?

a. potassium
b. arterial blood gases
c. serum magnesium
d. blood hemoglobin level

17.26 The most common sites for arterial puncture are:
I.     radial artery
II.    femoral artery
III.   brachial artery
IV.    carotid artery

a. I and III             c. I, II, and III
b. I, III, and IV        d. I, II, III, and IV

17.27 Which of the following arterial puncture sites are most often chosen in the infant?

a. radial and temporal
b. brachial and femoral
c. carotid and radial
d. popliteal and brachial

17.28 All of the following statements regarding femoral artery puncture sites selection are true *except:*

a. femoral artery may be felt just below inguinal ligament
b. it has a large diameter, thus making it an easy target
c. femoral artery punctures are usually reserved for emergencies
d. use of a 1/2–inch needle is recommended

17.29 Potential complications of arterial puncture may include:
I.     thrombosis
II.    hemorrhage
III.   hematoma formation
IV.    vasovagal response

a. IV only               c. I, III, and IV
b. I and IV              d. I, II, III, and IV

17.30 A mechanically ventilated patient requires an arterial blood gas. Which of the following cognitive abilities must any RCP have in order to perform the procedure?
I.     ability to review and understand the patient medical record
II.    ability to perform puncture in a poorly lit room
III.   ability to perform and interpret assessment skills
IV.    functional understanding of institution infection control policies

a. I and III             c. I, III, and IV
b. II, III, and IV       d. I, II, III, and IV

17.31 The usual waiting period necessary to allow the effects of a patient's status change or therapy to be reflected in arterial blood gases is:

a. 2–5 minutes
b. 20–30 minutes
c. 45–50 minutes
d. 60 minutes

17.32 During capillary sampling in neonates, arterialization of the capillary beds can be achieved by warming the skin using which of the following methods?
I.     vasoactive drugs
II.    warm compresses
III.   a water bath
IV.    a heat lamp

a. I, II, and III        c. II, III, and IV
b. III and IV            d. I, II, III, and IV

17.33 All of the following statements concerning point of care (POC) ABG testing are true *except:*

a. POC cost effectiveness needs to be better established
b. POC systems are simple and may be used by untrained staff
c. some POC systems can also measure electrolytes
d. POC systems require rigid quality control measures

17.34 Devices that monitor gas exchange of oxygen at the transcutaneous or tissue level rely on which of the following technology principles to be true?

I. gas diffusion varies with perfusion of blood beneath skin
II. all gases diffuse through the skin
III. sensor equilibration time is relatively short after electrode placement
IV. required electrode position changes are rare

a. I and II
b. I, II, and III
c. II and IV
d. I, II, III, and IV

17.35 All of the following factors limit the clinical utility of transcutaneous monitoring *except:*

a. skin color
b. membrane condition
c. skin thickness
d. age

17.36 A RCP is asked to explain the possible limitations of pulse oximetry in the critical care setting. Which of the following conditions might the RCP need to consider?

I. motion of extremity
II. sunlight or high–intensity light interference
III. abnormal hemoglobin species
IV. low perfusion states

a. I and IV
b. I, II, and III
c. II, III, and IV
d. I, II, III, and IV

17.37 A RCP notices that an intubated patient with a mainstream capnograph in place is coughing frequently with large amounts of secretions reaching the ventilator circuit tubing. End–tidal $CO_2$ values may be in question because:

a. $N_2O$ values may be increased on the monitor
b. mainstream monitors typically have a slow response time
c. secretions may block the sensor window
d. real–time readings will show cardiac activity

# Basic Pulmonary Function Measurements

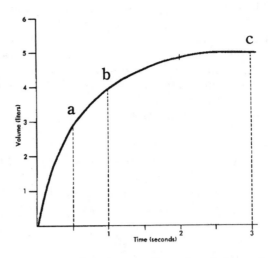

**Figure 18–2** Forced expiratory volumes

## CONTENT EXERCISES

**Labeling:** Match the diagram components listed on the right to the letter labels in each of the following figures:

18.2

a. _____ FEV$_3$

b. _____ FEV$_1$

c. _____ FEV$_{0.5}$

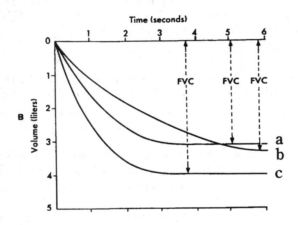

**Figure 18–1** Forced vital capacity curves

18.1

a. _____ normal curve

b. _____ obstructive curve

c. _____ restrictive curve

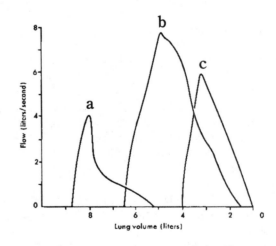

**Figure 18–3** Maximum expiratory flow-volume curves

18.3

a. _____ normal curve

b. _____ obstructive curve

c. _____ restrictive curve

**True/False:** For each of the following statements, indicate whether it is mainly true or mainly false by circling the corresponding letter (T=True, F=False):

18.4   T   F   The role of pulmonary function testing is limited to diagnostic assessment.

18.5   T   F   Pulmonary function testing can be helpful in selecting or modifying a specific therapeutic approach to patient care.

18.6   T   F   Compliance is decreased in all restrictive disease processes.

18.7   T   F   A lung capacity consists of two or more lung volumes.

18.8   T   F   In general, the inspiratory capacity will be reduced in both restrictive and obstructive lung diseases.

18.9   T   F   The expiratory reserve volume is always reduced in both obstructive and restrictive lung diseases.

18.10  T   F   Characteristic of restrictive lung diseases is a decrease in vital capacity.

18.11  T   F   The RV must be known in order to measure the TLC and FRC.

18.12  T   F   Both the RV and FRC are usually elevated in obstructive lung diseases.

18.13  T   F   In patients with severe obstructive lung disease, helium equilibration during an FRC measurement occurs more quickly than normal.

18.14  T   F   Assessment of a patient's degree of cooperation is essential in interpreting most pulmonary function test results.

18.15  T   F   The $FEF_{25-75}$ may detect changes in the lung function that are not apparent from the $FEF_{200-1200}$.

18.16  T   F   Normally, airway resistance is higher during inspiration and lower during exhalation.

18.17  T   F   Restrictive lung diseases reduce lung compliance as a result of the stiffness of the lung tissue.

18.18  T   F   Closing volume cannot be measured accurately in disorders characterized by severe airway obstruction.

**Short Answer:** Complete each statement by filling in the correct information in the space(s) provided:

18.19 Pulmonary function testing _____ programs are designed to detect lung change caused by disease in the general population or in high–risk groups.

18.20 The primary factor in obstructive airway disease is an increase in _____.

18.21 The primary factor in restrictive lung disease is a decrease in _____.

18.22 The normal vital capacity represents approximately _____ % of the total lung capacity.

18.23 To be significant, the difference between the vital capacity and the forced vital capacity should be greater than _____ %.

18.24 Normal helium equilibration time during an FRC measurement is less than _____ minutes.

18.25 The FVC will be less than the normal slow vital capacity when _____ and _____ are present.

18.26 At a standardized flow of 0.5 L/sec, normal airway resistance ranges between _____ cm $H_2O$/L/sec.

18.27 The volume of a gas per minute that will transverse the alveolar–capillary membrane for a given partial pressure gradient is termed _____ _____.

18.28 Lung function studies that use radioactive materials to assess gas distribution and blood flow in the lungs are referred to as _____ _____.

18.29 When determining the compliance of the lung and thorax together ($C_{LT}$), one must measure both the _____ and the specific lung _____.

18.30 The volume of gas remaining in the lung when the small airways begin to collapse during a maximum exhalation is the _____.

18.31 In normal individuals, V/Q scans will show ventilation and perfusion _____ in the bases of the lung and ventilation and perfusion _____ in the apices.

**Multiple Choice:** Circle the letter corresponding to the single best answer from the available choices:

18.32 You observe pulmonary function testing being conducted on an asthmatic patient. The technologist performs one set of tests, then administers a drug, then repeats the same tests. For which purpose is this assessment most likely being conducted?

a. to screen this patient for pulmonary disease
b. to evaluate this patient for surgical risk
c. to assess the progression of this patient's disease
d. to help select a therapeutic approach for the patient

18.33 You observe pulmonary function testing being conducted on an elderly, obese patient who has been scheduled for elective thoracic surgery. For which purpose is this assessment most likely being conducted?

a. to screen this patient for pulmonary disease
b. to assist in determining this patient's disability
c. to help select a therapeutic approach for the patient
d. to evaluate this patient for surgical risk

18.34 Pulmonary function parameters that signify obstructive disease processes include which of the following?
I.    increased airway resistance
II.   decreased lung volumes
III.  decreased forced expiratory flows
IV.   air trapping

a. I, II, and III        c. I, III, and IV
b. II and IV             d. I, II, III, and IV

18.35 Most restrictive lung diseases are characterized by:

a. decreased flows and increased airway resistance
b. decreased compliance and increased airway resistance
c. increased compliance and increased airway resistance
d. decreased lung volumes and decreased compliance

18.36 In which of the following conditions may lung volumes be reduced (restrictive process) without a reduction in lung or chest wall compliance?

a. fibrotic lung disease
b. kyphoscoliosis
c. chronic lung inflammation
d. neuromuscular diseases

18.37 "Combined" lung disease is characterized by:

a. decreased flows and decreased volumes
b. increased flows and decreased volumes
c. decreased flows and normal volumes
d. normal flows and decreased volumes

18.38 Which of the following volumetric divisions of the lung *cannot* be measured by simple spirometry?
I.    FRC
II.   ERV
III.  RV
IV.   TLC

a. I, III, and IV        c. I and II
b. II, III, and IV       d. I, II, III, and IV

18.39 A patient has a vital capacity of 4200 ml, a functional residual capacity of 5500 ml, and expiratory reserve volume of 1200 ml. What is her residual volume?

a. 9700 ml
b. 3000 ml
c. 4300 ml
d. 6700 ml

18.40 A patient has an expired minute ventilation of 10,700 ml and a ventilatory rate of 21/min. What is his average tidal volume?

a. 440 ml
b. 635 ml
c. 725 ml
d. 510 ml

18.41 In patients with severe obstructive lung diseases, the vital capacity is generally reduced. In these patients, the most probable mechanism causing the decrease in vital capacity is:

a. an increase in inspiratory capacity
b. a decrease in chest wall compliance
c. an increase in lung compliance
d. an increase in residual volume

18.42 A patient with COPD has a normal VC of 3300 ml and an FVC of 2600 ml. Which of the following mechanisms best explains this difference?

a. muscle fatigue during the forced expiration
b. airway collapse during the forced expiration
c. decreased compliance during the forced expiration
d. failure to close the glottis during the forced expiration

18.43 You observe an FRC measurement on a patient using the helium dilution method. The technologist firsts bleeds in 300 ml of He and obtains an initial reading of 5.00% ($He_1$). After patient equilibration, the second He reading is 3.00% ($He_2$). The patient has a BTPS corrected (BTPS factor 20 C = 1.102) ERV of 1200 ml. What is the patient's RV (rounded to the nearest 10 ml)?

a. 4410 ml
b. 3210 ml
c. 5610 ml
d. 4800 ml

18.44 You observe an FRC measurement on a patient using the nitrogen washout method. After equilibration is reached, the technologist records an expired volume (BTPS corrected) of 42.0 liters ($V_2$) and a final $N_2$ concentration of 4.50% ($N_2$). The patient has a BTPS corrected ERV of 1000 ml. What is the patient's RV?

a. 2400 ml
b. 5300 ml
c. 1400 ml
d. 3800 ml

18.45 In both the helium dilution test and nitrogen washout FRC determinations, the patient should be connected to the system at:

a. full forced inspiration
b. end–tidal expiration
c. end–tidal inspiration
d. full forced expiration

18.46 A patient has an FRC via helium dilution of 2400 cc and an FRC via body plethysmography (body "box") of 3400 cc. Which of the following statements could help explain this difference?

a. the body box tends to overestimate actual FRC
b. the helium dilution test was obviously in error
c. the body box measures the entire thoracic gas
d. airway obstruction causes low results via helium dilution

18.47 In addition to the actual results of lung volume and capacity measurements, which of the following factors must be considered in interpreting the results of such tests?
I.  the patient's history
II.  the patient's degree of cooperation
III.  the patient's predicted values

a. I and II
b. II and III
c. I and III
d. I, II, and III

18.48 Within three seconds after initiating a forced vital capacity (FVC) maneuver, a patient with normal lungs should be able to exhale what percent of the FVC?

a. 35–50% of the FVC
b. 50–70% of the FVC
c. 70–83% of the FVC
d. 94–97% of the FVC

18.49 All spirometric values obtained under ambient conditions should be converted to:

a. ambient temperature and pressure, saturated (ATPS)
b. body temperature, ambient pressure, saturated (BTPS)
c. standard temperature and pressure, dry (STPD)
d. ambient temperature and pressure, dry (ATPD)

18.50 Which of the following statements are true regarding the forced expiratory flow 25%–75% ($FEF_{25-75}$)?
I.  it is sensitive to early changes in obstructive lung disease
II.  it is a very good indicator of patient effort (effort-dependent)
III.  it mainly measures the function of the smaller airways
IV.  it is normally greater than 4 liters/sec (240 L/min)

a. I, II, and III
b. III and IV
c. I, III, and IV
d. I, II, III, and IV

18.51 Which of the following tests of airflow volumes tends to be the most responsive to bronchodilator therapy?

a. forced expiratory flow, 25%–75% ($FEF_{25-75}$)
b. peak expiratory flow (PEF)
c. maximum voluntary ventilation (MVV)
d. forced expiratory flow, 200–1200 ($FEF_{200-1200}$)

18.52 Which of the following are true regarding the maximum voluntary ventilation (MVV)?

I.   the MVV may be normal in restrictive conditions
II.  test results are highly dependent on patient effort
III. test results reflect airway resistance and muscle status
IV.  normal values vary substantially in the population

a. I, II, and III
b. I and IV
c. I, III, and IV
d. I, II, III, and IV

18.53 The most common method for measuring airway resistance is:

a. body plethysmography
b. nitrogen washout
c. helium dilution
d. radioxenon scan

18.54 Compliance of the lung is measured using:

a. an esophageal balloon
b. body plethysmograph
c. X–Y plotter/recorder
d. water-sealed spirometer

18.55 Which of the following would cause a reduction in lung compliance?

I.   diseases of the bones/joints
II.  severe obesity
III. destruction of lung support tissues
IV.  stiffness of the lung tissue

a. II and III
b. II and IV
c. IV only
d. I, II, III, and IV

18.56 Closing volume is measured using:

a. the single–breath nitrogen test
b. body plethysmography
c. the helium dilution method
d. the nitrogen washout test

18.57 Physiologically, the onset of phase IV during the single breath nitrogen test represents:

a. the mixing of deadspace gas and alveolar gas
b. the changeover to deadspace gas only
c. the collapse of the basal small airways
d. the collapse of the larger central airways

18.58 In which of the following patient groups would you expect to find an abnormal increase in closing volume?

I.   those with early obstructive airway disease
II.  those with a persistent smoking history
III. older or elderly patients

a. I and II
b. II and III
c. I and III
d. I, II, and III

18.59 Which portion of the maximum expiratory flow-volume curve (MEFV) is most effort–independent and reproducible?

a. the first third
b. the first quarter
c. the latter two–thirds
d. the peak flow portion

18.60 A normal $D_{LCO}$ (single breath method) is about:

a. 10 ml/min/mm Hg
b. 100 ml/min/mm Hg
c. 40 ml/min/mm Hg
d. 60 ml/min/mm Hg

18.61 Which of the following factors can influence the results of a diffusing capacity test?

I.   the integrity of the alveolar capillary membrane
II.  the pulmonary capillaries' blood flow and volume
III. the surface area of the lung available for diffusion
IV.  the amount of hemoglobin (Hb) in the blood
V.   alteration in the ventilation–perfusion ratio (V/Q)

a. II, III, IV, and V
b. II, IV, and V
c. III and IV
d. I, II, III, IV, and V

**Interpretation of Pulmonary Function Test Results:**

Each of the following sets of patient data were obtained from conventional pulmonary function tests administered in the pulmonary laboratory of a respiratory care department (all volumes are expressed in liters). For each data set:

1. Determine the predicted values for the patient's forced vital capacity measurements, using the nomograms provided in Figure 18–13 in the text.

2. Calculate the % predicted value for each measurement using the following formula:

$$\%PRED = \frac{ACTUAL}{PRED} \times 100$$

3. Identify and note in the space provided any significant deviations from normal. For purposes of this exercise, consider a value to be significantly abnormal if the %PRED is below 80% or above 120%.

4. Using the "decision trees" in Figure 18–17 in the text, provide your conclusions regarding the test results.

b. Significant Deviations From Normal (List):

_____

_____

_____

_____

c. Conclusions:

_____

_____

_____

_____

18.62 The following data were obtained from a 24–year–old 70–kg male patient admitted for elective surgery. The patient is 65 in (165 cm) tall.

a.

| Lung Volumes | ACTUAL | PRED | %PRED |
|---|---|---|---|
| TLC | 6.39 | 6.50 | _____% |
| FRC | 2.95 | 2.88 | _____% |
| RV | 1.35 | 1.32 | _____% |
| VC | 5.04 | 4.78 | _____% |

Forced Vital Capacity

| | ACTUAL | | %PRED |
|---|---|---|---|
| FVC | 5.05 | _____ | _____% |
| FEV$_1$ | 4.10 | _____ | _____% |
| FEV$_1$% | _____% | 83% | |
| FEF$_{200-1200}$ | 8.05 | _____ | _____% |
| FEF$_{25-75}$ | 4.38 | _____ | _____% |

18.63 The following data were obtained from a 47–year–old 55–kg female patient admitted for pulmonary complications arising from kyphoscoliosis. The patient is 60 in (152 cm) tall.

a.

| Lung Volumes | ACTUAL | PRED | %PRED |
|---|---|---|---|
| TLC | 3.13 | 4.09 | _____% |
| FRC | 1.44 | 1.96 | _____% |
| RV | 0.85 | 1.09 | _____% |
| VC | 2.28 | 2.92 | _____% |

Forced Vital Capacity

| | ACTUAL | | %PRED |
|---|---|---|---|
| FVC | 2.28 | _____ | _____% |
| FEV$_1$ | 1.75 | _____ | _____% |
| FEV$_1$% | _____% | 78% | |
| FEF$_{200-1200}$ | 4.32 | _____ | _____% |
| FEF$_{25-75}$ | 2.83 | _____ | _____% |

b. Significant Deviations From Normal (List):

_____

_____

_____

_____

c. Conclusions:

_____

_____

_____

_____

18.64 The following data were obtained from a 68–year–old 76–kg male patient being screened for participation in the pulmonary rehabilitation program. The patient has a history of 25 pack–years of smoking, exhibits an increase in his AP chest dimensions, and uses his accessory muscle at rest. The patient is 66 in (168 cm) tall.

a.

| Lung Volumes | ACTUAL | PRED | %PRED |
|---|---|---|---|
| TLC | 7.33 | 6.58 | _____% |
| FRC | 5.10 | 3.50 | _____% |
| RV | 4.30 | 2.33 | _____% |
| VC | 3.03 | 3.83 | _____% |

Forced Vital Capacity

| | | | |
|---|---|---|---|
| FVC | 2.67 | _____ | _____% |
| $FEV_1$ | 1.67 | _____ | _____% |
| $FEV_1\%$ | _____% | 83% | |
| $FEF_{200-1200}$ | 3.89 | _____ | _____% |
| $FEF_{25-75}$ | 1.45 | _____ | _____% |

b. Significant Deviations From Normal (List):

_____

_____

_____

_____

c. Conclusions:

_____

_____

_____

_____

18.65 The following data were obtained from a 32–year–old 61–kg female patient who admits to "occasional smoking" but otherwise reveals no past history of pulmonary problems. The patient is 63 in (160 cm) tall.

a.

| Lung Volumes | ACTUAL | PRED | %PRED |
|---|---|---|---|
| TLC | 4.75 | 4.90 | _____% |
| FRC | 2.31 | 2.21 | _____% |
| RV | 1.28 | 1.20 | _____% |
| VC | 3.48 | 3.63 | _____% |

Forced Vital Capacity

| | | | |
|---|---|---|---|
| FVC | 2.96 | _____ | _____% |
| $FEV_1$ | 2.55 | _____ | _____% |
| $FEV_1\%$ | _____% | 78% | |
| $FEF_{200-1200}$ | 4.33 | _____ | _____% |
| $FEF_{25-75}$ | 1.95 | _____ | _____% |

b. Significant Deviations From Normal (List):

_____

_____

_____

_____

c. Conclusions:

_____

_____

_____

_____

b. Significant Deviations From Normal (List):

_____

_____

_____

_____

c. Conclusions:

_____

_____

_____

_____

18.66 The following data were obtained from a 54–year–old 130–kg male coal miner whose chief complaint is shortness of breath at rest and on exertion. His dyspnea has worsened in the past 6 months, so much so that he is no longer able to work. Additional symptoms include a dry cough, and he admits to some sputum production when he has a "chest cold." He has smoked one pack of cigarettes a day since age 25. The patient is 72 in (183 cm) tall.

a.

| Lung Volumes | ACTUAL | PRED | %PRED |
|---|---|---|---|
| TLC | 4.89 | 6.73 | _____% |
| FRC | 1.73 | 1.99 | _____% |
| RV | 0.98 | 1.44 | _____% |
| VC | 3.91 | 5.07 | _____% |

Forced Vital Capacity

| | ACTUAL | PRED | %PRED |
|---|---|---|---|
| FVC | 3.51 | _____ | _____% |
| $FEV_1$ | 2.10 | _____ | _____% |
| $FEV_1\%$ | _____% | 83% | |
| $FEF_{200-1200}$ | 5.67 | _____ | _____% |
| $FEF_{25-75}$ | 2.32 | _____ | _____% |

# 19

## Systematic Analysis of the Chest Radiograph

## CONTENT EXERCISES

**True/False:** For each of the following statements, indicate whether it is mainly true or mainly false by circling the corresponding letter (T=True, F=False):

19.1   T   F   X–rays are electromagnetic waves.

19.2   T   F   Dense objects like bone absorb fewer x–rays than air–filled objects like lung tissue.

19.3   T   F   Small amounts of patient rotation can make normal structures appear abnormal on the x–ray.

19.4   T   F   The right heart border is usually not seen on the normal chest x–ray.

19.5   T   F   On the lateral chest x–ray, the esophagus is located in front of the trachea.

19.6   T   F   The oblique fissures of the lungs are best seen on the lateral chest x–ray.

19.7   T   F   On the normal PA chest x–ray, the gastric bubble should appear on the patient's right side.

19.8   T   F   On a normal chest x–ray, the right hilum is always lower than the left.

19.9   T   F   The anterior air space (the area behind the sternum and in front of the heart) is best seen on the AP chest film.

19.10  T   F   Breast shadows overlying the lower portions of the lung can appear as an abnormal interstitial pattern.

19.11  T   F   A pneumomediastinum is best observed on the lateral chest x–ray view.

19.12  T   F   Pulmonary nodules less than 1 cm are usually benign.

19.13  T   F   The most common cause of calcifications seen in the lung are healed infections.

19.14  T   F   On the normal chest x–ray, the right lung should appear smaller than the left.

19.15  T   F   Computed tomography (CT) is used to evaluate the resectability of a lesion prior to surgical repair.

**Short Answer:** Complete each statement by filling in the correct information in the space(s) provided:

19.16 The ability of x–rays to penetrate matter is dependent on the _____ of the matter.

19.17 X–rays that pass through air–filled or low–density objects create a _____ image on the film.

19.18 If a patient has his or her back to the x–ray tube with the anterior chest pressed against the film cassette, a _____ view is being taken.

19.19 The cardiothoracic (C/T) ratio is abnormal if it is greater than _____ the distance across the lungs at the level of the diaphragms.

19.20 The right diaphragm is usually about _____ rib interspace(s) higher than the left.

19.21 The top of the gastric bubble should be no more than _____ centimeters from the top of the dome of the diaphragm.

19.22 The most important indirect sign of collapse of part of the lung is displacement of the _____ _____.

19.23 The presence of an interstitial infiltrate can be confirmed by looking at the _____ _____.

19.24 The presence of Kerley B line suggests _____ _____.

19.25 The _____ is the part of the chest that is found between both lungs.

19.26 A condition in which air gets into the mediastinum best describes _____.

19.27 If the chest radiograph film has been taken properly and inspiration has been deep enough, the diaphragm will descend to the bottom of the _____ rib anteriorly or the _____ rib posteriorly.

19.28 The right middle lobe is seen best with a _____ view.

**Multiple Choice:** Circle the letter corresponding to the single best answer from the available choices:

19.29 Which of the following can be "seen" on a chest radiograph film?
I.     bone
II.    soft tissue
III.   fat
IV.    air

a. II and IV                     c. III and IV
b. I, II, and III                d. I, II, III, and IV

19.30 If a patient requiring a chest x–ray is in bed and cannot be moved, the film is placed behind the patient's back, and the x–ray tube positioned in front. This position produces which of the following views?

a. left oblique
b. posterior–anterior (PA)
c. apical lordotic
d. anterior–posterior (AP)

19.31 A prominent abnormal white patch seen in a lung field on the chest x–ray most likely indicates an area of:

a. hyperinflation
b. cavitation
c. underperfusion
d. consolidation

19.32 Which of the following normally appear as areas of high density on the chest x–ray?
I.     heart/mediastinum
II.    lung fields
III.   lymph nodes

a. I and II                      c. I and III
b. II and III                    d. I, II, and III

19.33 A standard AP x–ray film shows the trachea deviated to the left side. Which of the following conditions could explain this finding?
I.     left–sided pulmonary fibrosis
II.    an incorrectly rotated film
III.   volume loss on the left side
IV.    left–sided hyperinflation

a. II and IV                     c. III and IV
b. I, II, and III                d. I, II, III, and IV

19.34 A standard AP x–ray film shows the space between the ribs narrower on the right side than on the left. Which of the following conditions best explains this finding?

a. right–sided muscle paralysis
b. right tension pneumothorax
c. Goodpasture's syndrome
d. left–sided muscle paralysis

19.35 On a standard AP x–ray film, the bones appear "washed out" or of lower than normal density. Which of the following conditions could explain this finding?
I.     renal disease
II.    steroid therapy
III.   aging

a. I and II                      c. II only
b. II and III                    d. I, II, and III

19.36 The two bulges making up the right heart border on a chest x–ray represent which of the following structures?
I.     superior vena cava
II.    right ventricle
III.   right atrium
IV.    inferior vena cava

a. II and IV                     c. I and III
b. I and IV                      d. I, II, III, and IV

19.37 On a standard AP x–ray film, the right heart border is not clearly observed. Which of the following conditions could explain this finding?
I.     right middle lobe collapse
II.    right–sided pneumothorax
III.   right middle lobe pneumonia
IV.    pulmonary hypertension

a. I, II, and III                c. II, III, and IV
b. II and IV                     d. I, II, III, and IV

19.38 On a standard PA x–ray film, the heart is observed to be about 2/3 as wide as the distance across the lungs at the diaphragm. Which of the following conditions would best explain this finding?

a. tension pneumothorax
b. congestive heart failure
c. pulmonary emphysema
d. right middle lobe collapse

19.39 On a standard AP x-ray film, you observe that the right hilum is displaced farther to the right than normal. Which of the following conditions could explain this finding?
I.    hyperinflation of the left lung
II.   collapse of an area of the right lung
III.  a right–sided tension pneumothorax

a. I and II
b. II and III
c. I and III
d. I, II, and III

19.40 On a standard AP x-ray film, you observe enlargement of the hilar area. Which of the following conditions are associated with this finding?
I.    cancer metastasis
II.   immunologic diseases
III.  pulmonary infection
IV.   sarcoidosis

a. II and IV
b. I, II, and III
c. I and III
d. I, II, III, and IV

19.41 Causes of lobar collapse include which of the following?
I.    an intrinsic mass
II.   lymph node enlargement
III.  bronchial injury
IV.   mucous plugging

a. I, II, and III
b. II and IV
c. I and III
d. I, II, III, and IV

19.42 A radiology report specifies the presence of a collapsed right middle lobe in a 25–year–old asthmatic. In inspecting this patient's x-ray, which of the following would you expect to find?
I.    deviation of the trachea to the left
II.   elevation of the right diaphragm
III.  overaeration on the left side
IV.   shifting of the heart to the right

a. II and IV
b. I, II, and III
c. II, III, and IV
d. I, II, III, and IV

19.43 Which of the following are potential causes of overaeration as observed on a chest radiograph?
I.    pneumothorax
II.   bullous emphysema
III.  pneumonia
IV.   pneumatocele

a. II and IV
b. I, II, and III
c. I, II, and IV
d. I, II, III, and IV

19.44 On a standard AP x-ray film, you cannot clearly identify the right costophrenic angle. This finding most strongly suggests which of the following?

a. pleural effusion
b. pulmonary emphysema
c. phrenic nerve paralysis
d. sarcoidosis

**Matching:**

19.45 The dotted areas in the following drawings represent locations of infiltrates in various lung segments. Match the location of each infiltrate area with the letter of the corresponding lung segment listed on the right (R=right; L=left; U=upper; M=middle; W=lower).

_____1.

a. apical segment right upper lobe

b. medial segment right middle lobe

_____2.

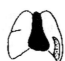

c. superior segment right lower lobe

d. anterior segment left lower lobe

_____3.

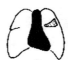

e. anterior–medial segment left lower lobe

_____4.

_____5.

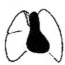

# Synopsis of Cardiopulmonary Diseases

## CONTENT EXERCISES

**True/False:** For each of the following statements, indicate whether it is mainly true or mainly false by circling the corresponding letter (T=True, F=False):

20.1 T  F  Compared with pneumococcal pneumonia, staphylococcal pneumonia responds more quickly to antibiotics.

20.2 T  F  The prognosis for patients with gram–negative nosocomial pneumonias generally is good.

20.3 T  F  Any patient in whom tuberculosis is suspected should initially be isolated.

20.4 T  F  Viral infections of the respiratory tract are more common in adults than in children.

20.5 T  F  Clinical manifestations of most common fungal infections closely resemble those in tuberculosis.

20.6 T  F  Airway collapse is the primary factor causing airway obstruction in chronic bronchitis.

20.7 T  F  Hypersensitivity pneumonitis is caused by exposure to inorganic dusts.

20.8 T  F  Most of the morbidity and mortality of AIDS is associated with the disease itself.

20.9 T  F  Severe obesity causes mechanical restriction to ventilation.

20.10 T  F  Chronic neuromuscular disorders are associated with a decrease in the compliance of both the lungs and thorax.

20.11 T  F  Reversible unilateral diaphragmatic paralysis may occur following cardiac surgery.

20.12 T  F  The use of both the diaphragm and intercostal muscles is possible following spinal transection below C4.

20.13 T  F  The mortality rate for the Guillain–Barre syndrome is over 50%.

20.14 T  F  Antibiotics such as gentamicin, streptomycin, or neomycin can cause muscle weakness or paralysis.

20.15 T  F  Pleural exudates have a lower protein content than do transudates.

20.16 T  F  Reabsorption of pleural air can be expedited by oxygen administration.

20.17 T  F  Oxygen therapy can reduce myocardial work, especially when hypoxemia is present.

20.18 T  F  Right ventricular failure is the most common cause of cardiogenic pulmonary edema.

20.19 T  F  The most common cause of acute noncardiogenic pulmonary edema is damage to the alveolar–capillary membrane.

20.20 T  F  Anaphylactic shock can cause death within 5 to 10 minutes.

20.21 T  F  Obstruction of a large pulmonary artery by an embolus is manifested predominantly by respiratory signs.

20.22 T  F  A normal $P_{O_2}$ generally excludes massive pulmonary embolism.

20.23 T  F  The presence of fat embolism is confirmed by fat globules in the sputum and urine and elevated serum lipase values.

20.24 T  F  Aspiration is the most common postoperative pulmonary complication.

20.25 T  F  Most patients with tracheostomies show evidence of one or more incidents of aspiration.

**Short Answer:** Complete each statement by filling in the correct information in the space(s) provided:

20.26 Antibiotic treatment of most gram–negative pneumonias involves use of a broad–spectrum _____

_____.

20.27 The primary antibiotic used in the treatment of Legionnaires' disease is _____.

20.28 Infection by *Mycobacterium tuberculosis* normally occurs by inhalation of organisms carried on

_____.

20.29 A positive tuberculin skin test is evident with induration of _____ or more in diameter.

20.30 _____ is the primary antibiotic for coccidioidomycosis, histoplasmosis, and blastomycosis.

20.31 Air spaces greater than 1 cm in size that may develop in endstage emphysema are called _____ _____.

20.32 Type I, or immediate–type, hypersensitivity is produced when IgE antibodies fixed to _____ _____ react with antigens.

20.33 A prolonged asthma attack that does not respond to standard therapeutic measures is termed _____ _____.

20.34 A condition in which the normal posterior curve of the spine is exaggerated best describes _____ _____.

20.35 Nocturnal airway obstruction associated with severe obesity is often treated with continuous _____ delivered by nasal mask.

20.36 Patients with neuromuscular abnormalities have an inability to generate normal _____

20.37 _____ represents a polyneuritis of unknown cause which commonly develops 1 to 2 weeks after a mild upper respiratory infection or episode of gastroenteritis.

20.38 A diagnosis of myasthenia gravis may be confirmed using the _____ test.

20.39 A hereditary disorder causing progressive degeneration of the skeletal muscles, resulting in severe muscle weakness, best describes _____ _____.

20.40 Abnormal amounts of plasma fluid may accumulate in the pleural space when either hydrostatic pressures _____ or oncotic pressures _____.

20.41 Definitive diagnostic evaluation of pleural effusion is made by _____.

20.42 In patients with a _____ , positive pressure develops in the pleural space, causing compression of the affected lung.

20.43 When left ventricular failure is associated with both a high left ventricular filling pressure and low cardiac output, _____ therapy can improve myocardial performance.

20.44 Conditions caused by massive pulmonary capillary leakage with normal hydrostatic pressure are grouped together under the general diagnosis of _____.

20.45 Pulmonary hypertension exists when the mean pulmonary artery pressure exceeds _____ mm Hg.

20.46 The lungs respond to shock with increased movement of protein and water into the _____ _____.

20.47 Septic shock is due to the presence of _____ _____ in the blood stream.

20.48 In DIC, occlusion of capillaries and arterioles with fibrin causes _____.

**Multiple Choice:** Circle the letter corresponding to the single best answer from the available choices:

20.49 The pattern of arterial blood gases most typical of bacterial pneumonias is:

a. hypoxemia and respiratory acidosis
b. hypoxemia and metabolic acidosis
c. hyperoxia and respiratory alkalosis
d. hypoxemia and respiratory alkalosis

20.50 All of the following statements regarding Legionellosis are true *except*:

a. infection may occur by inhaling contaminated aerosols
b. the infection is highly communicable between patients
c. nausea, vomiting, and diarrhea may occur as early symptoms
d. the mortality rate for infected individuals is high

20.51 The organism most closely associated with hospital–acquired infections due to contaminated respiratory care equipment is:

a. *Pseudomonas aeruginosa*
b. *Staphylococcus aureus*
c. *Klebsiella pneumoniae*
d. *Escherichia coli*

20.52 The primary factor determining the outcomes of tuberculosis treatment is the:

a. dosage of drugs (isoniazid, rifampin, and pyrazinamide)
b. degree of patient compliance with the drug regimen
c. length of patient hospitalization after diagnosis
d. frequency of exposure to other infected individuals

20.53 Which of the following statements regarding influenza are true?
I. the incidence of influenza varies widely
II. most influenza infections are self–limiting
III. bacterial superinfections may complicate influenza
IV. principle symptoms are fever and myalgia

a. I and III
b. I and IV
c. II, III, and IV
d. I, II, III, and IV

20.54 Which of the following are common causes of bronchiectasis?
I. repeated episodes of pneumonitis
II. aspiration of a foreign body
III. pulmonary vascular hypertension
IV. bronchial obstruction by neoplasm

a. I and IV
b. I, II, and IV
c. II and IV
d. I, II, III, and IV

20.55 Causes of lung abscess include which of the following?
I. bacteremia (blood sepsis)
II. pulmonary aspiration of infected material
III. obstruction of a bronchus
IV. pulmonary ischemia (e.g., pulmonary infarction)
V. prolonged or repeated episodes of pneumonias

a. I, II, and III
b. III, IV, and V
c. II and IV
d. I, II, III, IV, and V

20.56 Clinical manifestation of hypersensitivity pneumonitis (extrinsic allergic alveolitis) include which of the following?
I. eosinophilia
II. acute onset of fever
III. dyspnea
IV. dry cough
V. malaise

a. II, III, IV, and V
b. I and IV
c. III and V
d. I, II, III, IV, and V

20.57 Pathophysiologic features common to an acute asthma attack include:
I. excessive bronchial secretions
II. spasm of the bronchial musculature
III. increased alveolar–capillary permeability
IV. destruction of the alveolar septa
V. edema of the bronchial mucosa

a. II, III, IV, and V
b. I, II, and V
c. I and III
d. I, II, III, IV, and V

20.58 Common clinical manifestations of acute asthma include which of the following?
I. severe dyspnea
II. expectoration of tenacious mucus
III. high fever
IV. audible expiratory wheezing
V. anxiety

a. I and IV
b. II, IV, and V
c. I, II, IV, and V
d. I, II, III, IV, and V

20.59 The most common secondary infection affecting patients with AIDS or AIDS–related complex is:

a. *Pneumocystis carinii* pneumonia
b. cytomegalovirus infections
c. cryptococcosis
d. atypical tuberculosis

20.60 Generalized airway obstruction that is *not* fully reversible with treatment is termed:

a. extrinsic or atopic asthma
b. hypersensitivity pneumonitis
c. chronic obstructive pulmonary disease (COPD)
d. extrinsic allergic alveolitis

20.61 Compared with a patient with chronic bronchitis, an emphysematous patient would tend to exhibit which of the following?
I. an increased total lung capacity
II. a decreased diffusing capacity
III. an increased compliance
IV. chronic hypercapnea

a. II and III
b. I and IV
c. I, II, and III
d. I, II, III, and IV

20.62 The destruction of elastic tissue that occurs in emphysema has which of the following effects on the lung?
I.    a decrease in elastic recoil force
II.   a decrease in lung compliance
III.  loss of small airway anatomic support
IV.   an increased total lung capacity

a. I, III, and IV      c. II and III
b. I, II, and III      d. I, II, III, and IV

20.63 The diagnostic procedure most likely to confirm bronchogenic carcinoma is:

a. a normal chest radiograph
b. cytologic examination of sputum
c. tissue biopsy via bronchoscopy
d. computerized axial tomography

20.64 Which of the following statements regarding bronchial adenomas are true?
I.    these tumors usually arise in the proximal bronchi
II.   bronchial adenomas are highly malignant
III.  hemoptysis is common with bronchial adenomas
IV.   symptoms are similar to bronchogenic carcinoma
V.    examination of the sputum is helpful in diagnosis

a. II, IV, and V      c. I, III, and IV
b. I and III      d. I, II, III, IV, and V

20.65 When the amount of pleural effusion fluid is large, or it continues to accumulate despite treatment of the primary disease process, the recommended treatment approach is:

a. therapeutic thoracentesis
b. open chest thoracotomy
c. postural drainage/percussion
d. chest tube drainage

20.66 On physical examination of a patient with a large pleural effusion, you would expect to find which of the following signs (on the affected side)?
I.    increased breath sounds on the affected side
II.   egophony on the affected side
III.  decreased vocal fremitus on the affected side
IV.   displacement of the trachea away from the effusion
V.    a flat percussion note on the affected side

a. II, III, IV, and V      c. I, IV, and V
b. I and III      d. I, II, III, IV, and V

20.67 A patient with a neuromuscular condition has an accompanying hypoxemia. The presence of this hypoxemia suggests:

a. worsening of the primary restrictive process
b. progressive inspiratory muscle weakness
c. the presence of a complication like atelectasis
d. an increase in physiologic deadspace

20.68 Factors commonly complicating morbid obesity include:
I.    pulmonary hypertension
II.   chronic hypercapnea
III.  cor pulmonale
IV.   obstructive sleep apnea
V.    polycythemia

a. II, IV, and V      c. I, II, IV, and V
b. I, II, III, and IV      d. I, II, III, IV, and V

20.69 The accumulation of purulent fluid in the pleural space may be due to:
I.    the direct spread of a bacterial pneumonia
II.   invasion from a subdiaphragmatic infection
III.  traumatic penetration of the thorax
IV.   rupture of a lung abscess into the pleural space

a. II, III, and IV      c. I and III
b. I, II, and III      d. I, II, III, and IV

20.70 A condition in which the vertebral bodies and the costovertebral joints become fused, causing a decrease in thoracic wall compliance, best describes:

a. ankylosing spondylitis
b. Duchenne's muscular dystrophy
c. the Pickwickian syndrome
d. kyphoscoliosis

20.71 A patient with a large tension pneumothorax will usually exhibit:
I.    acute shortness of breath (dyspnea)
II.   reduced chest expansion and breath sounds
III.  dullness to percussion note on the affected side
IV.   mediastinal shift toward the affected side
V.    hypotension and shock

a. I, II, and V      c. II, III, and V
b. I, II, III, IV, and V      d. II, III, IV, and V

20.72 A condition in which excessive amounts of plasma enter the pulmonary interstitium and alveoli best describes:

a. pulmonary hypertension
b. pulmonary thromboembolism
c. cor pulmonale
d. pulmonary edema

20.73 Primary categories of disorders associated with ventricular failure include which of the following?
I. myocardial weakness/inflammation
II. increased CNS stimulation
III. excessive ventricular work load
IV. shock/hypotension

a. I and III
b. III and IV
c. II, III, and IV
d. I, II, III, and IV

20.74 The use of digitalis (or its derivatives) in some forms of left ventricular failure is based on its ability to:
I. increase myocardial contractility
II. slow AV node conduction
III. prolong diastolic filling time
IV. increase cardiac output

a. I, III, and IV
b. I and III
c. II, III, and IV
d. I, II, III, and IV

20.75 Supportive therapy for ventricular failure aims to accomplish which of the following objectives?
I. to increase the efficiency of contractions
II. to increase the afterload on the ventricles
III. to decrease the work load on the myocardium
IV. to reduce the retention of sodium and water

a. I, II, and III
b. I, III, and IV
c. II, III, and IV
d. I, II, III, and IV

20.76 Signs of right ventricular failure include which of the following?
I. jugular venous distention
II. an enlarged liver (hepatomegaly)
III. gravity–dependent edema
IV. right upper abdominal pain

a. III only
b. II, III, and IV
c. I and II
d. I, II, III, and IV

20.77 Which of the following clinical signs and symptoms are most useful in differentiating pulmonary embolism from pneumonia?
I. presence of a fever, cough, and chills
II. collateral patient history
III. chest physical examination
IV. respiratory rate

a. II, III, and IV
b. I, II, and III
c. I and II
d. I, II, III, and IV

20.78 The pattern of arterial blood gases most commonly seen with pulmonary thromboembolism is:

a. compensated respiratory acidosis without hypoxemia
b. hypoxemia in the presence of respiratory acidosis
c. hypoxemia in the presence of respiratory alkalosis
d. combined respiratory and metabolic acidosis

20.79 The general management of shock involves which of the following approaches?
I. drug therapy
II. cardiac support
III. fluid resuscitation
IV. ventilatory support

a. II, III, and IV
b. III and IV
c. I, III, and IV
d. I, II, III, and IV
e. II and IV

20.80 The clinical and laboratory features of pulmonary thromboembolism depend mainly on the:

a. origin of the clot causing the embolus
b. coagulation state of the blood
c. efficiency of myocardial contractions
d. level at which the obstruction occurs

20.81 Epinephrine, aminophylline, and hydrocortisone are common drug agents used to treat which form of shock?

a. neurogenic shock
b. cardiogenic shock
c. anaphylactic shock
d. hyperdynamic shock

20.82 Early signs of hypovolemic shock include which of the following?

I. postural changes in blood pressure
II. cool and clammy skin
III. distended neck veins
IV. concentrated urine
V. weak/irregular pulse

a. I, II, and IV
b. II, III, IV, and V
c. III, IV, and V
d. I, II, III, IV, and V

20.83 A burn patient has the following clinical signs: fever; agitation; a rapid, bounding strong pulse; slightly decreased blood pressure; tachypnea; normal neck veins; dry and warm skin; and a normal urine output. What is the most likely cardiovascular diagnosis?

a. hyperdynamic septic shock
b. anaphylactic shock
c. neurogenic shock
d. cardiogenic shock
e. hypovolemic shock

20.84 The extent of pulmonary injury caused by post-operative aspiration of gastric contents is determined by the:

I. frequency of aspiration
II. length of surgical procedure
III. volume of material aspirated
IV. pH of the aspirated material

a. II, III, and IV
b. I, III, and IV
c. I and IV
d. I, II, III, and IV

20.85 Two days after abdominal surgery, a patient develops a low-grade fever, tachypnea, and signs of consolidation in the lower lobes. The most likely cause of this problem is:

a. pleural effusion
b. atelectasis
c. pulmonary aspiration
d. postoperative pneumonia

20.86 Once a patient develops postoperative atelectasis, which of the following treatments may be applied?

I. chest percussion, drainage, and coughing
II. hyperinflation therapy (e.g., IS or IPPB)
III. therapeutic bronchoscopy
IV. nasotracheal/endotracheal suctioning

a. II and III
b. II, III, and IV
c. III and IV
d. I, II, III, and IV

**Matching:**

20.87
Below are several brief admitting notes taken from patients' medical records. Following those are listed several possible diagnoses. In the space provided to the left of each admitting note, write the letter corresponding to the most likely diagnosis.

_____ History: 65 y.o. male, 15–pack–year smoker with persistent cough; mucopurulent sputum for last 4 months; recurrent pneumonia for last 2 years. Physical: mildly obese with pronounced rhonchi and rales on auscultation, mild hepatomegaly, and pedal edema. PFTs: decreased FEV1% , FEF$_{25-75}$ not responsive to bronchodilators; normal TLC and compliance; slight increase in RV; normal D$_{LCO}$. ABGs: pH 7.34, Pco$_2$ 60, Po$_2$ 58 (room air). X–ray: evidence of right ventricular hypertrophy.

_____ History: 28 y.o. white female with a chief complaint of progressive daily syndrome fatigue; difficulty swallowing; double vision. Physical: normal lungs; slurred speech; "lazy" left eye; drooping eye lids. PFTs: marked decrease in IC and VC. Lab: normal chemistry and hematology. X–ray: normal lung fields, but minimal diaphragmatic motion. Other: positive Tensilon test.

_____ History: 73 y.o. Hispanic male with chief complaint of general fatigue; severe shortness of breath while lying in bed; and nightly coughing with frequent urination. Physical: increased strength and leftward displacement PMI; gallop rhythm with accentuated P$_2$ ; cool extremities. X–ray: increased vascular markings upper lung fields; enlarged heart.

_____ History: 17 y.o. male student with 5th ER admission for acute SOB, cough with thick sputum. Physical: patient agitated and in distress; severe wheezing and rales on auscultation. ABGs: pH 7.57, Pco$_2$ 28, Po$_2$ 68 (cannula at 6 L/min). Lab: mucoid sputum contains plugs and spirals; WBC dif: eosinophilia. X–ray: mild hyperinflation.

_____ History: 5 y.o. female child received tetanus anti-toxin in ER and immediately began choking, wheezing, and coughing. Physical: child is unconscious with a BP of 62/36; pupils dilated but reactive; temp of 103° F; face edematous; hives on chest/arms; central cyanosis on room air.

_____ History: 28 y.o. female with sudden onset of chills, high fever, pain during inspiration, cough with blood streaked sputum. Physical: tachypnea, diminished chest excursions and breath sounds on right side, fine inspiratory crackles. Lab: gram stain: gram$^+$ cocci in pairs. CBC: leukocytosis. ABG: pH 7.54, $P_{CO_2}$ 31 mm Hg, $P_{O_2}$ 53 mm Hg (room air). X–ray: increased density right lower/middle lobes.

a. left ventricular failure

b. chronic bronchitis

c. Guillain–Barre

d. anaphylactic shock

e. pneumococcal pneumonia

f. asthma

g. cor pulmonale

h. myasthenia gravis

i. septic shock

j. tuberculosis

# Pharmacology for Respiratory Care

## CONTENT EXERCISES

**True/False:** For each of the following statements, indicate whether it is mainly true or mainly false by circling the corresponding letter (T=True, F=False):

21.1 T F The kidneys are the major route of excretion for most drugs.

21.2 T F Urinary excretion of a drug is enhanced when it is in ionized form.

21.3 T F The majority of drugs used by respiratory care practitioners act at specific receptor sites.

21.4 T F Sympathetic innervation causes the release of epinephrine from the adrenal gland into the blood.

21.5 T F At effector organs, sympathetic fibers release acetylcholine.

21.6 T F An increase in the cellular level of cGMP causes smooth muscle relaxation.

21.7 T F Anticholinergic drugs, like atropine, block the adenyl cyclase receptor site.

21.8 T F The majority of an aerosolized drug is either exhaled or swallowed.

21.9 T F In contrast to atropine, ipratropium bromide does not elicit any subjective drying of oral secretions.

21.10 T F Bronchial glands can be stimulated either directly (by topical cholinergic drugs) or indirectly (by agents that evoke a vagal response).

21.11 T F A normal saline aerosol can provoke bronchospasm in patients with reactive airways.

21.12 T F Large mucoid molecular chains tend to break in alkaline environments.

21.13 T F Steroids can increase the effectiveness of adrenergic bronchodilators, especially when tolerance has developed.

21.14 T F Cromolyn sodium is an effective agent against existing bronchospasm.

21.15 T F The aerosol application of antibiotics is an effective substitute for the systemic route.

21.16 T F Common antibiotics are not effective against viral infections.

21.17 T F Ribavirin (Virazole) administered via an unmodified ventilator circuit can cause jamming of valve mechanisms.

21.18 T F To prevent bronchospasm in patients with hyperreactive airways, aerosolized acetylcysteine should always be administered with an adrenergic bronchodilator.

21.19 T F Terbutaline is twice as potent as metaproterenol and has a longer duration of action.

21.20 T F Atropine and ipratropium bromide are both anticholinergic bronchodilators and act by inhibiting increases in intracellular cyclic GMP.

21.21 T F Patients on long–term steroids may exhibit "cushingoid" features and possibly develop osteoporosis.

**Short Answer:** Complete each statement by filling in the correct information in the space(s) provided:

21.22 A _____ represents any effect produced by a drug other than its desired effect.

21.23 _____ is a measure of how rapidly a drug is inactivated or excreted from the body.

21.24 The _____ is responsible for the metabolism and inactivation of most drugs.

21.25 Repeated use of a specific drug may result in a decreased response to the same dose. This is phenomenon is known as _____ _____.

21.26 _____ is the type of interaction whereby coadministration of two drugs results in each increasing the effect of the other.

21.27 The tendency a drug has to combine with a receptor is termed _____.

21.28 If a drug has affinity and produces an effect, it is termed an _____.

21.29 A drug which blocks the effect of other agents by forming reversible bond with a receptor is termed a _____ antagonist.

21.30 The balance of influence on receptor function between the sympathetic and parasympathetic components of the autonomic nervous system is referred to as _____.

21.31 Adrenergic agents produce bronchodilation by causing stimulation of _____ which in turn is responsible for the increased production of cyclic AMP from ATP.

21.32 The chemical transmitter at the ganglia of both the sympathetic and parasympathetic systems is _____.

21.33 Drugs that act like adrenaline are known as _____ agents.

21.34 Drugs with effects similar to those of the parasympathetic nervous system are called _____ agents.

21.35 The agent of choice for sputum induction is _____.

21.36 Therapeutic levels of theophyllines range between _____ µg/ml in blood plasma.

21.37 Atrovent is best classified as an _____ _____ bronchodilator.

21.38 Of all the agents used to modify the character of respiratory tract secretions, none is more important than _____.

21.39 Half–normal saline is _____ % sodium chloride.

21.40 _____ lyse the material found in purulent sputum.

21.41 Steroids are used in respiratory care basically because of their _____ action.

21.42 Intal, Nasalcrom, and Opticrom are all brand name preparations of _____ , used in the prevention of allergic/asthmatic responses.

21.43 _____ has emerged as a mainstay of therapy in the management of AIDS patients having *Pneumocystis carinii* pneumonia. This drug is classified as an _____ agent.

Listing: Complete each list as directed in its statement.

21.44 List at least five (5) physiologic side effects of glucocorticoid production or administration:

1. _____

2. _____

3. _____

4. _____

5. _____

**Compare and Contrast:**

21.45 Compare and contrast the sympathetic and parasympathetic components of the autonomic nervous system by completing the following table:

| | Sympathetic Nervous System | Parasympathetic Nervous System |
|---|---|---|
| a. Origin | | |
| b. Preganglionic Fibers | | |
| c. Postganglionic Fibers | | |
| d. Transmitter at Ganglia | | |
| e. Receptor at Ganglia | | |
| f. Transmitter at Effector Organ | | |
| g. Receptor at Effector Organ | | |
| h. Major Effect | | |

**Multiple Choice:** Circle the letter corresponding to the single best answer from the available choices:

21.46 Which of the following are possible disadvantages associated with the administration of drugs via the inhalation route?
I. requires patient cooperation
II. requires special equipment
III. risk of overdose or untoward side effects

a. II only  
b. I and III  
c. II and III  
d. I, II, and III

21.47 All of the following are required on a patient's prescription *except*:

a. patient's name  
b. contraindications  
c. drug name and dose  
d. frequency of administration

21.48 Which of the following are examples of nonreceptor drugs, i.e., those which act by diffusion at many tissue sites?
I. alcohol
II. general anesthetics
III. bronchodilators
IV. mucus–diluting agents

a. I and II  
b. I and III  
c. I, II, and IV  
d. I, II, III, and IV

21.49 Which of the following represent strategies used to enhance mucokinesis?
I. simple dilution of the mucus with liquid agents
II. contracting arterioles, muscle fibers
III. stimulation of serous secretion within the airways
IV. actual chemical breakdown of secretion components

a. I, III, and IV  
b. I and IV  
c. II and III  
d. I, II, III, and IV

21.50 Proper monitoring of a patient receiving an adrenergic bronchodilator should include which of the following?

I.   pre/post–assessment of pulse and respiratory rate
II.  pre/post–assessment of pulmonary function values
III. pre/post–auscultation of lung fields
IV.  continual monitoring for systemic side effects

a. I and IV                    c. II and III
b. II, III, and IV             d. I, II, III, and IV

21.51 Which of the following can impair mucokinesis by inhibiting ciliary activity?
I.   dehydration
II.  cigarette smoke
III. alcohol
IV.  anticholinergic drugs

a. I and IV                    c. II and III
b. I, II, and III             d. I, II, III, and IV

21.52 When a saline solution is administered with a beta agonist, it is being used as a:

a. diluting agent
b. wetting agent
c. mucolytic agent
d. proteolytic agent

21.53 The most common side effect of aerosolized steroids administration is:

a. hypocalcemia
b. candidiasis
c. hypertension
d. tachyphylaxis

21.54 Adverse effects of pentamidine include which of the following?
I.   anemia
II.  neutropenia
III. azotemia
IV.  abnormal blood glucose levels

a. II, III, and IV             c. II and III
b. I and IV                    d. I, II, III, and IV

21.55 Bronchodilation is most commonly achieved via the use of which of the following agents?

a. cholinergic
b. parasympathetic
c. adrenergic
d. anticholinergic

21.56 Which one of the following is an anticholinergic bronchodilator?

a. ipratropium bromide
b. isoproterenol hydrochloride
c. metaproterenol sulfate
d. terbutaline sulfate

21.57 The generic name for Alupent is:

a. epinephrine
b. isoproterenol
c. metaproteronol
d. salbutamol

21.58 Which of the following are possible side effects associated with the administration of adrenergic bronchodilators?
I.   tachycardia
II.  skeletal muscle tremor
III. insomnia
IV.  decreased $PaO_2$

a. I and II                    c. III and IV
b. I, II, and III             d. I, II, III, and IV

21.59 Which of the following are responses produced by methylxanthines?
I.   CNS stimulation
II.  bronchodilation
III. pulmonary vasoconstriction
IV.  diuresis

a. I, II, and IV              c. III and IV
b. II only                    d. I, II, III, and IV

21.60 Which of the following will require the patient to increase dosage of theophylline?
I.   cigarette smoking
II.  marked hypoxemia
III. marked obesity
IV.  high caffeine intake

a. I and IV                    c. II and IV
b. II, III, and IV            d. I, II, III, and IV

21.61 This agent is both hygroscopic and a solvent for bronchodilators. However, it can inhibit the growth of fungi and mycobacteria and should not be used for sputum induction when the goal is to culture either of these organisms. Which agent is it?

a. propylene glycol
b. ethanol
c. normal saline
d. sodium bicarbonate
e. half–normal saline

21.62 This mucolytic chemically replaces the disulfide bonds of mucoproteins with weaker sulfhydryl bonds, and this action disrupts the molecular structure, thus lowering the viscosity of mucus. Which is it?

a. sodium bicarbonate
b. tyloxapol
c. N–acetylcysteine
d. propylene glycol
e. pancreatic dornase

21.63 Which of the following are inhalant steroids (available in MDI form) used in the treatment of bronchial asthma?
I.    dexamethasone sodium phosphate
II.   beclomethasone dipropionate
III.  triamcinolone acetonide
IV.   cromolyn sodium

a. I and IV            c. II and III
b. I, II, and III      d. I, II, III, and IV

21.64 This agent is effective in the treatment of bronchiolitis associated with the respiratory syncytial virus and appears to be effective against both DNA and RNA viruses. Which agent is it?

a. pentamidine
b. amantidine
c. interferon
d. ribavirin

**Solute Computations:**

**Quantitative Classification of Solutions.** There are six methods whereby the amount of solute in a solution may be quantified. These include the ratio solution, the weight per volume (W/V) solution, the percent solution, the molar solution, the normal solution, and the molal solution.

1. **Ratio solution.** The relationship of the solute to the solvent is expressed as a proportion (e.g., 1:100, parts per thousand, etc.). This is used frequently in describing concentrations of pharmaceuticals.

2. **Weight per volume (W/V) solution.** Often erroneously referred to as a "percent solution," the W/V solution is the one most commonly used in pharmacy and medicine for solids dissolved in liquids. It is calibrated in *weight of solute per volume of solution as grams of solute per 100 ml of solution*. Therefore, 5 g of glucose dissolved in 100 ml of solution is properly called a 5% (W/V) solution. In contrast, a liquid dissolved in a liquid is measured as volumes of solute to volumes of solution (V/V solution).

3. **Percent solution (% or W/W).** Used in chemistry, a percent solution is calibrated as *weight of solute per weight of solution* (weight/weight or W/W solution). Five grams of glucose dissolved in 95 g of water is a true percent solution since the glucose is 5% of the total solution weight of 100 g.

4. **Molar solution.** Physiologically, the molar solution and the normal solution are the most important of all solutions. A molar solution has *1 mol of solute per liter of solution* (or 1 mmol per ml of solution). A 1 mol/L solution of sodium chloride contains 58.5 g per liter of solution; a 0.5 mol/L solution has 29.25 g/L of solution; a 2 mol/L solution has 117 g/L of solution, etc. The solute is measured into a container, and the solvent is added to the total solution volume desired. The molar solution is chemically important because equal volumes of solutions of equal molarity contain the same number or fractions of solute moles.

5. **Normal solution (N).** Widely used in chemistry and biochemistry, the normal solution has *1 gram equivalent weight of solute per liter of solution* (or 1 mEq/ml of solution). Accordingly, 1 mol of HCl, or 1/2 mol of $H_2SO_4$, each dissolved in 1 liter of solution, make 1 N solutions of the respective solutes. For all monovalent solutes, normal and molar solutions are the same because the equivalent weights of such solutes equal their gram formula weights. Equal volumes of

solutions of the same normality contain chemically equivalent amounts of their solutes. If the solutes react chemically with one another, then equal volumes of the solutions will react completely, and neither substance will remain in excess. Solutions of known normality are often used as standard solutions in an analytic process known as titration for determining the concentrations of other solutions.

6. **Molal solution.** Less frequently used in physiologic chemistry than are the molar solution and the normal solution, a molal solution contains *1 mole of solute per kilogram of solvent* (or 1 mmol per gram of solvent). With its solvent measured in weight, the concentration of a molal solution is independent of temperature.

**Calculating Solute Content.** The amount of solute present in any W/V, W/W, or V/V solution can be computed as follows:

Solute content (weight or volume) = Total volume x concentration (%)

In each case (W/V, W/W, or V/V), one must first know the total volume of the solution *and* its concentration in percent (%). For W/V and W/W solutions, the concentration is usually given as a percent, e.g., 3% (W/V) or 5% (W/W). On the other hand, when one is dealing with a ratio solution (like 1:200), one must first compute the percent equivalent.

Converting ratio solutions to their percent equivalent is complicated by the fact that in clinical practice some ratio solutions express a *true* volume/volume relationship, while others are equivalent to a weight/volume solution. For example, a 1:3 ratio solution of alcohol (solute) in water (solvent) is a true volume/volume solution. To convert a 1:3 ratio solution of alcohol in water (true V/V) to a percent solution, one must go through the following steps (example A):

Total volume: 1 (alcohol) + 3 (water) = 4

$$\% \text{ alcohol} = \frac{\text{volume alcohol (1)}}{\text{total volume (4)}} \times 100$$

$$\% \text{ alcohol} = 25\% \ (0.25)$$

On the other hand, it is common practice to express *dilute* W/V solutions in the ratio format, e.g., a 1:1000 solution of epinephrine in water. In this case, the ratio of 1:1000 indicates that 1000 ml of the solution contain 1 gram of epinephrine (a solid). To convert this ratio to a percent, one simply multiplies the ratio times 100 (example B):

$$\% \text{ solution (epinephrine)} = \frac{1}{1000} \times 100$$

$$= 0.1\% \ (0.001)$$

As a rule of thumb, when computing the percent concentration of true V/V solutions (in which one volume is added to another), one must take into account the *total* volume by adding the constituent parts (example A). On the other hand, when the ratio format simply is expressing the ratio of W/V in a dilute solution, the direct percent conversion (example B) is appropriate. In any case, once the percent concentration and total volume are known, the total solute content is computed as below:

Solute content (weight or volume) = Total volume x concentration (%)

**Example 1.** For example, to compute the solute content of a 1.5 L of a 1:4 V/V solution of the solute glutaraldehyde (a disinfectant) in water (the solvent):

Total volume: 1 (glutaraldehyde) + 4 (water) = 5

$$\% \text{ glutaraldehyde} = \frac{\text{volume glutaraldehyde (1)}}{\text{total volume (5)}} \times 100$$

$$= 20\% \ (0.20)$$

solute content (volume) = total volume x concentration (%)

$$= 1.5 \text{ L} \times 0.20$$

$$= 0.30 \text{ L or } 300 \text{ ml}$$

**Example 2.** To compute the amount of solute in 50 ml of a 10% W/V solution of glucose in water:

solute content (weight) = total volume x concentration (%)

$$= 50 \text{ ml} \times 0.10$$

$$= 5 \text{ grams}$$

**Example 3.** To compute the amount of solute in 2 ml of a 1:200 W/V solution of isoproterenol in water:

$$\% \text{ solution} = \frac{1}{200} \times 100$$

$$= 0.5\% \ (0.005)$$

solute content (weight) = total volume x concentration (%)

$$= 2 \text{ ml} \times 0.005$$

$$= 0.01 \text{ grams or } 10 \text{ mg}$$

Example # 3 (computing the amount of solute in a small volume of a dilute W/V solution of a drug) is probably the most common computation in respiratory pharmacology. To aid in solving these types of problems, it is useful to commit to memory some of the most common solute content relationships:

| Percent Strength | Solute Content (mg/ml) |
|---|---|
| 20% | 200 mg/ml |
| 10% | 100 mg/ml |
| 5% | 50 mg/ml |
| 1% | 10 mg/ml |
| 0.5% | 5 mg/ml |
| 0.1% | 1 mg/ml |
| 0.05% | 0.5 mg/ml |

For example, to compute the amount of solute in 3 ml of a 1:100 W/V solution of isoetharine in water, compute the percent strength:

$$\% \text{ solution} = \frac{1}{100} \times 100$$

$$= 1.0\%$$

Then, by reference to the pertinent relationship in the above table (1% solution = 10 mg/ml), multiply the volume x the solute content/ml:

$$3 \text{ ml} \times 10 \text{ mg/ml} = 30 \text{ mg isoetharine}$$

21.65 Convert the following dilute W/V ratios solutions into their equivalent percent (%) strengths:

a. 1:200 = _____

b. 1:1000 = _____

21.66 For each of the following W/V solutions, compute (1) the total grams of solute in the given volume of the solution and (2) the number of milligrams of solute in each milliliter of the solution (mg/ml):

| | Solution Volume in ml | Concentration of Solution (W/V) | Total Solute Content in grams | Solute Content in mg/ml |
|---|---|---|---|---|
| a. | 5 | 1.00% | _____ | _____ |
| b. | 2 | 3.00% | _____ | _____ |

21.67 A W/V solution that is 0.1% strength contains how many mg/ml of active ingredient? _____ _____

21.68 You have a 0.5% W/V solution. The physician wishes to administer 2.5 mg of the drug to the patient. How many ml would you need? _____ _____

**Dilution Computations:**

It is often necessary to make a dilute solution from a stock preparation. This can be done accurately if the concepts of solution concentrations are understood. Such dilution problems usually involve medications and are based on the pharmacologic weight per unit volume (W/V) percent principle defined earlier. Diluting a solution increases its volume without changing the amount of solute it contains but reduces its concentration. Therefore the amount of solute in a given sample after dilution is the same as was present in the smaller original volume. In diluting a solution, then, the initial volume times the initial concentration equals the final volume times the final concentration. This can be simplified with the following formula:

$$V_1 C_1 = V_2 C_2$$

When three of the data are known, the fourth can be calculated.

**Example 1.** If 50 ml of water are added to 150 ml of a 3% solution, what is the final percent concentration?

$$V_1 C_1 = V_2 C_2$$

$$V_1 C_1 = V_2 C_2$$

$$C_2 = V_1 C_1 / V_2$$

$$C_2 = 150 \times 3 / 200$$

$$C_2 = 2.25\%$$

**Example 2.** If 50 ml of a .33% solution are diluted to a 0.1% concentration, what is the final volume?

$$V_1 C_1 = V_2 C_2$$

$$V_2 = V_1 C_1 / C_2$$

$$V_2 = 50 \times 0.33 / 0.1$$

$$V_2 = 167 \text{ ml}$$

**Example 3.** How much water must be added to 10 ml of a 2% solution to obtain concentration of 0.5%?

First the final volume must be found:

$$V_1 C_1 = V_2 C_2$$

$$V_2 = V_1 C_1 / C_2$$

$$V_2 = 10 \times 2 / 0.5$$

$$V_2 = 40 \text{ ml}$$

Then the original volume must be subtracted from the final volume:

$$V_2 - V_1 = 40 \text{ ml} - 10 \text{ ml}$$

$$= 30 \text{ ml}$$

Thus 30 ml of water must be added to 10 ml of 2% solution to make 40 ml of a 0.5% solution.

21.69 You dilute 30 ml of a 20% solution with 20 ml water. What is the final percent concentration? _____

_____

21.70 What is the final percent concentration when 0.5 ml of a 1.0% solution is mixed with 3.0 ml of normal saline? _____

_____

21.71 How much solvent ($H_2O$) must be added to 10 ml of a 1.0% solution to create a 0.4% solution? _____

_____

# 22

# Airway Care

## CONTENT EXERCISES

**True/False:** For each of the following statements, indicate whether it is mainly true or mainly false by circling the corresponding letter (T=True, F=False):

22.1  T  F  Suctioning of a patient's airway should be performed at least every hour.

22.2  T  F  Use of too large a suction catheter can result in atelectasis.

22.3  T  F  Patient oxygenation can decrease after five seconds of suctioning.

22.4  T  F  Artificial airways are commonly used to bypass obstruction occurring distal to the trachea.

22.5  T  F  Loss of airway protective reflexes generally proceeds up from the trachea to the pharynx.

22.6  T  F  Accidental extubation is most common with tracheostomy tubes.

22.7  T  F  The purpose of a endotracheal tube stylet is to aid in extubation.

22.8  T  F  Capnography is a good way to determine if an endo tube is misplaced in a mainstem bronchus.

22.9  T  F  Nasotracheal tubes are more difficult to insert than orotracheal tubes.

22.10  T  F  Nasotracheal tubes are better tolerated by conscious patients.

22.11  T  F  A tracheostomy tube is the device of choice for overcoming upper airway obstruction or trauma.

22.12  T  F  Some forms of airway damage may take months to develop.

22.13  T  F  Movement of endotracheal tubes is a primary cause of damage to the larynx and the trachea.

22.14  T  F  Endotracheal and tracheostomy tubes should be changed at least every 48 hours.

22.15  T  F  Overinflation of a high–volume, low–pressure cuff changes its performance to a high–pressure cuff.

22.16  T  F  The minimal leak technique negates the need for monitoring cuff pressures.

22.17  T  F  Use of high–volume cuffs prevents aspiration of pharyngeal contents.

22.18  T  F  The major complication associated with extubation is laryngospasm.

22.19  T  F  The primary use of a tracheal button is to maintain a tracheostomy stoma during the decannulation process.

22.20  T  F  Epiglottitis and/or croup are absolute contraindications for nasotracheal suctioning.

**Short Answer:** Complete each statement by filling in the correct information in the space(s) provided:

22.21 The most common complication of airway suctioning is _____.

22.22 Bradycardia during suctioning results from _____ originating at the larynx or carina.

22.23 The external diameter of suction catheters should never exceed _____ the internal diameter of the airway.

22.24 One should continue to insert a suction catheter until either the patient coughs or _____ is felt.

22.25 Stagnant secretions present an ideal medium for _____.

22.26 Endotracheal tube sizes are normally expressed in metric units, corresponding to the _____ diameter of the tube.

22.27 The _____ laryngoscope blade lifts the epiglottis indirectly as the tip of the blade is advanced into the vallecula.

22.28 The tip of an endotracheal tube should be advanced until the cuff has passed the cords by _____ centimeters.

22.29 The first and simplest technique used to confirm endotracheal tube placement following endotracheal intubation is _____.

22.30 The emergency route of choice to establish a tracheal airway in a patient with spinal or jaw injuries is _____.

22.31 A rare life–threatening complication of tracheotomy that occurs when the tracheal tube is placed too low is _____.

22.32 When used to secure an endotracheal tube, tape may adhere to the skin better if one applies _____ _____.

**Listing:** Complete each list as directed in its statement.

22.33 List at least six (6) complications of airway suctioning:

1. _____
2. _____
3. _____
4. _____
5. _____
6. _____

22.34 List the equipment necessary for airway suctioning (aspiration):

1. _____
2. _____
3. _____
4. _____
5. _____
6. _____
7. _____

22.35 For each patient listed on the left, indicate the size oral endotracheal tube you would select.

| Patient | Tube Size in mm |
| --- | --- |
| a. newborn infant | _____ |
| b. 6–month–old | _____ |
| c. 5–year–old | _____ |
| d. 12–year–old | _____ |
| e. adult female | _____ |
| f. adult male | _____ |

**Labeling:** Match the components or structures listed on the right to the letter labels in the following figure:

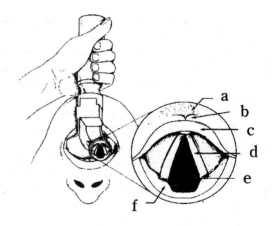

**Figure 22–1** Laryngoscopic view of larynx

22.36
a. _____ glottis

b. _____ vocal cord

c. _____ tongue

d. _____ arytenoid cartilage

e. _____ vallecula

f. _____ epiglottis

**Multiple Choice:** Circle the letter corresponding to the single best answer from the available choices:

22.37 Retention of secretions can cause which of the following?
I.   increased work of breathing
II.  atelectasis/alveolar collapse
III. hypoxemia and hypercapnea
IV.  pulmonary infection
V.   increased airway resistance

a. I, III, and IV      c. I, II, IV, and V
b. II, III, and IV     d. I, II, III, IV, and V

22.38 To prevent hypoxemia when suctioning a patient, the respiratory care practitioner should initially do which of the following?

a. manually ventilate the patient with a resuscitator
b. preoxygenate the patient with 50% oxygen
c. preoxygenate the patient with 100% oxygen
d. give the patient a bronchodilator treatment

22.39 While suctioning a patient, you observe an abrupt change in the ECG waveform being displayed on the cardiac monitor. Which of the following actions would be most appropriate?

a. stop suctioning and immediately administer oxygen
b. stop suctioning and report your findings to the nurse
c. decrease the amount of negative pressure being used
d. instill 10 cc normal saline directly into the trachea

22.40 Which of the following should be employed to minimize the likelihood of atelectasis occurring as a result of suctioning?
I.   limiting the amount of negative pressure
II.  using the largest possible catheter
III. limiting the duration of suctioning
IV.  pre/post hyperinflating the patient

a. I, II, and III      c. I, III, and IV
b. III and IV        d. I, II, III, and IV

22.41 The normal range of negative pressure to use when suctioning children is:

a. –80 to –100 mm Hg
b. –60 to –80 mm Hg
c. –100 to –120 mm Hg
d. –150 to –200 mm Hg

22.42 An unconscious patient has a large volume of secretions in her oropharynx. Which of the following procedures would you recommend as the best method to remove these secretions?

a. perform endotracheal suctioning
b. perform an emergency tracheostomy
c. perform a therapeutic bronchoscopy
d. use Yankauer (tonsillar) suction

22.43 Which of the following are contraindications for nasotracheal suctioning?
I.   occluded nasal passages
II.  nasal bleeding
III. epiglottitis or croup
IV.  larynogospasm

a. I, II, and III      c. I and III
b. II and IV        d. I, II, III, and IV

22.44 Before suctioning a patient you note that there is no vacuum being generated at the catheter thumbport. Which of the following is the most likely problem?

a. the selected catheter is too small
b. there is a leak in the suction system
c. the catheter end–tip is obstructed
d. the bulk oxygen source has failed

22.45 Total application time for endotracheal suction in adults should not exceed:

a. 3–5 seconds
b. 10–15 seconds
c. 20–25 seconds
d. 15–20 seconds

22.46 You are asked by a physician to assist him in monitoring a patient during a fiberoptic bronchoscopy procedure. Which of the following would you recommend?
I.   vital signs (pulse, respiratory rate)
II.  heart rhythm via electrocardiogram (ECG)
III. forced expiratory flow rates (e.g., $FEV_1$)
IV.  arterial oxygen saturations via oximetry

a. I, II, and III      c. II and III
b. I, II, and IV      d. I, II, III, and IV

22.47 Which of the following is *not* a cause of airway obstruction?

a. tumors within or outside the airway
b. decreased compliance of the lung/chest wall
c. changes in muscle tone or tissue support
d. edema or swelling of the airway mucosa

22.48 For which of the following is a *cuffed* artificial airway indicated?
I. to protect the lower airway from aspiration
II. to relieve airway obstruction
III. to facilitate removal of secretions
IV. to facilitate positive pressure ventilation

a. II and IV          c. I and IV
b. I, II, and III     d. I, II, III, and IV

22.49 Which of the following are true regarding artificial airways?
I. artificial airways increase airway resistance above normal
II. the larger the tube, the greater the increase in resistance
III. small tubes dramatically increase the work of breathing
IV. the imposed work load is lowest at high minute ventilations

a. I, II, and III     c. I and III
b. II and IV          d. I, II, III, and IV

22.50 A gag response is produced via which of the following reflexes?

a. laryngeal
b. pharyngeal
c. tracheal
d. J receptor

22.51 Which of the following features incorporated into most modern endotracheal tubes assist in verifying proper tube placement?
I. length markings on the curved body of the tube
II. an additional side port (Murphy eye) near the tube tip
III. an imbedded radiopaque indicator near the tube tip

a. I and III          c. III only
b. II and III         d. I, II, and III

22.52 The purpose of the pilot balloon on an endotracheal or tracheostomy tube is to:

a. help ascertain proper tube position
b. minimize mucosal trauma during insertion
c. protect the airway against aspiration
d. monitor cuff status and pressure

22.53 The removable inner cannula commonly incorporated into modern tracheostomy tubes serves which of the following purposes?
I. to aid in routine tube cleaning/tracheostomy care
II. to provide a patent airway should it become obstructed
III. to prevent the tube from slipping into the trachea

a. II and III         c. I and II
b. III only           d. I, II, and III

22.54 The purpose of a tracheostomy tube obturator is to:

a. provide a patent airway should the tube become obstructed
b. aid in the emergency removal of the tracheostomy tube
c. help ascertain the proper tube position by x–ray
d. minimize trauma to the tracheal mucosa during insertion

22.55 In the absence of neck or facial injuries, the procedure of choice to establish a patent tracheal airway in an emergency is:

a. surgical tracheotomy
b. nasotracheal intubation
c. cricothyrotomy
d. orotracheal intubation

22.56 You are about to suction a female patient who has an 8.0 mm (ID) endotracheal tube in place. What is the *maximum* size catheter you would use in this case?

a. 8 Fr
b. 10 Fr
c. 12 Fr
d. 16 Fr

22.57 *Before* beginning an intubation procedure, the practitioner should check and confirm the operation of which of the following?
I.     laryngoscope light source
II.    cardiac defibrillator
III.   suction equipment
IV.    endotracheal tube cuff

a. I, II, and III          c. I, III, and IV
b. II and IV               d. I, II, III, and IV

22.58 The maximum time devoted to any intubation attempt should be no more than:

a. 60 seconds
b. 2 minutes
c. 3 minutes
d. 30 seconds

22.59 After a physician intubates a patient in the emergency room, your partner begins manual ventilation with 100% $O_2$. On auscultation, you note the absence of breath sounds but hear gurgling over the epigastrium. Which of the following has most likely occurred?

a. a right–sided tension pneumothorax
b. intubation of the left mainstem bronchus
c. intubation of the patient's esophagus
d. intubation of the right mainstem bronchus

22.60 In order to prevent a patient from compressing an oral endotracheal tube between the teeth, you would recommend:

a. administration of a neuromuscular blocking agent
b. administration of a strong narcotic–analgesic
c. application of a Brigg's adapter ("T–tube")
d. use of a "bit block" or oropharyngeal airway

22.61 Serious complications of oral intubation include which of the following?
I.     tongue lacerations
II.    acute hypoxemia
III.   bradycardia
IV.    cardiac arrest

a. II and IV               c. II, III, and IV
b. I, II, and III          d. I, II, III, and IV

22.62 Which of the following injuries are *not* seen with tracheostomy tubes?
I.     tracheomalacia
II.    tracheal stenosis
III.   glottic edema
IV.    vocal cord granulomas

a. III and IV              c. I and IV
b. I, II, and III          d. I, II, III, and IV

22.63 The most common sign associated with the transient glottic edema or vocal cord inflammation that follows extubation is:

a. stridor
b. hoarseness
c. wheezing
d. orthopnea

22.64 Soon after endotracheal tube extubation, an adult patient exhibits a high–pitched inspiratory noise, heard without a stethoscope. Which of the following actions would you recommend?

a. a STAT heated aerosol treatment with saline
b. careful observation of the patient for 6 hours
c. immediate reintubation via the nasal route
d. a STAT racemic epinephrine aerosol treatment

22.65 A patient has had a tracheostomy tube in place for three weeks. Over the last ten days, it has required higher and higher pressures in order to obtain an effective cuff seal. What is the most likely problem?

a. T–E fistula
b. blown cuff
c. tracheomalacia
d. glottic edema

22.66 A physician is concerned about the potential for tracheal damage due to tube movement in a patient who recently underwent tracheotomy and is now receiving 40% oxygen via T–tube (Brigg's adapter). Which of the following would be the best way to limit tube movement in this patient?

a. switch from the T–tube to a tracheostomy collar
b. give a neuromuscular blocker to prevent patient movement
c. secure the T–tube delivery tubing to the bed rail
d. tape the T–tube to the tracheostomy tube connector

22.67 Despite manual hyperoxygenation/hyperinflation, a patient on mechanical ventilatory support with PEEP tends to easily develop hypoxemia during suctioning. Techniques that could help minimize this problem include:
I. performing hyperoxygenation/inflation through the ventilator
II. using an adapter that does not require ventilator disconnection
III. using a special catheter that provides both suction and oxygen

a. I and II
b. II and III
c. I and III
d. I, II, and III

22.68 The rationale underlying use of high residual volume, low–pressure cuffs on endotracheal and tracheostomy tubes is to:

a. make it possible for the patient to talk
b. lessen the incidence of tracheal damage
c. provide for better tube stability
d. aid in tube visualization on x–ray

22.69 The maximum recommended range of tracheal tube cuff pressures is:

a. 10–15 mm Hg
b. 15–20 mm Hg
c. 20–25 mm Hg
d. 25–30 mm Hg

22.70 An adult male patient on ventilatory support has just been intubated with a 7.0–mm oral endotracheal tube equipped with a high residual volume, low–pressure cuff. When sealing the cuff to achieve a minimal occluding volume, you note a cuff pressure of 45 cm $H_2O$. What is the most likely problem?

a. the cuff pilot balloon and line are obstructed
b. the pressure manometer is out of calibration
c. the tube chosen is too small for the patient
d. the tube is in the right mainstem bronchus

22.71 A patient with a tracheal airway exhibits severe respiratory distress. On quick examination you note the complete absence of breath sounds and no gas flowing through the airway. What is the most likely problem?

a. complete tube obstruction
b. partial tube obstruction
c. right–sided pneumothorax
d. tracheoinnominate fistula

22.72 After coming upon a patient with complete obstruction of an oral endotracheal tube, your efforts to relieve the obstruction by moving the patient's head and neck and deflating the cuff both fail. What should be your *next* step?

a. immediately extubate the patient
b. try to pass a suction catheter
c. perform an emergency cricothyrotomy
d. call for an emergency tracheotomy

22.73 A patient with a nasal endotracheal tube is receiving positive pressure ventilation via a volume ventilator. Over the last two minutes, both the volume delivered to the patient and the peak inspiratory pressure have decreased. In addition, breath sounds are decreased and air flow can be felt at the mouth. Which of the following problems is most likely?

a. a large leak in the endotracheal tube cuff
b. complete obstruction of the endotracheal tube
c. the development of a right–sided pneumothorax
d. partial obstruction of the endotracheal tube

22.74 A physician has requested your assistance in extubating an orally intubated patient. Which of the following should be done *before* the tube itself is removed?
I. suction the oro/laryngopharynx
II. preoxygenate the patient
III. confirm cuff inflation
IV. suction the endo tube

a. II and IV
b. I, II, and IV
c. III and IV
d. I, II, III, and IV

22.75 The major complication associated with endotracheal tube extubation is:

a. bradycardia
b. tracheomalacia
c. laryngospasm
d. aspiration

22.76 Which of the following statements are true regarding colorimetric carbon dioxide ($CO_2$) analyzers to confirm the tube placement during intubation?
I. the colorimetric device is portable
II. use during cardiac arrest needs careful attention
III. end–tidal $CO_2$ analysis is a reliable indicator of tracheal intubation
IV. one colorimetric device can be used on multiple patients

a. I only
b. I, II, and III
c. II and IV
d. I, II, III, and IV

# Emergency Life Support

## CONTENT EXERCISES

**True/False:** For each of the following statements, indicate whether it is mainly true or mainly false by circling the corresponding letter (T=True, F=False):

23.1 T F Accidents are the leading cause of sudden death in children.

23.2 T F Advanced cardiac life support requires the supervision of a physician.

23.3 T F If the primary incident is respiratory arrest, the heart will normally also stop functioning immediately.

23.4 T F Expired air ventilation usually is sufficient to maintain life until advanced life support is available.

23.5 T F If the victim has dentures, the practitioner should remove them before initiating basic life support airway maneuvers and ventilation.

23.6 T F Victims with tracheostomies or laryngectomies can be ventilated directly through the stoma or tube.

23.7 T F Gastric distention during mouth–to–mouth ventilation is usual, particularly in children.

23.8 T F Massive aspiration of stomach contents into the lungs is nearly always a fatal event.

23.9 T F The liver and spleen of younger children lie lower in the abdominal cavity than they do in adults.

23.10 T F CPR for victims with cardiac pacemakers is similar to the procedure described for other CPR victims.

23.11 T F Where advanced capabilities exist, basic life support should be delayed until the ACLS team arrives.

23.12 T F Oropharyngeal airways are contraindicated in conscious or semi–conscious patients.

23.13 T F The most common complication of esophageal obturator airway use is esophageal rupture.

23.14 T F Removal of the EOA is almost always followed by immediate regurgitation of stomach contents.

23.15 T F Tracheotomy is the preferred method of securing the airway during advanced life support.

23.16 T F Even with a cuffed tracheal tube in place, ventilation must be synchronized with chest compressions during CPR.

23.17 T F Single–rescuer bag–mask ventilation is less effective than either the mouth–to–mouth or mouth–to–mask technique.

23.18 T F A pressure manometer always should be used with a manual resuscitator when ventilating infants and small children.

23.19 T F Gas–powered resuscitators are acceptable for ventilating infants and small children during CPR.

23.20 T F Intra–aortic balloon counterpulsation is a useful adjunct to enhance perfusion during true cardiac arrest.

23.21 T F Sinus arrest is common during body manipulations that elicit a strong vagal reflex.

23.22 T F Third–degree heart block is always lethal.

23.23 T F Sodium bicarbonate should be administered every five minutes during cardiac arrest.

**Short Answer:** Complete each statement by filling in the correct information in the space(s) provided:

23.24 Among adults, _____ is the primary cause of sudden death.

23.25 When ventilation and circulation both cease, a condition of _____ exists.

23.26 During basic life support, the practitioner should allow about _____ seconds to confirm the presence or absence of a pulse.

23.27 During most basic life support efforts, the _____ is the most effective airway restoration maneuver.

23.28 During basic life support, exhaled air provides about _____ % oxygen.

23.29 External cardiac compression (ECC) can provide _____ of a normal cardiac output.

23.30 The likelihood of irreversible brain death is high if pupils have been dilated and fixed for _____ minutes or longer.

23.31 With single–practitioner CPR the cycle consists of _____ compressions to every _____ breaths.

23.32 The most frequent and least harmful of all cardiac arrhythmias is _____.

23.33 When ventricular rates fall below 60 per minute, as in third–degree heart block, an _____ is indicated.

23.34 The longer than normal refractory period occurring after a premature ventricular contraction is called a _____ .

23.35 The primary analgesic agent employed in advanced cardiac life support is _____.

23.36 The application of a synchronous shock to the myocardium is called _____.

**Multiple Choice:** Circle the letter corresponding to the single best answer from the available choices:

23.37 Which of the following are common causes of primary respiratory arrest?
I.      airway obstruction
II.     myocardial infarction
III.    unconsciousness
IV.    drug overdose
V.     drowning

a. I, III, and IV
b. II, III, IV, and V
c. I, III, IV, and V
d. I, II, III, IV, and V

23.38 Which of the following is the most common cause of cardiac arrest?

a. arrhythmias associated with myocardial infarction
b. interference with the heart's contractile force
c. interference with blood flow in the heart
d. electrolyte disturbances (e.g., hypokalemia)

23.39 You enter a female patient's room and find her collapsed on the floor near the bed. After shaking her shoulder and shouting "Are you okay?" you get no response. You next step should be to *immediately:*

a. open her airway
b. begin chest compressions
c. determine pulselessness
d. call for help (call a code)

23.40 In order to assess the circulatory status of an adult during basic life support, which of the following pulses is normally palpated?

a. brachial
b. ulnar
c. carotid
d. popliteal

23.41 After implementing procedures to open the airway, an unconscious victim is still not breathing. Your next step should be to:

a. feel for the victim's carotid pulse
b. begin external cardiac compressions
c. attempt to restore ventilation
d. apply back blows to the victim

23.42 At the onset of adult mouth–to–mouth ventilation, the practitioner should provide:

a. two 400–800 cc breaths (1/2–1.0 sec each), without deflation pause
b. two 800–1200 cc breaths (1–1.5 sec each), with deflation pause
c. four 400–800 cc breaths (1/2–1.0 sec each), with deflation pause
d. four 800–1200 cc breaths (1–1.5 sec each), without deflation pause

23.43 You are trying to apply mouth–to–mouth ventilation to an unconscious adult patient but are unable to maintain a tight seal at the lips. At this point you should:

a. place a handkerchief over the victim's mouth and continue
b. use the jaw thrust maneuver instead of the head tilt/chin lift
c. apply mouth–to–nose ventilation instead of mouth–to–mouth
d. immediately perform the Heimlich maneuver (abdominal thrusts)

23.44 Which of the following help confirm restoration of adequate ventilation during basic life support?
I.      observing the victim's chest rise and fall
II.     feeling resistance as the victim's lungs expand
III.    observing the return of normal skin color
IV.    hearing/feeling air escape during exhalation

a. II and IV
b. I, II, and III
c. III and IV
d. I, II, III, and IV

23.45 After two attempts at securing the airway and ventilating an adult in respiratory arrest, you still cannot confirm adequate air movement. At this point you should:

a. apply back blows, followed by chest thrusts
b. apply 6–10 strong abdominal thrusts
c. try to ventilate again at a higher rate
d. halt ventilation and decompress the stomach

23.46 The major hazard associated with the Heimlich maneuver is:

a. laceration or rupture of the abdominal or thoracic viscera
b. the possibility of forcing the object deeper into the airway
c. increased intracranial pressure and cerebral hemorrhage
d. pulmonary barotrauma, especially tension pneumothorax

23.47 The proper rate of external cardiac compressions for infants is:

a. 80–100/min
b. 70–80/min
c. > 100/min
d. 40–60/min

23.48 With the exception of intubation attempts, the maximum amount of time external cardiac compressions should be interrupted is:

a. 5 seconds
b. 10 seconds
c. 15 seconds
d. 20 seconds

23.49 The most reliable indicator of effective external cardiac compressions is:

a. contraction of previously dilated pupils
b. a large positive "spike" on the EKG monitor
c. greater ease of sternal compressions
d. a palpable pulse with each compression

23.50 During two–person CPR applied to an adult, the proper ratio of compressions to ventilation is:

a. 5 compressions for every 1 breath
b. 5 compressions for every 2 breaths
c. 15 compressions for every 1 breath
d. 15 compressions for every 2 breaths

23.51 Oropharyngeal and nasopharyngeal airways help restore airway patency by:

a. providing a secure route into the larynx and trachea
b. separating the tongue from the posterior pharyngeal wall
c. isolating/protecting the lower airway from aspiration
d. displacing the soft palate and uvula posteriorly

23.52 A patient in the emergency room exhibits signs of acute upper airway obstruction and is concurrently having severe seizures which make it impossible to open her mouth. In this case, the adjunct airway of choice would be a(n):

a. oropharyngeal airway
b. nasopharyngeal airway
c. esophageal obturator airway
d. oral endotracheal tube

23.53 During an attempt to insert a nasopharyngeal airway in a patient, you encounter an obstruction to further movement. What is the most appropriate action at this time?

a. use a stylet to force the nasopharyngeal airway in place
b. attempt to pass the airway through the opposite naris
c. insert the nasopharyngeal airway through the oral cavity
d. use a tongue depressor to push the airway posteriorly

23.54 An unconscious patient is admitted to the ER with an esophageal obturator airway (EOA) in place. The attending physician wants to "pull" the EOA and intubate the patient orally. Which of the following would you recommend?

a. not remove the EOA until a nasogastric tube is passed around it
b. not remove the EOA until the cuffed endotracheal tube is placed
c. place the patient in a side–lying position before removing the EOA
d. remove the EOA, suction the oropharynx, then intubate the patient

23.55 During CPR, a properly positioned endotracheal tube can:
I. isolate and protect the lower airway from aspiration
II. permit suctioning of the trachea and mainstem bronchi
III. facilitate positive pressure ventilation and oxygenation
IV. provide a route for administration of selected drug agents

a. III and IV
b. I, II, and III
c. I and IV
d. I, II, III, and IV

23.56 An "ideal" manual resuscitator should have which of the following characteristics?
I. have standard 15/22 mm connections
II. be easy to clean and disinfect
III. limit delivered pressure to 60 cm $H_2O$
IV. deliver 100% $O_2$ at high volumes/rates

a. II and IV
b. I, II, and III
c. I, II, and IV
d. I, II, III, and IV

23.57 In order to deliver as high a concentration of oxygen as possible with a manual resuscitator, you would:
I. use the highest recommended $O_2$ input flow
II. use the shortest possible refill time
III. connect an oxygen reservoir to the bag

a. I and II
b. II and III
c. I and III
d. I, II, and III

23.58 An "ideal" gas–powered resuscitator should:
I. have standard 15/22 mm connections
II. limit delivered pressure to 60 cm $H_2O$
III. free both hands to maintain a mask seal
IV. deliver 100% $O_2$ at flows $\geq$ 40 L/min

a. II and IV
b. I, II, and III
c. I and III
d. I, II, III, and IV

23.59 On inspection of an ECG rhythm strip from an adult patient, you note the following: rate of 150; regular rhythm; normal P waves, P–R intervals, and QRS complexes. The most likely problem is:

a. atrial flutter
b. sinus tachycardia
c. ventricular tachycardia
d. paroxysmal atrial tachycardia

23.60 Which of the following are potential causes of sinus tachycardia?
I. parasympathetic stimulation
II. increased metabolic demand
III. arterial hypoxemia
IV. sympathetic stimulation

a. II and IV
b. I, II, and III
c. II, III, and IV
d. I, II, III, and IV

23.61 Which of the following are treatment options in patients suffering from paroxysmal supraventricular tachycardia (PSVT)?
I. vagal stimulation via carotid sinus massage
II. administration of an adrenergic antagonist
III. synchronous electrical stimulation (cardioversion)

a. I and II
b. II and III
c. I and III
d. I, II, and III

23.62 On inspection of a patient's ECG strip, you note no identifiable P waves; rapid irregular undulations of the isoelectric line; and an irregular ventricular rhythm. In addition, the precordial cardiac rate is greater than the peripheral pulse rate. The most likely problem is:

a. 2° (Wenckebach) heart block
b. premature atrial contractions
c. ventricular fibrillation
d. atrial fibrillation

23.63 Distinguishing features of premature ventricular contractions (PVCs) include which of the following:
I. a compensatory pause following depolarization
II. a widened (0.10 sec) and distorted QRS complex
III. a greater than normal (0.20 sec) P–R interval

a. I and II
b. II and III
c. I and III
d. I, II, and III

23.64 Which of the following arrhythmias are considered potentially lethal?
I. ventricular fibrillation
II. ventricular tachycardia
III. third–degree heart block
IV. supraventricular tachycardia

a. I, II, and III
b. I and II
c. II, III, and IV
d. I, II, III, and IV

23.65 Which of the following drugs can be administered through an endotracheal tube during emergency life support?

I.    lidocaine HCl
II.   sodium nitroprusside
III.  epinephrine HCl
IV.  atropine sulfate

a. II and IV
b. I, III, and IV
c. III and IV
d. I, II, III, and IV

23.66 The initial energy level for the defibrillation of an adult patient is:

a. 25 joules
b. 100 joules
c. 200 joules
d. 300 joules

23.67 Physiologic factors that can thwart efforts to convert ventricular fibrillation include:

I.   renal failure
II.  hypoxia
III. acidosis

a. I and II
b. II and III
c. I and III
d. I, II, and III

**ECG Interpretation:** For each of the ECG rhythm strips pictured below, first assess the rate, rhythm, P waves, P–R interval, and QRS complexes. Then use this information to provide your interpretation.

23.68

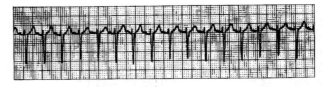

**Figure 22–1**

Rate: _____    Rhythm: _____

P Waves: _____    P–R Interval: _____

QRS Complexes: _____

Interpretation: _____

23.69

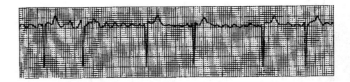

**Figure 22–2**

Rate: _____    Rhythm: _____

P Waves: _____    P–R Interval: _____

QRS Complexes: _____

Interpretation: _____

23.70

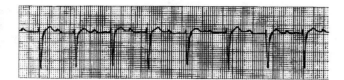

**Figure 22–3**

Rate: _____     Rhythm: _____

P Waves: _____     P–R Interval: _____

QRS Complexes: _____

Interpretation: _____

23.71

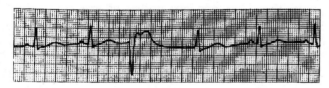

**Figure 22–4**

Rate: _____     Rhythm: _____

P Waves: _____     P–R Interval: _____

QRS Complexes: _____

Interpretation: _____

23.72

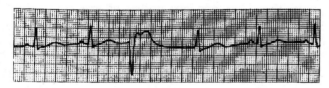

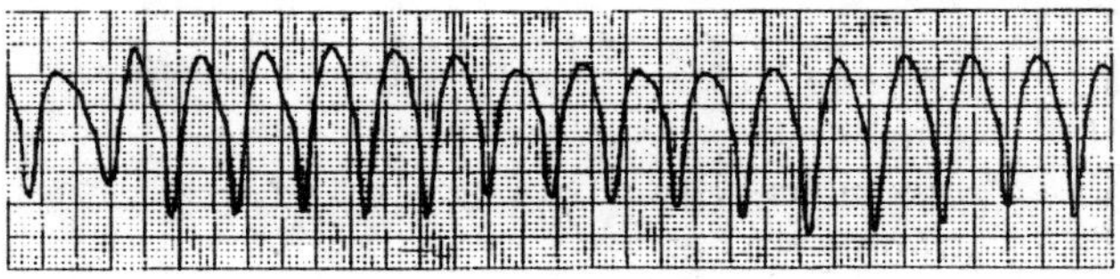

**Figure 22–5**

Rate: _____     Rhythm: _____

P Waves: _____     P–R Interval: _____

QRS Complexes: _____

Interpretation: _____

# 24

## Production, Storage, and Delivery of Medical Gases

## CONTENT EXERCISES

**True/False:** For each of the following statements, indicate whether it is mainly true or mainly false by circling the corresponding letter (T=True, F=False):

24.1  T F  Regulatory agencies often adopt the voluntary standards developed by recommending agencies as their legal requirements.

24.2  T F  Small home compressors can power some equipment at unrestricted flows at 50 psig.

24.3  T F  Medical gas cylinder color codes are internationally standardized.

24.4  T F  The only means of positive identification of the gas in a cylinder is by reading the attached label.

24.5  T F  Medical gases with critical temperatures below room temperature can be stored in cylinders as liquids at room temperature.

24.6  T F  Cylinder pressures for medical gases stored in the liquid form at room temperature are considerably higher than those for vaporous gases.

24.7  T F  A full cylinder of nitrous oxide will contain the same volume of gas as a cylinder of carbon dioxide.

24.8  T F  One of the greatest risks in medical gas therapy is the inadvertent administration of the wrong gas to a patient.

24.9  T F  No gases share an identical American Standard Safety System (ASSS) connection.

24.10  T F  "Quick–Connect" DISS connectors made by different manufacturers are usually compatible with each other.

**Short Answer:** Complete each statement by filling in the correct information in the space(s) provided:

24.11 The Food and Drug Administration (FDA) purity standard for oxygen is _____.

24.12 Small, portable devices used as remote emergency sources of low–pressure oxygen generated by chemical reaction are called _____.

24.13 Large compressor systems used to provide air to a hospital unit must be capable of maintaining flows of at least _____ at pressures of _____.

24.14 The Food and Drug Administration (FDA) purity standard for helium is _____.

24.15 The color code for a gas cylinder of carbon dioxide is _____.

24.16 The color code for a gas cylinder of compressed air is _____.

24.17 Cylinders of medical gases with critical temperatures above room temperature are filled according to the _____ specified for that gas.

24.18 The pressure in a cylinder of gas stored in its liquid form represents the _____ of the gas over its surface.

24.19 The pressure of medical gases in a bulk supply system is reduced to a standard working pressure of

_____

24.20 When the pressure on the primary side of a manifold cylinder system falls to a set pressure, a control valve should automatically switch over to a

_____

24.21 To prevent the liquid oxygen from reverting back to its gaseous form, the liquid must be kept well below oxygen's _____.

24.22 Liquid oxygen from a cryogenic container must be converted to the gaseous phase by a device called a

_____

24.23 Primary consideration in distribution and regulation of medical gases should always be _____

_____

24.24 Valves in hospital gas piping systems that can be closed for system maintenance or in case of fire are called _____.

24.25 The purpose of an indexed safety system is to make certain connections between cylinders and delivery systems are _____.

24.26 The Diameter–Indexed Safety System (DISS) was established specifically to prevent accidental interchanging among _____ connectors used for medical gas administration.

24.27 The most common application of the adjustable pressure reducing valve is in combination with a _____ flow gauge.

24.28 When more precision and smoothness in flow control are necessary, one would use a _____ _____ pressure reducing valve.

24.29 The only factor limiting the use of the pressure compensated Thorpe tube is _____.

**Multiple Choice:** Circle the letter corresponding to the single best answer from the available choices:

24.30 The regulating agency which has the authority to establish purity standards for medical gases and efficacy of medical devices is the:

a American National Standards Institute (ANSI)
b. National Fire Protection Association (NFPA)
c. Food and Drug Administration (FDA)
d. Compressed Gas Association

24.31 The regulating agency responsible for the standards governing the design, construction, and testing of gas cylinders is the:

a. National Fire Protection Association (NFPA)
b. Department of Transportation (DOT)
c. Food and Drug Administration (FDA)
d. Compressed Gas Association

24.32 The recommending agency responsible for the standards governing the storage of flammable and oxidizing gases is the:

a. National Fire Protection Association (NFPA)
b. Department of Transportation (DOT)
c. Food and Drug Administration (FDA)
d. Compressed Gas Association

24.33 Which of the following medical gases are classified as combustion supporting?
I. oxygen
II. carbon dioxide
III. compressed air
IV. nitrous oxide

a. I only          c. I, III, and IV
b. I and III       d. I, II, III, and IV

24.34 Which of the following medical gases are classified as flammable?
I. oxygen
II. cyclopropane
III. ethylene
IV. nitrous oxide

a. II and III      c. I, III, and IV
b. I and III       d. I, II, III, and IV

24.35 The density of oxygen at STPD (0° Celsius and one atmosphere pressure) is:

a. 0.179 g/L
b. 1.340 g/L
c. 1.429 g/L
d. 1.980 g/L

24.36 The most common and least expensive method for commercial production of oxygen is:

a. fractional distillation of air
b. electrolysis of water
c. chemical decomposition of sodium chlorate
d. physical separation by molecular sieves

24.37 Air for in–hospital use is most often produced by:

a. filtering by molecular sieves
b. compression of atmospheric air
c. combustion of natural gas
d. pumping from deep wells

24.38 The key property of helium which makes it useful as a therapeutic gas is its:

a. low solubility
b. low density
c. chemical inertness
d. low cost

24.39 A high pressure 3AA oxygen cylinder which has a filling pressure of 2015 psig marked on its shoulder can legally be filled to what pressure?

a. 2015 psig
b. 2200 psig
c. 2400 psig
d. 3300 psig

24.40 As specified in DOT regulations, every 5 or 10 years compressed gas cylinders are
I.    hydrostatically tested for leaks
II.   hydrostatically tested for cylinder expansion
III.  inspected internally and cleaned

a. II only          c. I and III
b. I and II         d. I, II, and III

24.41 According to the National Institute of Standards and Technology of the U.S. Department of Commerce, a gas cylinder that is color coded green should contain:

a. air
b. helium
c. oxygen
d. carbon dioxide

24.42 According to the National Institute of Standards and Technology of the U.S. Department of Commerce, a gas cylinder that is color coded brown and green contains:

a. an $O_2/N_2$ mixture
b. an $O_2/He$ mixture
c. an $O_2/CO_2$ mixture
d. carbon dioxide

24.43 In order to accurately determine the remaining contents of liquid–filled cylinder of carbon dioxide, nitrous oxide, or cyclopropane, you would:

a. multiply the pressure times the cylinder factor
b. weigh the contents of the cylinder
c. divide the pressure by the cylinder factor
d. carefully read the cylinder label and test dates

24.44 Under what conditions will the gauge pressure of a cylinder of carbon dioxide, nitrous oxide, or cyclopropane accurately represent its contents?
I.    when the liquid in the cylinder has completely vaporized
II.   when the filling density is less than 1.0 (water–filled)
III.  when the ambient temperature exceeds the critical temperature

a. I only          c. I and III
b. I and II        d. I, II, and III

24.45 One cubic foot of any gas is equivalent to how many liters of gas?

a. 3.79
b. 7.48
c. 12.6
d. 28.3

24.46 A cylinder factor is expressed in what units of measure?

a. psig
b. liters/psig
c. psig/liters
d. liters

24.47 One cubic foot of liquid oxygen is the equivalent of how many cubic feet of gaseous oxygen?

a. 187.5
b. 244.0
c. 360.4
d. 860.6

24.48 The NFPA standard for bulk oxygen systems requires that the reserve supply be:

a. equal to the average gas usage of one day
b. a fixed cylinder bank of 75 "H" cylinders
c. 100 cubic feet of gaseous oxygen for each bed
d. at least 3000 cubic feet of gaseous oxygen

24.49 The indexed safety system for threaded high–pressure connections between large compressed–gas cylinders and their attachments is the:

a. Pin–Indexed Safety System (PISS)
b. American Standard Safety System (ASSS)
c. Diameter–Index Safety System (DISS)
d. Compressed Gas Association System (CGAS)

24.50 To which of the following compressed gas cylinder sizes would a PISS connection apply?
I.    E
II.   G
III.  AA
IV.   D

a. I only          c. I, III, and IV
b. II and III      d. I, II, III, and IV

24.51 The PISS index hole position for oxygen is:

a. 1–5
b. 1–6
c. 2–5
d. 3–5

24.52 A device used to control both the pressure and flow of a medical gas is a:

a. Bourdon gauge
b. flowmeter
c. regulator
d. reducing valve

24.53 A low–cost flowmetering device which can deliver accurate gas flow rates to low–resistance equipment and cannot be inadvertently adjusted by a practitioner or patient is the:

a. Bourdon regulator
b. Thorpe tube flowmeter
c. second–stage reducing valve
d. flow restrictor

24.54 A device classified as a fixed–orifice, variable-pressure flowmetering device best describes a:

a. Bourdon gauge
b. reducing valve
c. flow restrictor
d. Thorpe tube flowmeter

24.55 Which of the following flowmeters is unaffected by gravity and therefore could be used in any position?
I.      flow restrictor
II.     Bourdon gauge
III.    Thorpe tube

a. I only                    c. I and II
b. II only                   d. I, II, and III

24.56 Of the three common flowmeters, the only device which truly measures flow is the:

a. Bourdon gauge
b. Thorpe tube flowmeter
c. reducing valve
d. flow restrictor

24.57 The increase in downstream resistance which can affect flowmeters is caused by:

a. changes in the size of the outlet orifice
b. changes in the source driving pressure
c. effects of gravity in the upright position
d. connection of jet nebulizers and other equipment

24.58 Concerning a Bourdon gauge, any increase in resistance to flow through the calibrated orifice will cause the gauge to indicate a flow which is:

a. lower than the actual flow
b. equal to the actual flow
c. higher than the actual flow
d. zero flow

24.59 Mrs. Brown needs an extended length oxygen tubing (25 feet) so that she can walk to the bathroom. The tubing is attached to a pressure–compensated, Thorpe tube flowmeter set at 8 L/min. This tubing causes 15 psig of back pressure. What flow of oxygen will she receive?

a. 4 L/min
b. 6 L/min
c. 8 L/min
d. 10 L/min

24.60 Mrs. Brown is now being taken to the x–ray department. You connect the extended length tubing (25 psig back pressure) to a portable E cylinder with a Bourdon gauge flowmeter which is set at 8 L/min. Approximately what flow of oxygen will she now receive?

a. 9 L/min
b. 6 L/min
c. 8 L/min
d. 10 L/min

24.61 Mrs. Brown is transferred to an older part of the hospital which has old uncompensated Thorpe tube flowmeters. Her extended length tubing (25 psig back pressure) is attached to a flowmeter which is then set for 8 L/min. Approximately what flow of oxygen will she now receive?

a. 6 L/min
b. 8 L/min
c. 7 L/min
d. 11 L/min

**Computations:**

24.62 Given the gas or gas mixture on the left and the specified gauge pressure and flow rate, compute the duration of flow from each cylinder in hours and minutes: (Hint: You must first determine the appropriate cylinder factor.)

| Gas or Mixture | Cylinder Size | Cylinder Factor | Gauge Pressure | Flow Rate | Duration of Flow Hours | Minutes |
|---|---|---|---|---|---|---|
| oxygen | H/K | _____ | 1500 | 8 | _____ | _____ |
| oxygen | H/K | _____ | 600 | 3 | _____ | _____ |
| oxygen | G | _____ | 2200 | 2 | _____ | _____ |
| oxygen | E | _____ | 1100 | 6 | _____ | _____ |
| oxygen | E | _____ | 500 | 9 | _____ | _____ |
| $O_2/CO_2$ | H/K | _____ | 1900 | 15 | _____ | _____ |
| $O_2/CO_2$ | G | _____ | 650 | 10 | _____ | _____ |
| $O_2/He$ | H/K | _____ | 1350 | 8 | _____ | _____ |
| $O_2/He$ | E | _____ | 1500 | 11 | _____ | _____ |

**Labeling:** Match the components or structures listed on the right to the letter labels in each of the following figures:

24.63

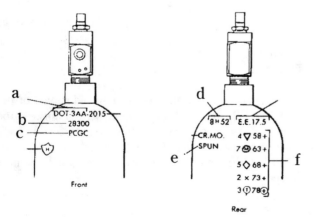

a. _____ retesting information

b. _____ ownership mark

c. _____ serial number

d. _____ spinning process used

e. _____ original hydrostatic test

f. _____ DOT specs/service pressure

**Figure 24–1** Typical markings for cylinders containing medical gases

24.64

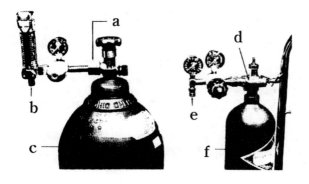

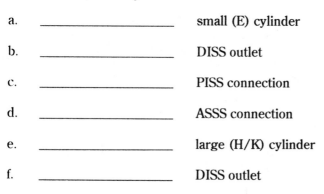

**Figure 24–2** Comparison of safety systems used for compressed gases

a. _____ small (E) cylinder

b. _____ DISS outlet

c. _____ PISS connection

d. _____ ASSS connection

e. _____ large (H/K) cylinder

f. _____ DISS outlet

24.65

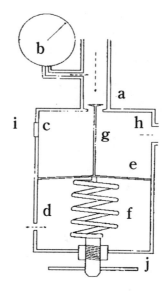

**Figure 24–3** Diagram of an adjustable, high–pressure reducing valve

a. _____ spring

b. _____ gas outlet

c. _____ cylinder pressure gauge

d. _____ valve stem/seat

e. _____ high–pressure (2200 psi) inlet

f. _____ high–pressure chamber

g. _____ ambient pressure chamber

h. _____ safety vent

i. _____ adjustable hand control

j. _____ flexible diaphragm

# Humidity and Aerosol Therapy

## CONTENT EXERCISES

**True/False:** For each of the following statements, indicate whether it is mainly true or mainly false by circling the corresponding letter (T=True, F=False):

25.1 T F In patients whose upper airways have been bypassed, heat and water vapor needs can be satisfactorily met by the lower airway.

25.2 T F The operating temperatures of unheated humidifiers are several degrees warmer than ambient conditions.

25.3 T F The smaller the surface area available for evaporation, the greater the amount of water vapor added to gas.

25.4 T F In transit from a heated humidifier, cooling will cause half of the original water vapor to "rain out" into the delivery tubing.

25.5 T F Hygroscopic condenser humidifiers can cause hyperpyrexia and overhydration.

25.6 T F In terms of humidification, well–designed hygroscopic condenser humidifiers outperform the human nose.

25.7 T F Bubble–diffusion humidifiers do not produce aerosols capable of carrying bacteria.

25.8 T F The penetration of aerosol particles into the respiratory tract is inversely related to their size.

25.9 T F As aerosol particle size drops below 2 microns, a larger percentage of the aerosol is exhaled.

25.10 T F The kinetic activity of a carrier gas affects mainly the largest particles in an aerosol suspension.

25.11 T F Only an aerosol can effectively supply additional water (beyond BTPS) to the airway.

25.12 T F Bland water aerosols are beneficial for patients whose upper airways are intact.

25.13 T F When the aim is to help mobilize secretions, cool water aerosols are preferable.

25.14 T F Unheated large reservoir jet nebulizers can fully overcome a humidity deficit in patients whose upper airways have been bypassed.

**Short Answer:** Complete each statement by filling in the correct information in the space(s) provided:

25.15 Mucociliary clearance can be impaired when water vapor content drops below _____ % body humidity.

25.16 In transit from an unheated humidifier to the patient, the relative humidity of gases _____ as the temperature _____.

25.17 A _____ is an electronic mechanism sensor that automatically keeps a heated humidifier's temperature within a preset range.

25.18 Water continually rises in a wick humidifier due to _____.

25.19 Airway temperatures substantially greater than 37°C can result in _____.

25.20 Most commercially available hygroscopic condenser humidifiers are capable of providing between _____ mg/L water vapor to the airway or, between _____ % body humidity.

25.21 The ability of aerosol to remain in suspension over time is referred to as its _____.

25.22 The measure of the actual weight of aerosol particles carried in a given volume of gas is called _____.

25.23 The point on an aerosol distribution curve that represents that particle size above and below which 50% of aerosol mass lies is referred to as the _____.

25.24 _____ occurs when aerosol particles become unstable and "fall out" on a nearby surface.

25.25 Particles that tend to absorb water are said to be _____.

25.26 The speed with which an aerosol particle settles out due to gravity is called the _____.

25.27 A _____ is a physical surface on which aerosol particles may impact, causing either further fragmentation or removal from the suspension.

25.28 The ultrasonic nebulizer employs a _____ _____ to convert electrical energy into the physical energy of high–frequency vibrations.

25.29 The most clinically significant hazard of aerosol therapy is _____.

**Listing:** Complete each list as directed in its statement.

25.30 List the three (3) key factors that determine the efficiency with which a humidifier vaporizes liquid water:

1. _____

2. _____

3. _____

25.31 List five (5) major factors that determine the penetration and deposition of aerosols in the lung:

1. _____

2. _____

3. _____

4. _____

5. _____

**Multiple Choice:** Circle the letter corresponding to the single best answer from the available choices:

25.32 Therapeutic gases being delivered to patients need to be humidified because they:

a. have low specific gravities
b. become less combustible when humidified
c. are supplied at low critical temperatures
d. are supplied in the anhydrous state

25.33 Among hospitalized patients, especially those who are dehydrated, inhalation of dry therapeutic gases can result in:
I.   increases in viscosity of secretions
II.  impaired mucociliary clearance
III. inspissated secretions

a. I and II          c. II and III
b. III only          d. I, II, and III

25.34 In order to prevent secretions from causing problems in the management of patients with artificial tracheal airways, one should:

a. suction as frequently as possible
b. reposition the patient every 15 minutes
c. provide 100% relative humidity at 32–34°C
d. clean the inner cannula every two hours

25.35 Which of the following devices would be contraindicated for a patient whose upper airway has been bypassed?

a. a heated wick–type humidifier
b. a simple bubble humidifier
c. a heated large–volume jet nebulizer
d. a hygroscopic condenser humidifier

25.36 According to ANSI standards, the minimum level of absolute humidity used to deliver therapeutic gases to a patient whose upper airway has been bypassed is:

a. 5 mg/L
b. 10 mg/L
c. 15 mg/L
d. 30 mg/L

25.37 Providing saturated gas to the airway at temperatures greater than 37°C can result in which of the following?
I.   hyperpyrexia
II.  overhydration
III. weight loss

a. I and II          c. II and III
b. III only          d. I, II, and III

25.38 Potential risks of long–term humidity therapy with a large–volume heated humidifier include which of the following?
I.      alterations in normal heat and water exchange
II.     the possibility of infection
III.    the possibility of electrical shock

a. I and II
b. III only
c. II and III
d. I, II, and III

25.39 You note that the servocontroller mechanism on a large–volume heated humidifier intermittently cycles on and off very rapidly. The most appropriate action in this situation would be to:

a. remove the temperature monitoring probe from the tubing
b. disable the servocontroller mechanism by turning it off
c. reconnect it to an appropriately grounded power receptacle
c. immediately take the equipment out of service and replace it

25.40 The single most important factor determining a humidifier's performance is:

a. surface area
b. time of contact
c. flow of carrier gas
d. temperature

25.41 The humidity output of a simple unheated humidifier is always:

a. greater than saturated air at ambient temperature
b. equal to saturated air at body temperature
c. greater than saturated air at body temperature
d. less than saturated air at ambient temperature

25.42 Which of the following occur as gas leaving a heated humidifier travels to a patient through unheated delivery tubing?
I.      water condenses out of the gas onto the tubing
II.     the relative humidity of the gas decreases
III.    the temperature of the gas decreases
IV.     the absolute humidity of the gas increases

a. II and IV
b. I, II, and III
c. I and III
d. I, II, III, and IV

25.43 A patient has been supported by a mechanical ventilator using a hygroscopic condenser humidifier (heat and moisture exchanger) for the last three days. Suctioning reveals an increase in the amount and tenacity of secretions. Which of the following actions are indicated?

a. increase the hygroscopic condenser humidifier temperature
b. switch the patient to a large–volume heated humidifier
c. switch the patient to continuous ultrasonic nebulization
d. reassess the patient's secretions over the next 24–48 hours

25.44 In terms of their penetration and deposition in the respiratory tract, what is the primary fate of particles greater than 5 to 10 mm in size?

a. most are deposited in the upper airway
b. most are deposited in the conducting zones
c. most are deposited in the alveolar region
d. most are cleared during exhalation

25.45 A physician has ordered pentamidine isothionate by aerosol for an AIDS patient with *Pneumocystis carinii* pneumonia. *Pneumocystis carinii* tends to localize in the alveolar region of the lungs. Which of the following nebulizers would you select to deliver this drug agent?

a. nebulizer A – MMD of 50–80 μm
b. nebulizer B – MMD of 3–4 μm
c. nebulizer C – MMD of 30–50 μm
d. nebulizer D – MMD of 1–2 μm

25.46 Which of the following conditions or factors will increase aerosol deposition by inertial impaction?
I.      low–velocity gas flow
II.     variable/irregular tubing
III.    turbulent gas flow
IV.     particles of low mass

a. II and III
b. II, III, and IV
c. II and IV
d. I, II, III, and IV

25.47 Objectives of aerosol therapy include which of the following?
I.      to provide humidification to the respiratory tract
II.     to serve as an adjunct for mobilization of secretions
III.    to provide a route for drug administration

a. I and II
b. I and III
c. I only
d. I, II, and III

25.48 The *primary* objective of cool (unheated) water aerosol therapy in the treatment of inflammatory obstructions like laryngitis or croup is to:

a. increase the inspired $O_2$ concentration
b. soothe inflamed tissues and reduce edema
c. overcome a physiologic humidity deficit
d. force coughing and expectoration

25.49 A patient with COPD is receiving heated water aerosol via a jet nebulizer in order to aid in mobilizing retained secretions. While auscultating you note an increase in rhonchi. Which of the following recommendations would you make to the physician?

a. discontinue the heated water aerosol
b. aid coughing and postural drainage
c. perform a therapeutic bronchoscopy
d. consider treatments with a bronchodilator

25.50 All of the following statements regarding the aerosol route for drug administration are true *except:*

a. patient cooperation is necessary for optimum delivery
b. the aerosol route is a potential source of infection
c. the aerosol route results in a rapid therapeutic effect
d. most of the aerosolized drug reaches the alveoli

25.51 A jet nebulizer is set at an $O_2$ input flow of 10 L/min on the 100% setting. If the input flow remains constant when the air entrainment port is opened to the 40% $O_2$ setting, which of the following would occur?
I.     aerosol particle size would increase
II.    total aerosol output/min would increase
III.   aerosol weight density would decrease

a. I and III          c. III only
b. I and II           d. I, II, and III

25.52 In setting up a patient for home care, you connect a large–volume gas–powered jet nebulizer to a small air compressor capable of generating 35 psig. What will be the result of this action?

a. the upper limit of nebulizer input flow will exceed 15 L/min
b. the aerosol output per minute will be greater than normal
c. maximum nebulizer flow will be less than manufacturer's specs
d. air entrainment through an open chamber port will not occur

25.53 Which of the following occur when the water reservoir of a large–volume jet nebulizer is heated above ambient temperatures?
I.     increased condensation in the delivery tubing
II.    increased total aerosol output (ml/min)
III.   increased aerosol particle size (MMD)
IV.    increased aerosol particle stability

a. I, II, and III          c. I and II
b. II, III, and IV         d. I, II, III, and IV

25.54 A large–volume jet nebulizer is operating on 70% $O_2$ at 12 L/min. You observe that the aerosol comes out only intermittently and that there is a bubbling sound in the system. Which of the following actions would be most appropriate?

a. reduce the volume of water in the nebulizer reservoir
b. switch the nebulizer entrainment port to 40% oxygen
c. drain any excess condensate from the delivery tube
d. replace the large–bore tubing with small–bore tubing

25.55 A large–volume jet nebulizer is operating at the 100% $O_2$ setting with an input flow of 12 L/min. What effect will changing the entrainment port setting from 100% to 70% have on the system?

a. the input liter flow will increase by 30%
b. the total output liter flow will decrease
c. the aerosol weight density will increase
d. the total output liter flow will increase

25.56 A physician orders a potent bronchodilator drug for a patient via the aerosol route. Which of the following devices would be suitable for this task?
I.     microstat ultrasonic nebulizer
II.    small–volume jet nebulizer
III.   metered dose inhaler
IV.    hydronamics nebulizer

a. I, II, and III          c. II and III
b. II, III, and IV         d. I, II, III, and IV

25.57 A physician orders aerosol administration of a mucolytic drug Q.I.D. for a home care patient. Which of the following equipment would you select to provide this therapy?
I.     finger valve or Y–connector
II.    small–volume jet nebulizer
III.   small air compressor
IV.    compressed air cylinder/flowmeter

a. I and IV          c. I, II, and III
b. II, III, and IV   d. I, II, III, and IV

25.58 Techniques which maximize aerosol deposition with a metered dose inhaler (MDI) include:
I. slow and deep inspiration (flows < 30 L/min)
II. MDI activation before beginning inspiration
III. a breath hold at the end of inspiration
IV. a secure lip seal around delivery port

a. I and IV
b. I and III
c. II and IV
d. I, II, III, and IV

25.59 A physician has ordered administration of a steroid available only in a metered dose (MDI) preparation. In training the patient in its use, you cannot get her to coordinate MDI discharge with her breathing. Which of the following would you recommend to the ordering physician?

a. discontinue the steroid treatments altogether
b. adapt the MDI system with a spacer or holding chamber
c. substitute an oral steroid for the MDI preparation
d. substitute a bronchodilator via jet nebulization

25.60 A physician has ordered the antiviral agent ribavirin (Virazole) to be administered by aerosol to an infant with bronchiolitis. Which of the following devices would you recommend in this situation?

a. ultrasonic nebulizer
b. large–volume heated jet nebulizer
c. centrifugal (spinning disk) nebulizer
d. small particle aerosol generator

25.61 A physician orders a "cool mist" centrifugal nebulizer for room humidification for a patient being discharged to home care. In reviewing the order with the physician, you should:

a. suggest that the device be used only with an aerosol enclosure
b. recommend that only distilled water be used in the device
c. not recommend this device due to its potential to spread bacteria
d. suggest that the electrical system of the house be checked first

25.62 The aerosol output (in mg/L) of an ultrasonic nebulizer depends mainly on the which of the following?

a. couplant temperature
b. chamber baffling
c. signal frequency
d. signal amplitude

25.63 Which of the following are components of an ultrasonic nebulizer?
I. electronic module
II. air entrainment orifice
III. nebulizer chamber
IV. piezoelectric transducer
V. blower or fan

a. I, III, and IV
b. II, III, IV, and V
c. I, III, IV, and V
d. I, II, III, IV, and V

25.64 Which of the following types of nebulizers can produce the highest density aerosol suspension?

a. a heated jet nebulizer
b. a sidestream nebulizer
c. a metered dose inhaler
d. an ultrasonic nebulizer

25.65 Hazards of aerosol therapy include all of the following except:

a. airway reactivity/bronchospasm
b. spread of bacterial infections
c. pharmacologic side effects
d. loss of body fluids/dehydration

25.66 Which of the following procedures are recommended to reduce the likelihood of contamination and infection with nebulizer reservoir systems?
I. use disinfected or sterile water only
II. discard reservoir water before refilling
III. change nebulizer and circuit every 24 hours
IV. drain tubing condensate back into reservoir

a. I, II, and IV
b. III and IV
c. I, II, and III
d. I, II, III, and IV

25.67 A patient is receiving aerosol therapy with acetylcysteine to help mobilize his secretions. Although it is effective toward this end, the patient tends to develop persistent wheezing during the treatment sessions. Which of the following actions would you recommend to the ordering physician?

a. switch to a proteolytic enzyme aerosol
b. add a bronchodilator to the treatment regimen
c. administer a corticosteroid after treatments
d. discontinue the treatment regimen

# CHAPTER
## 26

# Medical Gas Therapy

## CONTENT EXERCISES

**True/False:** For each of the following statements, indicate whether it is mainly true or mainly false by circling the corresponding letter (T=True, F=False):

26.1 T F Therapeutic gases should be treated the same as any other pharmacological agent.

26.2 T F Hypoxemia caused by large physiologic shunts is usually responsive to supplemental oxygen therapy.

26.3 T F When hypoxemia exists with chronic hypercapnia, oxygen administration can stimulate the peripheral chemoreceptors.

26.4 T F Oxygen should be withheld from hypoxemic patients suspected of being susceptible to oxygen–induced hypoventilation.

26.5 T F The risk of absorption atelectasis in oxygen therapy is compounded when patients breathe at a minimal tidal volume.

26.6 T F CNS manifestations of oxygen toxicity become most apparent when breathing oxygen at hyperbaric pressures.

26.7 T F Prolonged exposure to high partial pressures of oxygen may interfere with the production of pulmonary surfactant.

26.8 T F High–flow oxygen delivery devices always perform as fixed–performance oxygen delivery systems.

26.9 T F Precise measurements of the $FIO_2$ delivered by low–flow oxygen delivery systems are neither practical nor necessary in the clinical setting.

26.10 T F Low–flow nasal oxygen devices are appropriate when the aim is to achieve oxygen concentration above 40% to 45%.

26.11 T F In general, reservoir devices are generally capable of providing a higher $FIO_2$ for a given oxygen input than low–flow systems.

26.12 T F Common disposable nonrebreathing masks should be considered variable–performance oxygen delivery systems.

26.13 T F The air to oxygen entrainment ratio for air entrainment devices is a constant mathematical value for each $O_2$ percentage.

26.14 T F Any enclosure, such as a tent with an oxygen–enriched atmosphere, is at increased risk of fire.

26.15 T F When oxygen analysis is indicated, monitoring should be conducted at least every 1 to 2 hours.

26.16 T F The physical (paramagnetic) oxygen analyzer actually measures the $Po_2$ and not the oxygen concentration.

26.17 T F Both the polarographic electrode and the galvanic fuel cell measure oxygen partial pressures according to a chemical reduction–oxidation reaction.

26.18 T F Breathing helium has little effect on the pressure gradients associated with flow in the small airways.

26.19 T F A simple mask is an acceptable device for administering helium mixtures.

26.20 T F 10% carbon dioxide mixtures should never be used for therapeutic purposes.

**Short Answer:** Complete each statement by filling in the correct information in the space(s) provided:

26.21 Oxygen is generally ordered either in _____ or as a _____ of oxygen.

26.22 The dose–response approach to oxygen therapy aims to provide the _____ amount of oxygen necessary to obtain the desired therapeutic objective.

26.23 The risk of oxygen–induced hypoventilation increases when $Paco_2$ has remained at or above _____ long enough for a compensatory acid–base response.

26.24 The likelihood of absorption atelectasis is greatest when the respiratory zones of the lung become _____.

26.25 100% oxygen breathed continuously for more than _____ hours can result in pulmonary damage.

26.26 It is believed that oxygen toxicity is mediated through the actions of chemical units known as ____ _____.

26.27 Excessive blood oxygen levels produce _____ of the retinal blood vessels.

26.28 A high–flow oxygen delivery device should provide at least _____ L/min total flow.

26.29 Low–flow oxygen delivery systems modified to reduce the waste of oxygen that typically occurs during the expiratory phase of breathing are called _____ _____.

26.30 As a rule of thumb, the practitioner may estimate that each L/min flow provided via a standard nasal low–flow device increases the inspired oxygen concentration by approximately _____ %.

26.31 With simple oxygen masks, a minimal flow of _____ L/min is necessary to ensure that the mask volume is replenished with oxygen at the end of exhalation.

26.32 The distinguishing features of the nonrebreathing oxygen mask are its series of _____ _____.

26.33 Air entrainment systems are indicated when the clinical objective is to provide stable or controlled $FIO_2$s between _____ and _____.

26.34 Ratios of air to oxygen in gas–powered nebulizers are altered by varying the size of the _____ _____.

26.35 Maximum oxygen inflow to gas–powered jet nebulizers is restricted to between _____ and _____ L/min at 50 psig.

26.36 The most convenient method of providing therapy to infants is the _____.

26.37 Primary safety concerns in the application of hyperbaric oxygenation are _____ and _____.

26.38 When using an oxygen flowmeter to deliver 80–20 helium–oxygen, one must multiply the displayed flow by a factor of _____ to obtain an accurate reading.

**Multiple Choice:** Circle the letter corresponding to the single best answer from the available choices:

26.39 Clinical objectives for the administration of supplemental oxygen include which of the following?
I. to prevent or correct arterial hypoxemia
II. to decrease myocardial work load
III. to decrease the work of breathing
IV. to prevent absorption atelectasis

a. II and III
b. III and IV
c. I, II, and III
d. I, II, III, and IV

26.40 Which of the physiologic causes of arterial hypoxemia are generally responsive to oxygen therapy alone?
I. hypoventilation
II. diffusion defects
III. moderate V/Q imbalances
IV. large physiologic shunt (25% of Q)

a. I and II
b. I, II, and III
c. II and IV
d. I, II, III, and IV

26.41 The compensatory response of the cardiopulmonary system to hypoxemia involves which of the following?
I. pulmonary vasodilation
II. increased ventilation
III. increased cardiac output

a. I only
b. I and III
c. II and III
d. I, II, and III

26.42 Which of the following represent possible hazards of oxygen therapy?
I. oxygen–induced hypoventilation
II. absorption atelectasis
III. oxygen toxicity
IV. retinopathy of prematurity

a. I and II
b. I and III
c. I, II, and III
d. I, II, III, and IV

26.43 The cause of oxygen–induced hypoventilation in patients with chronic hypercapnia is:

a. depression of the central nervous system
b. release of $CO_2$ from oxyhemoglobin (Haldane effect)
c. blunting of central chemoreceptor response
d. suppression of peripheral chemoreceptors ($PaO_2$ > 60 mm Hg)

26.44 A patient with chronic obstructive pulmonary disease and chronic $CO_2$ retention is admitted to the emergency room with an acute exacerbation of her condition. The most appropriate oxygen device to use initially would be which of the following?

a. nasal cannula at 2 liters/min
b. nasal cannula at 6 liters/min
c. simple mask at 2 liters/min
d. simple mask at 6 liters/min

26.45 The primary organ systems affected by oxygen toxicity are the:
I.    central nervous system
II.   cardiovascular system
III.  respiratory system

a. I only            c. II and III
b. I and III         d. I, II, and III

26.46 Which of the following represent manifestations of prolonged exposure to 100% oxygen at hyperbaric pressures?
I.    substernal chest tightness and burning
II.   shortness of breath (dyspnea)
III.  decreased vital capacity
IV.   decreased lung compliance

a. I and IV          c. I, II, and III
b. I and III         d. I, II, III, and IV

26.47 Which of the following are the primary factors determining the risk of oxygen's detrimental effects on the pulmonary parenchyma?
I.    concentration of oxygen ($FIO_2$)
II.   inspired partial pressure of oxygen ($PIO_2$)
III.  length of exposure to oxygen
IV.   other medical gases mixed with oxygen

a. I and II          c. II and III
b. I and III         d. I, II, III, and IV

26.48 Retinopathy of prematurity results in what physical problem?

a. dyspnea
b. blindness
c. pneumonia
d. atelectasis

26.49 The American Academy of Pediatrics has recommended maintaining what levels of $PaO_2$ to minimize the risk of retinopathy of prematurity in premature infants?

a. 20–30 mm Hg
b. 40–50 mm Hg
c. 50–70 mm Hg
d. 80–100 mm Hg

26.50 The $FIO_2$ delivered by a low–flow oxygen system depends on the:
I.    oxygen input in liters per minute
II.   patient's rate of breathing
III.  room temperature
IV.   patient's depth of breathing

a. II and III        c. II and IV
b. I, II, and IV     d. I, II, III, and IV

26.51 A patient receiving oxygen at 6 L/min via nasal cannula complains that he does not feel any oxygen coming out. The respiratory care practitioner should do which of the following?

a. increase the flow
b. check the equipment connections
c. tell the patient to relax
d. change the cannula

26.52 Which of the following devices attempt to meet the inspiratory demand of a patient by providing a reserve volume from which the patient can inspire?
I.    nonrebreathing mask
II.   nasal cannula
III.  venturi mask
IV.   simple mask

a. I and IV          c. I, III, and IV
b. II and IV         d. I, II, III, and IV

26.53 Disadvantages of a simple oxygen mask include all of the following *except:*

a. pressure necrosis on facial tissues
b. aspiration of gastric contents (comatose patients)
c. increased mechanical deadspace at low flows
d. difficult application

26.54 With a well–fitted partial rebreathing mask, adjusted so that the patient's inhalation does not deflate the bag (flows between 6 and 10 L/min), one can expect inspired oxygen concentrations of:

a. 25%–35%
b. 75% –85%
c. 85%–95%
d. 35%–60%

26.55 A doctor orders 2 liters of oxygen to be delivered via mask to a patient with chronic hypercapnea. The correct action at this time would be to:

a. carry out the doctor's order exactly as written
b. increase the flow to 6 L/min to wash out $CO_2$
c. recommend that the mask be changed to a cannula at 2 L/min
d. not carry out the order until you can contact the medical director

26.56 If you want to deliver an $F_{IO_2}$ of 80% to 100% with adequate flow to a 67–year–old tachypneic patient with pulmonary edema, which of the following systems would be most appropriate?

a. aerosol mask with nebulizer set to 100%
b. nonrebreathing mask at 12–15 L/min
c. nonrebreathing mask at 6–8 L/min
d. partial rebreathing mask at 12–15 L/min

26.57 A patient is receiving oxygen via a nonre-breathing mask at 8 L/min. The respiratory care practitioner notices that the reservoir bag on the mask empties completely before the end of inspiration. The practitioner should immediately do which of the following?

a. change to a partial rebreathing mask
b. remove the mask
c. increase the flow
d. intubate the patient

26.58 When a patient who is receiving oxygen via nonrebreathing mask inhales, the reservoir bag on the mask does not deflate. Probable causes of this situation include which of the following?
I.   the flowmeter setting is too low
II.  the mask is not tight enough
III. the one–way valve is sticking in the closed position

a. I only
b. III only
c. II and III
d. I, II, and III

26.59 Which of the following would decrease the total output flow of an air entrainment device?
I.   increasing the humidity of the source gas
II.  increasing the $F_{IO_2}$ of the source gas
III. increasing the resistance downstream of the jet
IV.  decreasing the flow to the jet

a. IV only
b. III and IV
c. II and IV
d. I, II, III, and IV

26.60 The oxygen concentration delivered by an air entrainment nebulizer to a patient's airway is usually higher than set. What is the reason for this discrepancy?

a. downstream resistance created by the delivery tubing
b. inaccuracy of the air entrainment system
c. air leaks in the tubing system
d. excessive forward velocity of the source gas

26.61 A patient with a tracheotomy tube and a minute ventilation of 10 L/min is connected via a T–tube to a jet nebulizer set at 70% oxygen with an input flow of 12 liters per minute. What assumptions regarding the application of this system to this patient can be drawn from the above information?
I.   the patient is not receiving 70% oxygen throughout inspiration
II.  the set–up, as described, is a high–flow oxygen delivery system
III. the oxygen input flow to the nebulizer is at or near its maximum

a. I only
b. II only
c. I and III
d. I, II, and III

26.62 How might you increase the likelihood of delivering 70% oxygen to this patient described in the situation above?
I.   increase the input flow to the nebulizer to 30 L/min
II.  add an open reservoir to the ambient side of the T–tube
III. hook two nebulizers in parallel, both at 12 L/min
IV.  place a one–way expiratory valve on the T–tube

a. II only
b. II and III
c. I and IV
d. III and IV

26.63 When using an oxyhood to provide supplemental oxygen to a premature infant, what is the minimum flow rate of source gas that should be set in order to prevent buildup of carbon dioxide in the hood?

a. 2–3 L/min
b. 3–4 L/min
c. 4–5 L/min
d. 10–12 L/min

26.64 Among the common commercially available oxygen analyzers for routine bedside use, which ones actually measure oxygen concentration as opposed to the partial pressure of oxygen?
I.    physical (paramagnetic) analyzer
II.   thermal conduction analyzer
III.  polarographic analyzer
IV.   galvanic cell analyzer

a. II only              c. I only
b. II and IV            d. I, II, III, and IV

26.65 The Clark polarographic oxygen electrode functions by:

a. utilizing oxygen to produce a reduction–oxidation reaction
b. measuring the magnetic properties of oxygen versus nitrogen
c. measuring the electrical potential across a Wheatstone bridge
d. measuring light absorption of oxygen compared with nitrogen

26.66 Continuous analysis of the $F_{IO_2}$ in controlled mechanical ventilation would be best achieved by the use of which of the following?

a. physical (paramagnetic) analyzer
b. thermal conduction analyzer
c. Sveringhaus electrode
d. polarographic analyzer

26.67 Which of the following conditions is best treated with hyperbaric oxygen?

a. skin graft
b. crush injury
c. carbon monoxide poisoning
d. sickle cell anemia crisis

26.68 If a patient is in a hyperbaric oxygen chamber breathing compressed air at a total pressure of 1900 mm Hg (1900 mm Hg absolute) in terms of partial pressure, this would be equivalent to breathing what concentration of oxygen at sea level?

a. 28%
b. 53%
c. 25%
d. 67%

26.69 Helium, in 60% or 80% mixtures with oxygen, is used clinically in specific situations. Which of the following descriptions of helium's characteristics or its physiological effects are a basis for its clinical use?
I.    $He/O_2$ is of lower viscosity compared with air or $O_2$
II.   $He/O_2$ is of lower density compared with air or $O_2$
III.  $He/O_2$ decreases the work of breathing in airway obstruction
IV.   $He/O_2$ is most effective in small airway obstruction

a. I only               c. II and III
b. II only              d. I, II, III, and IV

26.70 Which of the following are potential detrimental cardiovascular side effects of carbon dioxide therapy?
I.    increased heart rate (tachycardia)
II.   increased myocardial contractility
III.  elevation of systolic and diastolic blood pressure

a. I only               c. II and III
b. I and II             d. I, II, and III

## Computations:

26.71 Below are data on seven patients receiving supplemental oxygen via nasal cannula. Given the information provided, first estimate each patient's inspiratory flow. Then estimate the $F_{IO_2}$ each patient is receiving.

| | I:E ratio | Minute Vent (L/min) | Estimated Insp Flow (L/min) | $O_2$ Flow (L/min) | Estimated $F_{IO_2}$ |
|---|---|---|---|---|---|
| a. | 1:3 | 6 | _____ | 2 | _____ |
| b. | 1:5 | 5 | _____ | 4 | _____ |
| c. | 1:4 | 12 | _____ | 8 | _____ |
| d. | 1:1 | 7 | _____ | 3 | _____ |
| e. | 1:3 | 10 | _____ | 10 | _____ |
| f. | 1:2 | 4 | _____ | 3 | _____ |
| g. | 1:2 | 9 | _____ | 5 | _____ |

h. Can two patients have the same inspiratory flows but different $F_{IO_2}$s? Use specific examples from the above table to explain your answer.

_____

_____

_____

i. Can two patients have the same estimated $F_{IO_2}$ but at different $O_2$ input flows? Use specific examples from the above table to explain your answer.

_____

_____

_____

j. Can patients have the same minute ventilations and $O_2$ input flows but different $F_{IO_2}$s? Use specific examples from the above table to explain your answer.

_____

_____

_____

26.72 Compute the $F_{IO_2}$ resulting from mixing the following volumes of air and oxygen:

| | Air (liters) | Oxygen (liters) | Resulting $F_{IO_2}$ |
|---|---|---|---|
| a. | 7 | 3 | _____ |
| b. | 3 | 2 | _____ |
| c. | 8 | 5 | _____ |
| d. | 5 | 1 | _____ |
| e. | 1 | 3 | _____ |

26.73 For each oxygen percent listed on the left, first compute the ratio of air to oxygen needed to achieve this concentration. Then, given the oxygen input flow specified in the third column, compute the total output flow of the mixture in L/min.

| | Oxygen Percent | Air/$O_2$ Ratio | $O_2$ Input Flow (L/min) | Total Output Flow (L/min) |
|---|---|---|---|---|
| a. | 90 | _____ | 11 | _____ |
| b. | 70 | _____ | 12 | _____ |
| c. | 60 | _____ | 10 | _____ |
| d. | 50 | _____ | 8 | _____ |
| e. | 40 | _____ | 15 | _____ |
| f. | 35 | _____ | 6 | _____ |
| g. | 30 | _____ | 5 | _____ |
| h. | 28 | _____ | 4 | _____ |
| i. | 24 | _____ | 3 | _____ |

# 27

# Lung Expansion Therapy

## CONTENT EXERCISES

**True/False:** For each of the following statements, indicate whether it is mainly true or mainly false by circling the corresponding letter (T=True, F=False):

27.1  T  F  With all else constant, the greater the transpulmonary pressure gradient, the less the alveolar expansion.

27.2  T  F  A spontaneous deep breath increases the transpulmonary pressure gradient by decreasing the pleural pressure.

27.3  T  F  Positive alveolar pressure can increase pulmonary vascular resistance.

27.4  T  F  Pleural pressure never exceeds atmospheric pressure during IPPB.

27.5  T  F  Repetitive, shallow breathing is a major factor in the development of postoperative pulmonary complications.

27.6  T  F  The use of IPPB in pulmonary edema is based on its retarding effect on venous return to the right heart.

27.7  T  F  In using IPPB to treat cardiogenic pulmonary edema, the goal is to minimize intrathoracic pressures.

27.8  T  F  IPPB can result in bronchospasm and increased airway resistance in some patients.

27.9  T  F  An improperly administered IPPB treatment can increase the work of breathing.

27.10  T  F  Many of the reported failures associated with IPPB are due to the lack of adequate, skilled supervision.

27.11  T  F  Positive pressure in the thorax tends to decrease intracranial pressures.

27.12  T  F  A pressure–cycled IPPB device will not terminate inspiration if leaks in the system occur.

27.13  T  F  When applied to treat atelectasis, IPPB therapy should be volume–oriented.

27.14  T  F  Larger inspiratory volumes can be achieved if the patient is encouraged to breathe actively during IPPB.

27.15  T  F  Pulmonary barotrauma cannot occur during spontaneous breathing.

27.16  T  F  Proper equipment is essential in achieving the goals of incentive spirometry.

27.17  T  F  A forced exhalation should follow the inspiratory component of incentive spirometry.

27.18  T  F  CPAP is usually applied at lower levels than the peak pressures used with mechanical ventilation and IPPB.

27.19  T  F  PEP therapy uses a form–fitting face mask and an adjustable flow resistor.

**Short Answer:** Complete each statement by filling in the correct information in the space(s) provided:

27.20  The transpulmonary pressure gradient ($P_L$) is the difference between the _____ pressure and the _____ pressure.

27.21  During IPPB, positive pressure is transmitted from the alveoli to the pleural space, causing pleural pressures to _____.

27.22  The normal pattern of breathing includes intermittent sighs, occurring as often as every _____ minutes.

27.23  Lung tissue damage due to high pressures is called _____.

27.24  The esophageal opening pressure is estimated to range between _____ and _____ cm $H_2O$.

27.25  In some chronically hypercapnic patients, abrupt lowering of the $P_{CO_2}$ due to IPPB may cause post–treatment _____ and _____.

27.26  The use of expiratory retardation during IPPB _____ mean pleural pressures.

27.27  IPPB devices that end inspiration when a preset pressure is reached are called _____ ventilators.

27.28  Patient–cycled IPPB devices incorporate a _____ that responds directly to pressure differences during breathing.

27.29  Exact $F_{IO_2}$ control with an IPPB device requires an _____.

27.30 When applied to treat atelectasis, the IPPB pressure should be adjusted to deliver a volume equivalent to _____ per kg of body weight.

27.31 During a sustained maximal inspiration (SMI), a patient should inspire from the resting expiratory level up to his or her _____.

27.32 Volume achieved with a flow–oriented incentive spirometer is estimated as the product of _____ _____.

27.33 If a patient's postoperative vital capacity is less than 12 to 15 ml/kg of body weight, then _____ should be considered as the initial hyperinflation approach.

27.34 CPAP maintains the lungs at a greater _____ than normal.

27.35 The potential hazard of gastric insufflation during IPPB or intermittent CPAP can be eliminated by use of a _____.

27.36 EPAP therapy differs from PEP therapy because it uses a _____ resistor.

**Multiple Choice:** Circle the letter corresponding to the single best answer from the available choices:

27.37 Which of the following is *false* regarding intermittent positive pressure breathing (IPPB)?

a. during inspiration, pressure in the alveoli increases
b. the pressure gradients of normal breathing are reversed
c. during inspiration, alveolar pressure exceeds pleural pressure
d. during inspiration, pleural pressures decrease

27.38 All modes of hyperinflation therapy aid lung expansion by:

a. decreasing the transthoracic pressure gradient
b. increasing the pleural pressure
c. decreasing the alveolar pressure
d. increasing the transpulmonary pressure gradient

27.39 Hyperinflation methods that increase the transpulmonary pressure gradients by increasing alveolar pressure:
I.    expand the alveoli and airways
II.   decrease venous return to the heart
III.  increase pulmonary vascular resistance

a. I and II           c. I and III
b. II and III         d. I, II, and III

27.40 Which of the following patients is a poor candidate for IPPB therapy?

a. a post–op female patient with clinically diagnosed atelectasis
b. a chronically hypercapnic patient with full metabolic compensation
c. a patient with increased work of breathing due to kyphoscoliosis
d. a patient being treated for acute cardiogenic pulmonary edema

27.41 Which of the following are the best documented indications for IPPB?
I.    treatment of clinically diagnosed atelectasis
II.   management of impending hypercapnic respiratory failure
III.  treatment of decreased compliance in kyphoscoliosis
IV.   prevention of postoperative atelectasis

a. III and IV         c. I and III
b. I, II, and III     d. I, II, III, and IV

27.42 Which of the following patients would be most prone to pulmonary barotrauma during IPPB?

a. a patient with cardiac insufficiency
b. a patient with chronic hypercapnia
c. a patient with pulmonary fibrosis
d. a patient with bullous emphysema

27.43 Which of the following techniques can be used to minimize the likelihood of gastric insufflation during IPPB therapy?
I.    using only enough pressure to achieve the desired goal(s)
II.   using a mask to give the treatment instead of a mouthpiece
III.  properly instructing and supervising cooperative patients

a. I and III          c. I and II
b. II and III         d. I, II, and III

27.44 While you administer an IPPB treatment to a patient, she complains of dizziness and tingling in her fingers. What is the most likely cause of these symptoms?

a. pulmonary barotrauma
b. reactive bronchospasm
c. respiratory acidosis
d. hyperventilation

27.45 Air trapping in COPD patients during IPPB is most likely to occur when:

a. expiratory flows are mechanically retarded
b. the machine sensitivity is set too high
c. insufficient time is provided for inhalation
d. insufficient time is provided for exhalation

27.46 If exhalation is mechanically retarded during IPPB, which of the following will increase?
I.    mean pleural pressure
II.   expiratory time
III.  inspiratory time

a. I and II            c. II only
b. II and III          d. I, II, and III

27.47 What is the purpose of the venturi or air entrainment jet found on most IPPB devices?

a. to regulate the applied pressure level
b. to alter the sensitivity of the device
c. to enhance the device's flow capabilities
d. to provide precise control over $F_{IO_2}$

27.48 When adjusting the sensitivity control on an IPPB device, which of the following parameters are you changing?

a. the volume of gas delivered to the patient during inhalation
b. the effort required to cycle the device "off" (end inspiration)
c. the maximum pressure delivered to the patient during inhalation
d. the effort required to cycle the device "on" (begin inspiration)

27.49 Most IPPB devices cycle to end inspiration when:

a. a preset volume is reached
b. a preset pressure is reached
c. a preset time elapses
d. the gas source is depleted

27.50 In the Bird Mark 7 or 8 IPPB devices, bypassing the venturi (by pushing the "air–mix" control IN) will have which of the following effects?
I.    a decrease in available flow during inspiration
II.   an increase in the end–inspiratory pressure
III.  delivery of 100% source gas to the patient

a. II and III          c. I and III
b. I and II            d. I, II, and III

27.51 Which of the following are *false* regarding the Bennett AP–5 IPPB device?

a. the practitioner has limited control over the delivered flow
b. flow delivered to the patient decreases throughout inspiration
c. the practitioner can preset the end–inspiratory pressure limit
d. the practitioner can choose from a wide range of sensitivities

27.52 A physician orders IPPB therapy for a post–op patient exhibiting clinical signs and symptoms of atelectasis. Which of the following baseline measures would be most critical for this patient?

a. inspiratory or vital capacity
b. arterial blood gas analysis
c. forced expiratory flows
d. maximum minute ventilation

27.53 A physician orders IPPB therapy to enhance delivery of a bronchodilator aerosol to an asthmatic patient. Which of the following baseline measures would be most critical for this patient?

a. forced expiratory flows
b. inspiratory or vital capacity
c. arterial blood gas analysis
d. maximum minute ventilation

27.54 When checking a patient's IPPB breathing circuit prior to use, you note that the device will not cycle off, even when you occlude the mouthpiece. The most appropriate action in this case would be to:

a. secure a new IPPB ventilator
b. decrease the flow setting
c. check the circuit for leaks
d. increase the pressure setting

27.55 In administering IPPB therapy, which of the following breathing patterns would be most desirable?

a. 15–18 breaths/min, I:E ratio of 1:2
b. 6–8 breaths/min, I:E ratio of 1:2
c. 8–10 breaths/min, I:E ratio of 1:5
d. 12–15 breaths/min, I:E ratio of 1:2

27.56 During an IPPB treatment being given to a 72–year–old male patient with COPD, you note signs of further air trapping during exhalation. Which of the following changes in technique might you consider?
I.    coaching the patient to prolong exhalation
II.   increasing the inspiratory flow rate
III.  increasing the preset pressure limit
IV.   retarding exhalation via a restricted orifice

a. I, II, and III          c. I and IV
b. II and IV               d. I, II, III, and IV

27.57 After completing an IPPB session with a 61–year–old patient who recently underwent major thoracic surgery, you note a significant deterioration in his vital signs. Which of the following would you do at this time?

a. chart the patient's response in the respiratory notes
b. institute emergency cardiopulmonary resuscitation
c. remain with the patient and call for help
d. go to the nursing station and call the prescribing doctor

27.58 Which of the following generally occurs when an area of the lung develops atelectasis?
I.    the V/Q ratio increases
II.   intrapulmonary shunting increases
III.  arterial oxygen levels fall
IV.   compliance decreases

a. I, II, and III          c. II, III, and IV
b. I and III               d. I, II, III, and IV

27.59 The purpose of the breath hold at the end of a sustained maximum inspiration (SMI) is to:

a. increase the mean pleural pressure above atmospheric levels
b. improve gas distribution to lung units with abnormal time constants
c. lower airway resistance during the subsequent expiratory effort
d. decrease the transpulmonary pressure gradient $(P_{alv} - P_{pl})$

27.60 You visit a post–op cardiac patient whose nurse has given him the following instructions for performing incentive spirometry: "breath deeply; try hard to exhale but hold it in for a while; then exhale normally." What potential problem is likely to result from doing the incentive spirometry in this manner?

a. gastric insufflation
b. reactive bronchospasm
c. pulmonary barotrauma
d. compromised cardiac output

27.61 In observing a post–op female patient conduct incentive spirometry, you note repetitive performance of the SMI maneuver at a rate of about 10–12/min. Which of the following would you recommend to the patient?

a. that she increase her breathing rate to 12–15/min
b. that she decrease the treatment frequency to 4 times/day
c. that she take a 30–second rest period between breaths
d. that she ask her doctor if she needs further treatments

27.62 Which of the following are potential complications of intermittent CPAP administered by mask to treat atelectasis?
I.    hyperventilation
II.   barotrauma
III.  gastric insufflation
IV.   decreased venous return

a. I and III               c. II, III, and IV
b. II and III              d. I, II, III, and IV

27.63 Besides confirmation of clinically diagnosed atelectasis, which of the following patient criteria must be met in order to successfully apply CPAP to treat this disorder?

a. the patient must have a cuffed artificial airway in place
b. the patient must be able to use accessory muscles
c. the patient must have a vital capacity of at least 15 ml/kg
d. the patient must be able to maintain adequate ventilation

27.64 All of the following devices act as threshold resistors for EPAP therapy except:

a. spring–loaded diaphragms
b. one–way valves
c. gravity–weighted balls
d. reverse venturi systems

**Labeling:** Match the components or structures listed on the right to the letter labels in each of the following figures:

27.65

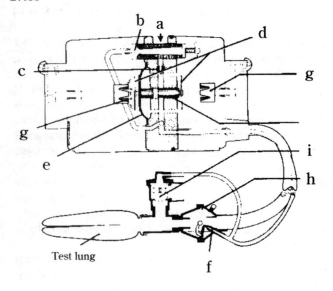

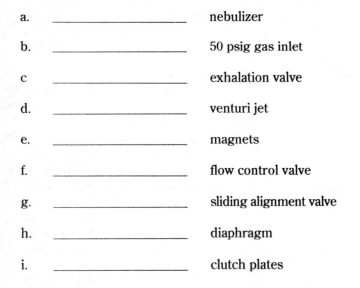

Figure 27–1 Structure of Bird Mark 7

a. _____ nebulizer

b. _____ 50 psig gas inlet

c _____ exhalation valve

d. _____ venturi jet

e. _____ magnets

f. _____ flow control valve

g. _____ sliding alignment valve

h. _____ diaphragm

i. _____ clutch plates

27.66

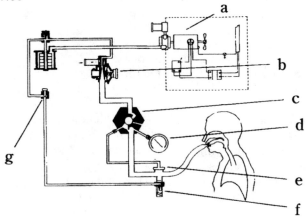

Figure 27–2 Functional diagram of AP series ventilators

a. _____ system pressure gauge

b. _____ nebulizer

c. _____ compressor/pump

d. _____ exhalation valve

e. _____ Bennett valve

f. _____ nebulizer control

g. _____ pressure control

# Chest Physical Therapy

## CONTENT EXERCISES

**True/False:** For each of the following statements, indicate whether it is mainly true or mainly false by circling the corresponding letter (T=True, F=False):

28.1  T  F  CPT after surgery can lower the risk of postoperative pulmonary complications in the elderly.

28.2  T  F  Patients with neuromuscular diseases tend to breathe at high lung volumes.

28.3  T  F  Postural drainage aids mucociliary clearance in normal subjects.

28.4  T  F  Adequate systemic and airway hydration is a prerequisite for effective postural drainage.

28.5  T  F  Modification of head–down drainage positions may be required in patients with orthopnea.

28.6  T  F  Auscultation should be conducted prior to initiating postural drainage.

28.7  T  F  Patients can be left alone during simple postural drainage treatments.

28.8  T  F  The effects of postural drainage on the patient may not be immediately evident.

28.9  T  F  In patients with unilateral infiltrates, the $Pa_{O_2}$ tends to fall when the "bad" lung is in the dependent position.

28.10  T  F  Percussion must never be performed directly over bony prominences.

28.11  T  F  Electrical and pneumatic percussors are more effective than manual techniques.

28.12  T  F  Properly directed coughing is as least as effective in clearing the respiratory tract as more complicated methods.

28.13  T  F  Proper positioning is an essential prerequisite for an effective cough.

28.14  T  F  In patients subject to bronchiolar collapse, a single strong cough is less fatiguing and more effective than several short bursts.

28.15  T  F  When used by patients with copious secretions, the forced expiration technique produces more sputum than traditional therapist–supervised intervention.

28.16  T  F  Diaphragmatic breathing exercises tend to result in faster rates of breathing.

28.17  T  F  With an adjustable flow resistor, the inspiratory muscle load is less when the patient breathes fast.

28.18  T  F  A threshold resistive breathing device can ensure a relatively constant load regardless of how fast or slow the patient breathes.

28.19  T  F  The changes in airway pressure during pursed–lip breathing may help diminish feelings of dyspnea.

28.20  T  F  Poorly conditioned skeletal muscle consumes more $O_2$/min for a given load than does properly conditioned muscle.

28.21  T  F  Chest physical therapy can decrease arterial $Pa_{O_2}$.

28.22  T  F  Forced exhalation abdominal breathing exercises are best taught with the patient in the sitting position.

**Short Answer:** Complete each statement by filling in the correct information in the space(s) provided:

28.23 Therapeutic positioning involves the application of _____ to achieve specific clinical objectives.

28.24 Postural drainage treatment times should be scheduled either before or at least _____ hours after meals or tube feedings.

28.25 In head–down postural drainage positions, the foot of the bed must be elevated by at least _____ inches to achieve the desired 25° angle.

28.26 A _____ allows precise postural drainage positioning at head–down angles up to 45°.

28.27 Total postural drainage treatment time should not exceed _____ minutes.

28.28 Forward flexion about the waist relaxes the abdominal muscles and facilitates descent of the

_____.

28.29 _____ is designed to facilitate movement of secretions toward the central airways during the expiratory phase of breathing.

28.30 The compression phase of a cough causes alveolar pressures to rise as high as _____ mm Hg.

28.31 A cough generally is an effective clearance mechanism only down to about the _____ branching of the tracheobronchial tree.

28.32 Coughing is not very effective in clearing secretions from the _____ airways.

28.33 _____ can mimic the normal cough mechanism by generating an increase in the velocity of the expired air.

28.34 One or two forced expirations from mid to low lung volume without closure of the glottis best describes the _____.

28.35 The goal of the forced expiration technique is to facilitate clearance of bronchial secretions with less likelihood of _____.

28.36 In most patients, V/Q ratios improve when the _____ lung is placed in the dependent or down position.

28.37 The primary purpose of "abdominal" breathing exercises is to promote greater use of the _____ _____.

28.38 _____ breathing exercises are a viable alternative to the diaphragmatic method, especially in patients having undergone abdominal surgery.

28.39 The purposeful imposition of extra work load on the inspiratory muscles during breathing best describes _____ exercises.

28.40 With an adjustable flow resistor, the pressure difference during inspiration varies directly with the _____.

28.41 Once an initial load is determined for inspiratory resistive breathing, the patient should progressively increase the _____ of the treatment sessions.

28.42 The primary purpose of walking exercises is to help minimize _____ during exertion.

28.43 The risk of hypoxemia during chest physical therapy can be minimized by providing _____.

**Listing:** Complete each list as directed in its statement.

28.44 List five (5) basic goals of chest physical therapy:

1. _____

2. _____

3. _____

4. _____

5. _____

28.45 Below are listed the four basic stages constituting the cough reflex. For each of the four stages, list at least three (3) conditions which could hinder or impair that cough component:

a. Irritation:

1. _____

2. _____

3. _____

b. Inspiration:

1. _____

2. _____

3. _____

c. Compression:

1. _____

2. _____

3. _____

d. Expulsion:

1. _____

2. _____

3. _____

# Matching:

8.46 Below on the left are five postural drainage positions. On the right is a listing of various lung segments. Match each position to the lung segment it would best drain.

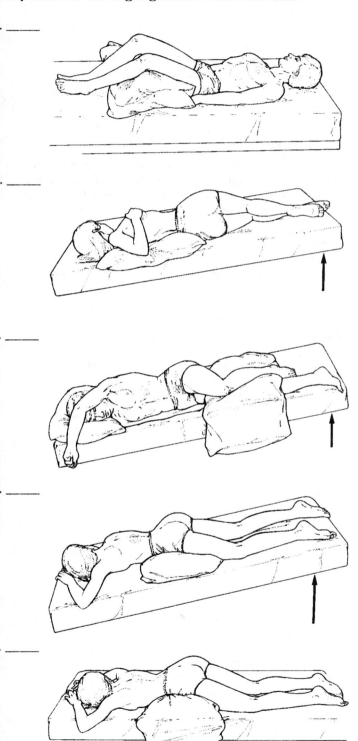

1. anterior basal left lower lobe

2. superior basal both lower lobes

3. posterior basal both lower lobes

4. lateral basal right lower lobe

5. lateral/medial right middle lobe

6. anterior segments upper lobes

**Multiple Choice:** Circle the letter corresponding to the single best answer from the available choices:

28.47 Major goals of chest physical therapy include which of the following?
I.    to facilitate clearance of airway secretions
II.   to promote more efficient breathing patterns
III.  to improve the distribution of ventilation
IV.   to improve cardiopulmonary exercise tolerance

a. I, II, and IV          c. II, III, and IV
b. I, II, and III         d. I, II, III, and IV

28.48 A physician orders postural drainage, chest percussion, and vibration for a 17–year–old male patient with cystic fibrosis. Which of the following is the most likely goal of this order?

a. to improve cardiopulmonary exercise tolerance
b. to promote a more efficient breathing pattern
c. to facilitate clearance of airway secretion
d. to improve the distribution of ventilation

28.49 Which of the following is considered a long–term goal of chest physical therapy, generally associated with comprehensive patient rehabilitation programs?

a. to promote a more efficient breathing pattern
b. to improve the distribution of ventilation
c. to improve cardiopulmonary exercise tolerance
d. to facilitate clearance of airway secretion

28.50 Which of the following conditions are associated with chronic production of large volumes of sputum?
I.    bronchiectasis
II.   pulmonary fibrosis
III.  cystic fibrosis
IV.   chronic bronchitis

a. II and IV          c. I and III
b. I, III, and IV     d. I, II, III, and IV

28.51 Patients with neuromuscular dysfunction tend to exhibit which of the following respiratory–related problems?
I.    ineffective cough and secretion retention
II.   progressive atelectasis due to small tidal volumes
III.  chronic production of large volumes of sputum

a. I and II           c. I only
b. II and III         d. I, II, and III

28.52 Special considerations in initial and ongoing patient assessment for chest physical therapy include which of the following?
I.    the patient's posture, muscle tone, and relaxation state
II.   the patient's breathing pattern and ability to cough
III.  the patient's sputum production (or lack thereof)
IV.   the patient's relative cardiovascular stability

a. II and IV          c. II and III
b. I, II, and III     d. I, II, III, and IV

28.53 If a physician's goal were to facilitate the mobilization of respiratory tract secretions in a patient with an ineffective cough, which of the following chest physical therapy techniques would you recommend?

a. relaxation positioning
b. inspiratory resistive breathing
c. pursed–lip breathing
d. postural drainage and percussion

28.54 In which of the following patients would you consider modifying any head–down positions used for postural drainage?
I.    a patient with unstable blood pressure
II.   a patient with a cerebrovascular disorder
III.  a patient with systemic hypertension
IV.   a patient with orthopnea

a. II and IV          c. II and III
b. I, II, and IV      d. I, II, III, and IV

28.55 If tolerated, a specified postural drainage position should be maintained for at least:

a. 3–5 minutes
b. 5–10 minutes
c. 10–20 minutes
d. 20–30 minutes

28.56 Strenuous patient coughing during postural drainage in head–down positions is contraindicated because it can:

a. markedly increase intracranial pressure
b. impair the mucociliary clearance mechanism
c. increase expiratory airway resistance
d. temporarily cause upper airway obstruction

28.57 Which of the following should be charted after completing a postural drainage treatment?
I.    amount/consistency of sputum produced
II.   patient tolerance of procedure
III.  position(s) used (including time)
IV.   any untoward effects observed

a. II and IV
b. I, II, and III
c. I and III
d. I, II, III, and IV

28.58 If a patient's chest x–ray shows infiltrates in the posterior basal segments of the lower lobes, postural drainage should be performed in which of the following positions?

a. head down, patient prone with a pillow under her abdomen
b. head down, patient supine with a pillow under her knees
c. patient prone with a pillow under her head, bed flat
d. patient supine with a pillow under her knees, bed flat

28.59 A patient under your care has x–ray and clinical evidence of severe unilateral right lung infiltrates. His $Po_2$ on a nonrebreathing mask is 49 mm Hg. The attending physician asks your advice on how best to improve this patient's oxygenation without committing to ventilatory support. Which of the following would you recommend?

a. place the patient on his left side (left lung down)
b. place the patient on his right side (right lung down)
c. turn the patient from the supine to prone position
d. institute a regimen of inspiratory resistive breathing

28.60 Percussion should not be performed over which of the following areas?
I.    trauma or surgery sites
II.   bony prominences
III.  fractured ribs

a. I only
b. I and II
c. I and III
d. I, II, and III

28.61 Properly performed chest vibration is applied:

a. throughout inspiration
b. throughout expiration
c. during breath holding
d. at the end of expiration

28.62 A patient still recovering from abdominal surgery is having difficulty developing an effective cough. Which of the following actions would you consider to aid this patient in generating a more effective cough?
I.    coordinating coughing with pain medication
II.   using the forced expiration technique
III.  "splinting" the operative site
IV.   applying manual chest compression

a. II and IV
b. I, II, and III
c. I and III
d. I, II, III, and IV

28.63 Strenuous expiratory efforts in some COPD patients limit the effectiveness of coughing. This is because:

a. strenuous expiration causes the abdominal pressure to fall
b. high expiratory pleural pressures compress the small airways
c. the accessory muscles of inspiration oppose the exhalation
d. all COPD patients have severe abdominal muscle weakness

28.64 During a session of coughing, an emphysematous patient suddenly appears unable to move air. As he strains to exhale, his neck veins distend and his face gets cyanotic. Which of the following actions would you take?

a. run to the nurses' station and call the attending physician
b. try to pass a suction catheter through the nasal passage
c. exert a series of compressions over the lateral costal margins
d. call a "code" and position the patient supine on the floor

28.65 A physician asks your advice on how best to improve bronchopulmonary clearance in a 17–year–old cystic fibrosis patient with copious secretions. Which of the following regimens would you recommend?

a. inspiratory resistive breathing, followed by directed coughing
b. postural drainage combined with manual chest compression
c. postural drainage combined with the forced expiration technique
d. percussion/vibration alone using a high–frequency pneumatic device

28.66 The best position for initiating diaphragmatic breathing exercises is:

a. supine with knees bent, head supported
b. sitting with feet supported on stool
c. semi–Fowler's position with knees bent
d. prone Trendelenburg with abdomen supported

28.67 Properly performed inspiratory resistive breathing imposes additional work load primarily on which of the following muscles/muscle groups?

a. abdominals
b. diaphragm
c. sternomastoids
d. scalenes

28.68 Upon a return visit to a home care COPD patient on an inspiratory resistive breathing exercise program, you note no increase in $P_{Imax}$ (maximum inspiratory force) since the last measure taken two weeks ago. No other changes are noted in the patient. What is the most likely cause of the lack of improvement in respiratory muscle strength?

a. rapid progression of the disease process
b. noncompliance with the exercise regimen
c. a faulty inspiratory resistive device
d. increased expiratory airway resistance

28.69 Which of the following are primary effects of pursed–lip breathing?
I.    moving the equal pressure point toward the larger airways
II.   decreasing expiratory flows and lengthening expiration
III.  decreasing the likelihood of bronchiolar collapse

a. I and II            c. II only
b. II and III          d. I, II, and III

28.70 A patient recovering from a neuromuscular disorder is having difficulty developing an effective cough due to weakness of the expiratory muscles. Which of the following breathing exercises would you recommend as a component of cough training for this patient?

a. breathing through pursed lips
b. force expiration abdominal breathing
c. bilateral costal breathing
d. graded exercises on a treadmill

28.71 A physician wants to increase a COPD patient's tolerance for simple physical activities around her home, such as gardening and walking to the mailbox. Which of the following methods would you recommend as best for this patient?

a. the forced expiration technique
b. postural drainage and percussion
c. force expiration abdominal breathing
d. simple coordinated walking exercises

28.72 Preconditions for applying a graded treadmill or ergometer exercise program include which of the following?
I.    the patient must be stable (not in the acute phase of illness)
II.   the patient must have mastered breathing control techniques
III.  the patient must not be in need of supplemental oxygen

a. I and II            c. III only
b. I and III           d. I, II, and III

28.73 Which of the following outcomes can be expected as a result of a properly conducted graded exercise program?
I.    an increased maximum ventilatory capacity
II.   decreased $O_2$ consumption for a given work load
III.  improved resting pulmonary function

a. I and II            c. II only
b. II and III          d. I, II, and III

28.74 During chest physical therapy, a patient develops hemoptysis. Which of the following actions would be appropriate at this time?

a. immediately discontinue the treatment and contact the physician
b. have the patient assume a sitting position and cough strenuously
c. place the patient in a head–down position and call the nurse
d. immediately institute tracheobronchial aspiration (suctioning)

28.75 Postural drainage in the Trendelenburg position for patients with head injuries is generally contraindicated. The primary concern in these patients is the risk of:

a. bronchiolar collapse
b. increased airway resistance
c. increased intracranial pressure
d. impaired cardiac output

28.76 In which of the following patient groups is arterial hypoxemia most likely to occur with application of chest physical therapy?
I.    patients with pulmonary emphysema
II.   patients with profuse bronchial secretions
III.  patients with cardiovascular instability

a. I and II            c. II only
b. II and III          d. I, II, and III

28.77 Which of the following patients would be considered at high risk for exhibiting a decreased cardiac output during chest physical therapy?
I.    patients with shock due to any cause
II.   patients lacking normal venomotor tone
III.  patients suffering from hypovolemia
IV.   patients with chronic airways obstruction

a. I, II, and III      c. III and IV
b. II and IV           d. I, II, III, and IV

# Respiratory Failure and the Need for Ventilatory Support

## CONTENT EXERCISES

**True/False:** For each of the following statements, indicate whether it is mainly true or mainly false by circling the corresponding letter (T=True, F=False):

29.1  T  F  Abnormalities of pulmonary gas exchange can occur in a wide variety of clinical disorders.

29.2  T  F  Acute respiratory failure is always present when the arterial $P_{CO_2}$ rises above 50 mm Hg.

29.3  T  F  Abnormalities of oxygen exchange can occur separately from inadequacies in ventilation or $CO_2$ excretion.

29.4  T  F  Hypoventilation is a cause of hypoxemic respiratory failure.

29.5  T  F  The $Pa_{O_2}$ in pure hypercapnic respiratory failure is less than would be expected for a given $FI_{O_2}$.

29.6  T  F  The $P(A-a)_{O_2}$ in hypercapnic respiratory failure is usually higher than normal.

29.7  T  F  A patient suffering from respiratory insufficiency may maintain normal or near normal blood gases.

29.8  T  F  Most neuromuscular disorders result in a primary hypoxemic respiratory failure.

29.9  T  F  Some patients with restrictive disorders of the chest wall or pleura actually hyperventilate.

29.10  T  F  ARDS is associated with an increase in the concentration of certain hormones and other chemical mediators.

29.11  T  F  An increase in the transpulmonary pressure gradient expands the alveoli in direct proportion to the pressure difference created.

29.12  T  F  High $Pa_{CO_2}$ values alone are an adequate reason for initiating ventilatory support.

29.13  T  F  The MVV measure can be performed on an unconscious or uncooperative patient.

29.14  T  F  Most respiratory muscle weakness is due to atrophy.

29.15  T  F  The treatment of severe hypoxemia requires mechanical ventilation.

29.16  T  F  Hypocapnia and alkalosis have additive effects in reducing cerebral blood flow.

29.17  T  F  Brief periods of apnea are normal during sleep.

29.18  T  F  PSV helps the patient overcome the added work associated with breathing through small endotracheal tubes.

**Short Answer:** Complete each statement by filling in the correct information in the space(s) provided:

29.19 The primary manifestation of hypoxemic respiratory failure is a lower than predicted _____ and a higher than predicted _____.

29.20 The hallmark of hypercapnic respiratory failure is an _____.

29.21 Situations in which hypoxemia and/or hypercapnea develop too rapidly to allow physiologic compensation best describes _____ respiratory failure.

29.22 "Acute–on–chronic" respiratory failure generally involves patients with _____.

29.23 Hypoxemia that does not respond well to oxygen therapy is termed _____ hypoxemia.

29.24 All modes of ventilatory support facilitate lung expansion by increasing the _____ pressure gradient.

29.25 The _____ is a more appropriate indicator of acute hypercapnic respiratory failure than is the $Pa_{CO_2}$.

29.26 Fatigued respiratory muscles typically take approximately _____ to _____ hours to fully recover.

29.27 Sustained breathing frequencies of _____ breaths/min or higher in the adult usually indicate a need for some form of ventilatory support.

29.28 A $\dot{V}_E$ of _____ L/min or less can be considered an acceptable ventilatory demand for most adult patients.

29.29 A $P_{(A-a)O_2}$ of _____ mm Hg or greater during breathing of 100% $O_2$ indicates severe hypoxemia.

29.30 The clinical benefits associated with hyperventilation in patients with closed head injuries are diminished after _____ to _____ hours.

29.31 The sleep apnea syndrome is defined as the occurrence of _____ or more apneic periods per hour, each lasting at least _____ seconds.

29.32 The most common factor associated with obstructive sleep apnea in men is _____.

**Listing:** Complete each list as directed in its statement.

29.33 List at least seven (7) causes of respiratory failure associated with intrinsic lung diseases:

1. _____

2. _____

3. _____

4. _____

5. _____

6. _____

7. _____

29.34 List at least six (6) pulmonary–related conditions associated with the Adult Respiratory Distress Syndrome:

1. _____

2. _____

3. _____

4. _____

5. _____

6. _____

29.35 Below on the left are listed some measurements used in determining the need for ventilatory support. In the space provided in the columns on the right, indicate (1) the adult normal range for that measurement and (2) the threshold value(s) indicating the need for ventilatory support:

| | Values | |
|---|---|---|
| Measurement | Adult Normal | Ventilatory Support |
| a. Vital capacity (VC) (ml/kg) | _____ | _____ |
| b. Respiratory rate (f) (breaths/min) | _____ | _____ |
| c. Maximum inspiratory force (MIF) (cm $H_2O$) | _____ | _____ |
| d. Minute ventilation ($\mathring{V}_E$), (L/min) | _____ | _____ |
| e. Maximum voluntary ventilation (MVV) (L/min) | _____ | _____ |
| f. Deadspace fraction ($V_D/V_T$) (%) | _____ | _____ |
| g. $Pa_{CO_2}$ (mm Hg) | _____ | _____ |
| h. $Pa_{O_2}$ (mm Hg) | _____ | _____ |
| i. Alveolar to arterial $P_{O_2}$ gradient; $P_{(A-a)O_2}$, breathing 100% $O_2$ (mm Hg) | _____ | _____ |

## Matching:

29.36 Below on the left are several definitions of various forms of ventilatory support. On the right are terms used to describe these modes. In the space provided above each definition, write the number corresponding to the correct term for that mode.

a. _____

| | |
|---|---|
| The maintenance of a pressure above atmospheric at the airway opening throughout a spontaneous breathing cycle. | 1. Control mode |

b. _____

| | |
|---|---|
| Continuous mandatory ventilation in which the rate of breathing is ventilation determined by the ventilator according to a preset cycling pattern without initiation by the patient. | 2. Pressure support ventilation |

c. _____

| | |
|---|---|
| Periodic ventilation with positive pressure, with the patient breathing spontaneously between breaths. These periodic breaths may be controlled or assisted. | 3. Continuous positive airway pressure |

d. _____

| | |
|---|---|
| Pressure–limited, flow–cycled, assisted ventilation designed to augment a spontaneously generated breath. The patient has primary control over the frequency of breathing, the inspiratory time, and the inspiratory flow. | 4. Assist–control mode |

e. _____

| | |
|---|---|
| Continuous mandatory ventilation in which the minimum frequency of breathing mandatory is predetermined by the ventilator ventilation controls, but the patient can initiate ventilation at a faster rate. | 5. Intermittent mandatory ventilation |

## Multiple Choice: Circle the letter corresponding to the single best answer from the available choices:

29.37 Hypoxemic respiratory failure is characterized by:
I. a lower than predicted $PaO_2$
II. alveolar hypoventilation
III. a normal or low $PaCO_2$
IV. a higher than predicted $P(A-a)O_2$

a. I, III, and IV     c. III and IV
b. I and IV     d. I, II, III, and IV

29.38 Hypoxemic respiratory failure may be caused by which of the following?
I. a diffusion impairment
II. intrapulmonary shunting
III. a low V/Q ratio
IV. L–R cardiac shunting

a. I, III, and IV     c. I and II
b. I, II, and III     d. I, II, III, and IV

29.39 Hypercapnic respiratory failure is characterized by:
I. a lower than normal $PaO_2$
II. alveolar hypoventilation
III. a higher than normal $PaCO_2$
IV. a normal/near normal $P(A-a)O_2$

a. I, III, and IV     c. III and IV
b. I and IV     d. I, II, III, and IV

29.40 A patient with an opiate drug overdose is unconscious and exhibits the following blood gas results breathing room air: pH = 7.21; $PcO_2$ = 85; $HCO_3$ = 26; $PO_2$ = 50. Which of the following best describes this patient's condition?

a. acute hypercapnic respiratory failure
b. chronic hypoxemic respiratory failure
c. chronic hypercapnic respiratory failure
d. acute hypoxemic respiratory failure

29.41 A 34–year–old male patient admitted to the emergency room with lung contusions exhibits the following blood gas results breathing 35% $O_2$: pH = 7.49; $PcO_2$ = 29; $HCO_3$ = 26; $PO_2$ = 44; $P(A-a)O_2$ = 170 mm Hg. Which of the following best describes this patient's condition?

a. acute hypercapnic respiratory failure
b. chronic hypoxemic respiratory failure
c. chronic hypercapnic respiratory failure
d. acute hypoxemic respiratory failure

29.42 A patient with a 10–year history of chronic bronchitis and an acute viral pneumonia exhibits the following blood gas results breathing room air: pH = 7.23; $P_{CO_2}$ = 65; $HCO_3$ = 26; $P_{O_2}$ = 40; $P(A - a)_{O_2}$ = 70 mm Hg. Which of the following best describes this patient's condition?

a. acute hypercapnic respiratory failure
b. chronic hypoxemic respiratory failure
c. chronic hypercapnic respiratory failure
d. combined hypercapnic/hypoxemic respiratory failure

29.43 Central nervous system (CNS) causes of respiratory failure include which of the following?
I.    brain, brainstem, or spinal cord trauma
II.   CNS infections (meningitis, encephalitis)
III.  obesity–related hypoventilation
IV.   brain or spinal cord tumors

a. II and IV                  c. I and III
b. I, II, and III             d. I, II, III, and IV

29.44 Disorders of the upper airway that can cause respiratory failure include which of the following?
I.    cystic fibrosis
II.   foreign body obstruction
III.  laryngotracheitis
IV.   epiglottitis

a. II and IV                  c. I and III
b. II, III, and IV            d. I, II, III, and IV

29.45 The most common cause of respiratory failure in neonates is:

a. foreign body aspiration
b. epiglottis
c. small airway obstruction
d. hyaline membrane disease

29.46 The common pathologic finding in all conditions leading to the Adult Respiratory Distress Syndrome (ARDS) is:

a. involuntary contraction of airway smooth muscle
b. a decreased alveolar–arterial $O_2$ gradient
c. a decreased CNS responsiveness to $CO_2$
d. damage to the alveolar–capillary membrane

29.47 In assessing the results of pulmonary function tests on a patient with ARDS, you would expect to find:
I.    an increase in lung volumes
II.   a decrease in lung compliance
III.  an increased work of breathing
IV.   evidence of muscle fatigue

a. I and IV                   c. III and IV
b. II, III, and IV            d. I, II, III, and IV

29.48 Ventilatory support may be indicated when the vital capacity (VC) falls below what level?

a. 65–75 ml/kg
b. 55–65 ml/kg
c. 45–55 ml/kg
d. 10–15 ml/kg

29.49 Ventilatory support may be indicated when the pulmonary R–L shunt fraction (Qs/Qt) rises above what level?

a. 3–5%
b. 5–10%
c. 10–15%
d. 20–30%

29.50 Which of the following patients has the most serious problem with oxygenation?

| Patient | $F_{IO_2}$ | $Pa_{O_2}$ |
| --- | --- | --- |
| a.  A | 1.00 | 85 |
| b.  B | 0.70 | 90 |
| c.  C | 0.40 | 95 |
| d.  D | 0.28 | 65 |

29.51 A patient is receiving positive pressure ventilation during every inspiration. The minimum frequency of breathing is preset at 10/min, but the patient can initiate ventilation at a higher rate. What mode of ventilatory support is being delivered?

a. continuous mandatory ventilation–control mode
b. pressure support ventilation (PSV)
c. continuous positive airway pressure (CPAP)
d. continuous mandatory ventilation assist–control mode

29.52 Pressure–limited, flow–cycled, assisted ventilation designed to augment a spontaneously generated breath best describes:

a. continuous mandatory ventilation–control mode
b. pressure support ventilation (PSV)
c. continuous positive airway pressure (CPAP)
d. intermittent mandatory ventilation (IMV)

29.53 The following arterial blood gases are obtained on four patients. Which of these patients is most in need of ventilatory support?

| Patient | pH | $P_{CO_2}$ | $HCO_3$ |
| --- | --- | --- | --- |
| a. A | 7.34 | 62 mm Hg | 32 mEq/L |
| b. B | 7.21 | 64 mm Hg | 25 mEq/L |
| c. C | 7.39 | 58 mm Hg | 34 mEq/L |
| d. D | 7.36 | 51 mm Hg | 27 mEq/L |

29.54 A drug overdose patient is suffering from acute hypercapnic respiratory failure due to a simple decrease in ventilatory drive. Which of the following ventilatory support modes would you suggest for this patient?

a. continuous positive airway pressure (CPAP)
b. CMV in the control or assist–control mode
c. pressure support ventilation (PSV)
d. intermittent mandatory ventilation (IMV)

29.55 A patient with a restrictive disorder develops hypercapnic respiratory failure. Prior to intubation, her breathing rate is 28/min. After being placed on CMV in the assist–control mode, her ABGs indicate respiratory alkalosis (pH=7.51). Which of the following would you recommend?

a. increase the minimum preset ventilator rate
b. switch the patient to CMV in the control mode
c. switch the patient to the IMV mode
d. decrease the minimum preset ventilator rate

29.56 Which of the following conditions could result in the development of respiratory muscle fatigue?
I.      pulmonary fibrosis
II.     acute asthma
III.    spinal cord trauma

a. I and II          c. II only
b. II and III        d. I, II, and III

29.57 You obtain a maximum inspiratory force (MIF; NIF) measurement of –13 cm $H_2O$ on a patient with Guillain–Barre syndrome. Based on this information, you may conclude that the patient has:

a. an excessive work of breathing
b. severe hypoxemia/hypoxia
c. inadequate alveolar ventilation
d. inadequate muscle strength

29.58 A patient recovering from myasthenia gravis has been receiving control mode CMV for 8 weeks and is now exhibiting signs of respiratory muscle atrophy. Which of the following approaches would you recommend to help "recondition" her muscles?

a. maintain control mode
b. changeover to CPAP
c. implement PEEP
d. switch to the IMV mode

29.59 Which of the following can result in excessive ventilatory demands being placed on a patient?
I.      an increase in physiologic deadspace ($V_D/V_T$)
II.     an increase in lung or thoracic compliance
III.    an increase in $CO_2$ production ($\dot{V}_{CO_2}$)

a. I and II          c. I and III
b. II and III        d. I, II, and III

29.60 A patient in respiratory failure exhibits a marked increase in the work of breathing due to poor lung expansion and decreased compliance. Which of the following modes of ventilatory support would you recommend for this patient?

a. control mode CMV
b. CMV with PEEP
c. simple IMV
d. assist–control CMV

29.61 A 200–lb male patient in hypoxemic respiratory failure is intubated with a 6–mm oral endotracheal tube and placed in the IMV mode at a rate of 6/min. Soon after, he exhibits signs of increased work of breathing. Which of the following is most likely causing his increased work of breathing?

a. the patient has severe restriction due to obesity
b. the rate selected for the IMV mode is too low
c. the endotracheal tube selected is too narrow
d. the gamma–efferent system is being stimulated

29.62 Deliberate hyperventilation via continuous mandatory ventilation (CMV) is sometimes applied to patients with closed head injuries in order to:

a. depress the medullary chemoreceptors
b. provoke dilation of the cerebral vasculature
c. reduce brain swelling and intracranial pressure
d. increase oxygen consumption of the brain

29.63 Which of the following is *false* regarding the management of flail chest?

a. only rarely is flail chest severe enough to demand vent support
b. flail chest is commonly cited as an indication for vent support
c. the size/location of the flail determines the clinical course
d. most patients with flail chest do not require vent support

29.64 In managing a patient suffering from an acute asthma attack with $O_2$ and bronchodilators, you note a rise in the $P_{CO_2}$ to 50 mm Hg, with a pH of 7.27. Although anxious, the patient remains alert and cooperative during therapy. Which of the following would you recommend at this time?

a. continuation of current management with careful monitoring
b. administration of a CNS respiratory depressant
c. intubation and mechanical ventilation in the IMV mode
d. intubation and mechanical ventilation in the CMV mode

29.65 Which of the following measures should be used in the initial treatment of a patient in acute respiratory failure due to an exacerbation of COPD?
I.     bronchodilator administration
II.    vigorous bronchial hygiene
III.   judicious oxygen therapy
IV.    intubation/mechanical ventilation

a. II and IV
b. I, II, and III
c. III and IV
d. I, II, III, and IV

29.66 A sleep study conducted on a 38–year–old adult male patient reveals the following: an average of 12 apneic periods/hr, each lasting at least 20 seconds. During the apneic episodes, the patient does not make any effort to breathe. The patient also complains of chronic daytime sleepiness. Which of the following is the most likely cause of this patient's problem?

a. obstructive sleep apnea
b. central sleep apnea
c. chronic hypothyroidism
d. high intracranial pressure

29.67 A physician requests your advice in managing a 49–year–old obese male patient with confirmed obstructive sleep apnea. Which of the following would you recommend?

a. placement of a tracheal button
b. night placement of a tongue retainer
c. use of respiratory stimulants
d. administration of CPAP at night

29.68 Which of the following is *false* regarding surfactant replacement in ARDS?

a. it should restore lung mechanics and limit injury
b. it should help rid the body of oxygen free radicals
c. research to date has failed to demonstrate any beneficial effects
d. questions related to safety, patient selection, and timing remain

# 30

## Physics and Physiology of Ventilatory Support

### CONTENT EXERCISES

**True/False:** For each of the following statements, indicate whether it is mainly true or mainly false by circling the corresponding letter (T=True, F=False):

30.1 T F All modes of ventilatory support aid lung expansion by increasing the transpulmonary pressure gradient.

30.2 T F A spontaneous inspiration increases the transpulmonary pressure gradient by increasing the pleural pressure.

30.3 T F CPAP maintains an increased alveolar pressure throughout both inspiration and expiration.

30.4 T F Positive pressure ventilation reverses the pressure gradients of normal spontaneous inspiration.

30.5 T F Alveolar pressure is greater than pleural pressure during positive pressure ventilation.

30.6 T F Pleural pressure never exceeds atmospheric pressure during positive pressure ventilation.

30.7 T F Continuous positive airway pressure (CPAP) alone provides some ventilation.

30.8 T F Controlled ventilation often requires patient sedation or induced neuromuscular paralysis to be successful.

30.9 T F In the control mode of ventilation, the patient initiates inspiration and determines the frequency of breathing.

30.10 T F In the assist–control mode of ventilation, the minimum rate of breathing is established by the patient.

30.11 T F The pressure pattern delivered by a flow generator varies with changes in patient compliance/resistance.

30.12 T F A volume–cycled ventilator provides gas under positive pressure until a set volume enters the patient's lungs.

30.13 T F The volume of gas delivered into a patient's lung by a positive pressure ventilator is always less than that expelled from the machine.

30.14 T F Pressure–cycled ventilators generally are better able to compensate for small leaks than volume ventilators.

30.15 T F Inspiratory–expiratory time ratios are most important in the intermittent mandatory ventilation (IMV) mode.

30.16 T F Positive pressure ventilation can increase a patient's work of breathing.

30.17 T F Hyperventilation is the preferred method to depress the respiratory drive of a patient who is fighting a ventilator.

30.18 T F High levels of PEEP increase the incidence of pulmonary barotrauma.

30.19 T F Air trapping during positive pressure ventilation can impede pulmonary blood flow.

30.20 T F Lung units prone to trapping air are those with short time constants, i.e., low resistance and/or low compliance.

30.21 T F The effects of moderate elevations in pleural pressure on cardiac output in normal subjects are minimal.

30.22 T F IMV allows the patient to breathe spontaneously between positive pressure breaths.

30.23 T F Negative end–expiratory pressure (NEEP) increases the FRC.

30.24 T F Short inspiratory times enhance the distribution of gases within the lung.

30.25 T F Negative pressure ventilation is an outdated means of ventilatory support.

**Short Answer:** Complete each statement by filling in the correct information in the space(s) provided:

30.26 An increase in the transpulmonary pressure gradient expands the alveoli in direct proportion to the _____ applied.

30.27 Airway pressure with CPAP is essentially _____ throughout the breathing cycle.

30.28 The means by which a positive pressure ventilator initiates the inspiratory phase of breathing is referred to as its _____ mechanism.

30.29 How much negative pressure is required to initiate a mechanical breath is determined by a _____ control.

30.30 How fast a ventilator responds to the patient's inspiratory effort is called the _____.

30.31 _____ is the only mode of cycling to inspiration that can provide precise and consistently predictable physiologic results.

30.32 The flow delivered by a constant pressure generator varies with respect to both time and the patient's _____.

30.33 The primary difference between a flow generator and a pressure generator is the amount of _____ available.

30.34 The maximum available value of a ventilator parameter is referred to as a _____.

30.35 Compressed volume loss is most critical when delivered volumes are _____.

30.36 A true threshold resistor maintains a given pressure level independent of changes in _____.

30.37 For a constant rate of positive pressure breathing, the greater the duration of _____ , the less the cardiovascular effect.

30.38 For a given positive pressure, the more compliant the lung, the _____ will be the increase in pleural pressure.

30.39 Positive pressure ventilation can reduce urinary output by as much as _____ %.

**Listing:** Complete each list as directed in its statement.

30.40 List five (5) devices that can be used to generate PEEP or CPAP:

1. _____

2. _____

3. _____

4. _____

5. _____

30.41 List five (5) factors affecting mean pleural pressure:

1. _____

2. _____

3. _____

4. _____

5. _____

**Matching:**

30.42 Below on the left are five patterns of airway pressure versus time. On the right is a listing of various ventilatory support mode acronyms. Match each pressure waveform to the correct mode.

a. _____

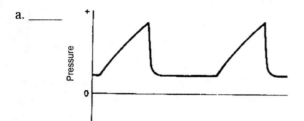

b. _____

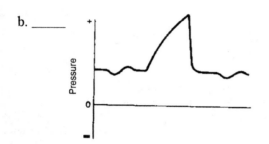

c. _____

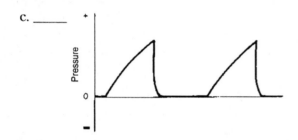

d. _____

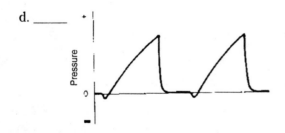

e. _____

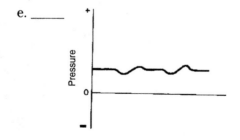

1. CMV control mode

2. CMV assist–control

3. IMV

4. IMV with PEEP

5. CPAP

6. CMV with PEEP

## Compare and Contrast:

30.43 In the table below, compare and contrast continuous mandatory ventilation (CMV) with intermittent mandatory ventilation (IMV) according to the criteria provided:

| Criterion | CMV | IMV |
|---|---|---|
| a. Spontaneous breathing | _____ | _____ |
| b. Patient determination of $V_T/f$ | _____ | _____ |
| c. Responsibility for minute ventilation ($\mathring{V}_E$) | _____ | _____ |
| d. Respiratory muscle use | _____ | _____ |
| e. Mean pleural pressure | _____ | _____ |

## Computations:

30.44 Five patients are receiving CMV in the control mode. In the following table, you are given each patient's frequency of breathing (f) and the expiratory time (te) in seconds. Calculate each patient's inspiratory time (ti) in seconds:

| Patient | f breaths/min | te seconds | ti seconds |
|---|---|---|---|
| a. | 12 | 2.50 | _____ |
| b. | 10 | 1.20 | _____ |
| c. | 15 | 2.40 | _____ |
| d. | 20 | 1.80 | _____ |
| e. | 8 | 3.00 | _____ |

## Multiple Choice: Circle the letter corresponding to the single best answer from the available choices:

30.45 The transpulmonary pressure gradient ($P_L$) can be increased by:
I.   increasing alveolar pressure
II.  decreasing transthoracic pressure
III. decreasing pleural pressure

a. I and II
b. II and III
c. I and III
d. I, II, and III

30.46 In which of the following types of ventilation is alveolar expansion during inspiration due to a decrease in pleural pressure?
I.   positive pressure ventilation
II.  negative pressure ventilation
III. spontaneous ventilation

a. I and II
b. II and III
c. I and III
d. I, II, and III

30.47 In which of the following types of ventilatory support does gas flow into and out of the lung depend on spontaneously generated changes in pleural pressure?
I.   positive pressure ventilation
II.  negative pressure ventilation
III. continuous positive airway pressure

a. I and II
b. II and III
c. III only
d. I, II, and III

30.48 In order for continuous positive airway pressure (CPAP) to be successful, the patient must have:

a. an adequate $Pao_2$ on less than 50% $O_2$
b. a secure artificial airway in place
c. adequate spontaneous ventilation
d. intact upper airway protective reflexes

30.49 An asthmatic patient is struggling to initiate inspiration on a Puritan–Bennett 7200 ventilator operating in the assist–control mode. Which of the following ventilator settings would you first check to determine the cause of this problem?

a. the pressure limit
b. the sensitivity
c. the tidal volume
d. the oxygen percent

30.50 A volume ventilator has an individual rate setting that determines the controlled frequency of breathing in breaths/min. Assuming this control remains set at 12/min, which of the following parameters will determine the normal length of inspiration and expiration?

I. flow
II. $FIO_2$
III. volume

a. I and II
b. II and III
c. I and III
d. I, II, and III

30.51 Which of the following are false regarding the assist–control mode of ventilatory support?

a. the minimum cycling frequency is preset on the ventilator
b. if the patient becomes apneic, the preset rate is delivered
c. the patient can override the preset minimum rate of breathing
d. the time interval between breaths will remain constant

30.52 A patient receiving continuous mechanical ventilation in the assist–control mode at a preset rate of 12/min stops breathing. Which of the following will occur?

a. the high pressure limit alarm will sound (if properly set)
b. the ventilator will switch over to the spontaneous mode
c. the low tidal volume alarm will sound (if properly set)
d. the patient will continue to be ventilated at 12 breaths/min

30.53 Which of the following are functional characteristics of a constant pressure generator?

I. flow starts out low but increases during inspiration
II. flow varies with both time and the patient's lung properties
III. the inspiratory pressure pattern is constant (a square wave)
IV. the patient's lung properties do not alter the pressure pattern

a. I, II, and III
b. II and IV
c. II, III, and IV
d. I, II, III, and IV

30.54 Which of the following are functional characteristics of a constant flow generator?

I. flow remains constant throughout inspiration (square wave)
II. pressure increases progressively throughout inspiration
III. the patient's lung properties alter the pattern of flow

a. II and III
b. I and II
c. I only
d. I, II, and III

30.55 Which of the following is *false* regarding the end–inspiratory pause or EIP (inflation hold, inspiratory hold, volume hold)?

a. during an EIP the ventilator exhalation valve remains closed
b. use of an EIP lengthens the time available for exhalation
c. when applied, an EIP creates an observable pressure "plateau"
d. an EIP normally occurs after delivery of the mechanical breath

30.56 The plateau pressure achieved during an end–inspiratory pause (EIP) maneuver provides a rough estimate of a patient's:

a. airway resistance
b. thoracic compliance only
c. lung compliance only
d. total lung–thorax compliance

30.57 In order to estimate the airway resistance of a patient receiving mechanical ventilatory support, which of the following measures would you use?

a. (plateau – baseline) pressure during an end–inspiratory pause
b. (peak + plateau) pressure during an end–inspiratory pause
c. plateau pressure after an end–inspiratory pause
d. (peak – plateau) pressure during an end–inspiratory pause

30.58 A ventilator delivers gas under positive pressure until an adjustable, preset pressure has been reached. Under these circumstances, which of the following parameters will always vary if the mechanical properties of the patient's lungs change?

a. the rate of breathing
b. the inspiratory flow rate
c. the expiratory time
d. the delivered volume

30.59 Which of the following is *false* regarding time–cycled ventilators?

a. time–cycled ventilators are not used on adults
b. the device cycles off when a preset time interval ends
c. the pressure, volume, and flow delivered may vary
d. essentially all infant ventilators are time–cycled

30.60 Flow–cycling has been incorporated as the means to end inspiration in which of the following modes of ventilation?

a. intermittent mandatory ventilation
b. continuous positive airway pressure
c. pressure support ventilation
d. mandatory minute ventilation

30.61 An infant ventilator is operating in the time–cycled, pressure–limited mode. Which of the following is *false* regarding this system?

a. a relief valve vents gases when a preset pressure is reached
b. inspiration will end as soon as the pressure limit is reached
c. volume will vary according to the patient's lung mechanics
d. the length of inspiration will be constant breath to breath

30.62 All adult volume–cycled ventilators incorporate a pressure limit as a safety backup to normal cycling modes. In these devices, if the pressure needed to deliver the volume rises to the preselected limit:

a. pressure will hold at the preset limit until end–inspiration
b. the ventilator will automatically cycle to end–inspiration
c. inspiratory time will increase to compensate for the lost volume
d. volume will increase to compensate for the loss of pressure

30.63 The volume of gas actually delivered to a patient by a positive pressure ventilator is always less than that expelled from the machine. Which of the following factors help explain this finding?
I.   the presence of built–in leaks in all ventilators
II.  gas compression occurring under positive pressure
III. expansion of the flexible ventilator circuitry

a. II and III          c. I and III
b. I and II            d. I, II, and III

30.64 After accounting for the compressed volume loss on an adult patient being ventilated by a volume–cycled ventilator at a preset volume of 1000 ml, you still note a 200–ml difference between the expected and actual delivered volume. Which of the following is most likely causing this problem?

a. absorption of gas across the alveolar membrane
b. an abnormal increase in the respiratory quotient
c. a large leak in the patient–ventilator system
d. an overinflated endotracheal tube cuff

30.65 An adult patient is being supported via a pressure–cycled ventilator. You find that you must continually increase the pressure in order to maintain the desired volume. Which of the following could explain this problem?
I.   decreased airway resistance
II.  decreased thoracic compliance
III. decreased lung elastance

a. I and II            c. I and III
b. II and III          d. I, II, and III

30.66 A post–op patient with an oral endotracheal tube in place is being ventilated with a pressure–cycled ventilator. You note that the ventilator will not cycle off at end–inspiration. The most likely problem is:

a. the ventilator sensitivity is set incorrectly
b. the tube is displaced into the right bronchus
c. the endotracheal tube cuff is overinflated
d. there is a large leak in the ventilator system

30.67 A time–cycled constant flow generator is set up with a flow of 50 L/min and an inspiratory time of 1.2 sec. What is the tidal volume?

a. 1000 ml (1.0 L)
b. 1500 ml (1.5 L)
c. 750 ml (0.75 L)
d. 1200 ml (1.2 L)

30.68 During time–cycled, pressure–limited ventilation, if the pressure limit is reached before the inspiratory time cycle is completed, which of the following will occur?
I.    the additional flow will vent to the atmosphere
II.   the pressure will be maintained at the preset limit
III.  the ventilator will cycle to end–inspiration

a. I and II
b. II and III
c. II only
d. I, II, and III

30.69 Which of the following parameters may be used to cycle a ventilator operating in the pressure support mode from the inspiratory into the expiratory phase?
I.    volume
II.   flow
III.  time

a. I and II
b. II and III
c. I and III
d. I, II, and III

30.70 Which of the following parameters would you change to alter the tidal volume being delivered to a patient receiving ventilatory support in the time–cycled, pressure–limited mode?

a. the trigger sensitivity
b. the pressure limit
c. the flow rate
d. the PEEP level

30.71 During simple positive pressure ventilation, gas movement during exhalation is due to:

a. negative pressure applied to the airway during exhalation
b. positive pressure applied to the chest wall after inspiration
c. active contraction of the expiratory muscles (abdominals)
d. the stored potential energy in the expanded lungs and thorax

30.72 A patient being supported by positive pressure ventilation can exhale passively to atmospheric pressure and is allowed to spontaneously breathe between mechanical breaths. Which mode of ventilatory support is this patient receiving?

a. simple CMV
b. IMV with PEEP
c. CMV with PEEP
d. simple IMV

30.73 Which of the following are true regarding the continuous mandatory ventilation (CMV) mode of ventilatory support?
I.    the ventilator provides the full minute ventilation
II.   spontaneous breathing by the patient is prohibited
III.  the patient's use of respiratory muscles is minimal
IV.   pleural pressures are higher than spontaneous breathing

a. II and III
b. I, II, and III
c. I, III, and IV
d. I, II, III, and IV

30.74 Which of the following will increase if you apply expiratory resistance or retard to a patient on positive pressure ventilation?
I.    the patient's expiratory time
II.   the patient's mean pleural pressure
III.  the patient's cardiac output

a. I and II
b. II and III
c. I and III
d. I, II, and III

30.75 The primary physiologic effect of PEEP is to:

a. increase the inspiratory reserve volume
b. decrease expiratory flow rates
c. increase the functional residual capacity
d. decrease the compliance of the lung

30.76 A patient receiving ventilatory support in the CMV mode has just been placed on 15 cm $H_2O$ positive end–expiratory pressure (PEEP). Which of the following potentially detrimental effects of this therapy should you be prepared for?
I.    decreased cardiac output
II.   pulmonary barotrauma
III.  increased lung compliance
IV.   decreased shunt fraction

a. II and IV
b. I, II, and III
c. I and II
d. I, II, III, and IV

30.77 A patient receiving continuous mandatory ventilation (CMV) with an $FIO_2$ of 0.70 has a $PaO_2$ of 52 mm Hg. When placed on 10 cm $H_2O$ PEEP, her $PaO_2$ increases to 135 mm Hg. Which of the following best explains the observed improvement in oxygenation?

a. increased alveolar ventilation
b. decreased work of breathing
c. decreased physiologic shunting
d. increased Hb affinity for $O_2$

30.78 Which of the following is not a potentially harmful pulmonary effect of positive pressure ventilation (PPV)?

a. respiratory alkalosis
b. increased insensible $H_2O$ loss
c. alteration in V/Q ratios
d. pulmonary barotrauma

30.79 When placed on positive pressure ventilation (PPV) at the same $F_{IO_2}$ he was breathing spontaneously, a patient exhibits an increase in the $P(A-a)O_2$. Which of the following best explains this finding?

a. an increase in V/Q due to redirection of blood flow
b. an increase in physiologic deadspace and $V_D/V_T$ ratio
c. a decrease in resistance to pulmonary blood flow
d. a decrease in V/Q due to redirection of blood flow

30.80 Which of the following detrimental effects may result from hyperventilating a patient receiving ventilatory support?
I. impaired $O_2$ unloading at the tissue
II. cardiac arrhythmias and/or tetany
III. impaired cerebral perfusion

a. I and II          c. I and III
b. II and III        d. I, II, and III

30.81 Which of the following patients are at high risk for developing pulmonary barotrauma as a complication of positive pressure ventilation?
I. a patient with normal lungs
II. a patient with bullous emphysema
III. a patient on high levels of PEEP

a. I and II          c. I and III
b. II and III        d. I, II, and III

30.82 An emphysematous patient receiving ventilatory support in the assist–control mode develops signs of air trapping. Which of the following actions would you recommend to resolve this problem?

a. extubate the patient and discontinue ventilatory support
b. decrease the length of time available for exhalation
c. increase the preset frequency of breathing by 30%
d. increase the length of time available for exhalation

30.83 Which of the following techniques can be used to overcome the increased work of breathing imposed by some IMV or CPAP circuit systems?
I. using pressure support ventilation (PSV) to "unload" the muscles
II. decreasing the response time of the ventilator demand valve
III. using continuous high flow through a low resistance circuit

a. I and II          c. II only
b. I and III         d. I, II, and III

30.84 Which of the following are potential effects of positive pressure ventilation (PPV) on the cardiovascular system?
I. increased pooling in the abdominal veins
II. decreased cranial perfusion pressures
III. decreased pulmonary blood flow
IV. decreased ventricular stroke volume

a. II and IV         c. III and IV
b. I, II, and III    d. I, II, III, and IV

30.85 Assuming a constant rate of breathing, which of the following I:E ratios would tend to most greatly impair a patient's cardiovascular performance?

a. 1:1
b. 1:2
c. 1:3
d. 1:4

30.86 Assuming equivalent total minute ventilations, which of the following modes of ventilatory support would tend to have the least deleterious circulatory effect?

a. CMV with PEEP
b. simple CPAP
c. IMV without PEEP
d. IMV with PEEP

30.87 Which of the following factors exerts the greatest influence on cardiac output during positive pressure ventilation (PPV)?

a. the length of expiration
b. the peak airway pressure
c. the mean pleural pressure
d. the mean inspiratory flow rate

30.88 Which of the following gastrointestinal conditions are commonly associated with long–term positive pressure ventilation?

I. bleeding
II. diarrhea
III. ulceration

a. I and II
b. II and III
c. I and III
d. I, II, and III

30.89 Positive pressure ventilation (PPV) can have all of the following effects *except:*

a. decreased left ventricular stroke volume
b. decreased right ventricular preload
c. increased pulmonary vascular resistance
d. decreased central venous pressure (CVP)

30.90 Which of the following patients are good candidates for negative pressure ventilation (NPV)?

a. patients with acute obstructive disorders of the upper airway
b. patients suffering acute exacerbations of chronic lung disease
c. patients with end–stage chronic obstructive pulmonary disease
d. patients with chronic neuromuscular disorders and normal airways

# 31

## Engineering Principles of Ventilatory Support Devices

## CONTENT EXERCISES

**True/False:** For each of the following statements, indicate whether it is mainly true or mainly false by circling the corresponding letter (T=True, F=False):

31.1  T  F  The most common forms of input power for a mechanical ventilator are electric and pneumatic.

31.2  T  F  An electrically powered ventilator uses voltage from an electrical line outlet to power its drive mechanism.

31.3  T  F  When compressed gas is used as the drive mechanism for a ventilator, its force is usually adjusted via a pressure reducing valve.

31.4  T  F  The Sine–wave flow pattern most closely resembles that occurring during spontaneous breathing.

31.5  T  F  The Siemens Servo 900C drive mechanism is based on a rotary vane compressor.

31.6  T  F  Many ventilators use more than one output control valve.

31.7  T  F  The elastic load is the pressure needed to overcome the elastance (or compliance) of the lungs and thorax.

31.8  T  F  Ventilator manufacturers often coin terms for modes without regard to consistency or theoretical relevance.

31.9  T  F  A ventilator must function as either a pressure, volume, or flow controller.

31.10 T  F  In ventilators, a transducer and electronic circuitry are needed to perform automatic open loop–control.

31.11 T  F  The advantage of fluidic control ventilators are that they have no moving parts to wear out.

31.12 T  F  Inspiration begins when some measured variable reaches a preset valve.

31.13 T  F  Inspiratory limit variables are frequently confused with cycle variables.

31.14 T  F  Most ventilator waveforms are either rectangular, exponential, ramp, or sinusoidal in shape.

31.15 T  F  Pressures measured at the outlet of a ventilator are always the same as when measured at the patient's airway opening.

31.16 T  F  Any variable that can be measured can potentially be used to trigger inspiration.

**Short Answer:** Complete each statement by filling in the correct information in the space(s) provided:

31.17 In the home care setting, a _____ for electrically powered ventilators is an essential life–saving feature in the event of a power outage.

31.18 An _____ is an electric motor with a rotating crank and piston rod.

31.19 The _____ valve regulates the flow of gas to the patient.

31.20 The patient effort required to trigger inspiration is determined by the ventilator's _____.

31.21 The _____ variable is the variable controlled during the expiratory time.

31.22 The _____ waveform is what many respiratory care practitioners call an "accelerating or decelerating flow waveform."

31.23 For a given ventilator output waveform display such as volume pressure and flow, a slower sweep speed will visually _____ the waveform.

**Multiple Choice:** Circle the letter corresponding to the single best answer from the available choices:

31.24 Which of the following represent the basic functions of a mechanical ventilator?
I. power input
II. power transmission or conversion
III. control scheme
IV. output

a. II and IV
b. II and III
c. I, III, and IV
d. I, II, III, and IV

31.25 In the United States, the line voltage of an electrically powered ventilator is normally:

a. 60–140 volts AC
b. 40–60 volts DC
c. 110–115 volts AC
d. 200–250 volts DC

31.26 The S–shaped or sigmoid airway pressure pattern is characteristic of a ventilator using a:

a. weighted energy reservoir
b. rotary driven piston
c. double–circuit drive
d. diaphragm or bellows

31.27 Commonly used output control valves on ventilators include:
I. pneumatic diaphragm
II. pneumatic poppet valve
III. electromagnetic poppet/plunger valve
IV. proportional valve

a. II and IV
b. I, II, and III
c. III and IV
d. I, II, III, and IV

31.28 Which of the following ventilators use a rotating crank and piston as their drive mechanism?
I. Siemens Servo 900C
II. Emerson 3–PV
III. Bennett Companion 2800
IV. Emerson IMV

a. I, III, and IV
b. II and IV
c. II, III, and IV
d. I, II, III, and IV

31.29 To qualify as a true volume controller, a ventilator must:
I. maintain consistent volume waveform during varying loads
II. measure volume and use this signal to control the volume waveform
III. alter inspiratory and expiratory times

a. I only
b. I and II
c. II and III
d. I, II, and III

31.30 Which of the following ventilators are controlled by fluidic logic systems?
I. Monaghan 225/SIMV
II. Sechrist IV–100B
III. Bio–Med MVP–10
IV. Bennett MA–1

a. III and IV
b. I, II, and III
c. I, III, and IV
d. I, II, III, and IV

31.31 Electronically controlled ventilators using preprogrammed microprocessors include which of the following?
I. Bear 1000
II. Puritan–Bennett 7200
III. Siemens Servo 900C
IV. Hamilton Veolar

a. I and II
b. II, III, and IV
c. I, II, and IV
d. I, II, III, and IV

31.32 The most common inspiratory trigger variables are:

a. time and pressure
b. pressure and flow
c. flow and time
d. pressure and inspiratory volume

31.33 The variable that is measured and used to end inspiration is called the:

a. cycle variable
b. limit variable
c. trigger variable
d. baseline variable

31.34 The main distinguishing feature of a ventilator classified as an oscillator is that:

a. it can generate positive transrespiratory pressure
b. it can generate negative transrespiratory pressure
c. it starts generating airway pressure at its peak valve
d. it generates flow waveforms which are truncated

31.35 Which of the following ventilator flow waveform patterns is most common?

a. rectangular
b. ascending ramp
c. descending ramp
d. sinusoidal

31.36 Disturbances that might affect the proper function of a ventilator's closed loop–control include:
I.    condensation or leaks in the patient circuit
II.   elevated minute ventilation
III.  endotracheal tube obstruction
IV.   changes in respiratory resistance and compliance

a. I and III              c. I, III, and IV
b. II, III, and IV        d. I, II, III, and IV

31.37 The control and limit variables during continuous mandatory ventilation (CMV) are:
I.    pressure
II.   volume
III.  time
IV.   flow

a. I, III, and IV         c. II, III, and IV
b. I, II, and IV          d. I, II, III, and IV

31.38 The control and limit variables during pressure support ventilation (PSV) breaths are:
I.    pressure
II.   volume
III.  flow
IV.   time

a. I only                 c. II, III, and IV
b. I and III              d. I, II, III, and IV

31.39 Spontaneous breaths which are augmented by pressure support ventilation can, depending on the ventilator, be triggered by:
I.    pressure
II.   volume
III.  flow
IV.   time

a. I and III              c. I, II, and III
b. II and IV              d. I, II, III, and IV

31.40 Compared with pressure, volume, and flow measured at the patient's airway opening, these same variables measured at the inspiratory outlet of a ventilator are:

a. always the same
b. never the same
c. sometimes lower
d. not affected by circuit compliance and resistance

31.41 When ventilating neonates, the effects of the patient circuit compliance can be as much as:

a. three times that of the respiratory system
b. five times that of the respiratory system
c. six times that of the respiratory system
d. eight times that of the respiratory system

31.42 Specifications for a ventilator alarm event should include which of the following features?
I.    conditions that trigger the alarm
II.   a response in the form of audible and/or visual message
III.  any associated response such as termination of inspiration
IV.   whether alarm must be manually reset or resets itself

a. I, II, and III         c. II, III, and IV
b. II and IV              d. I, II, III, and IV

31.43 A ventilator's low peak airway pressure alarm may be activated under which of the following patient conditions?

a. possible endotracheal tube obstruction
b. exhalation manifold obstruction
c. leak in the patient circuit
d. auto–PEEP development

31.44 Which of the following alarms may indicate a ventilator self–triggering situation?
I. high ventilatory frequency alarm
II. cumulative volume alarm
III. inspired gas alarm
IV. low baseline pressure

a. I and II
b. II and III
c. I, III, and IV
d. I, II, III, and IV

31.45 Potential causes of an inappropriate inspiratory time alarm include all of the following *except:*

a. patient circuit obstruction
b. exhalation manifold malfunction
c. heater/humidifier failure
d. inadequate tidal volume delivery

# CHAPTER
## 32

# Initiating and Adjusting Ventilatory Support

## CONTENT EXERCISES

**True/False:** For each of the following statements, indicate whether it is mainly true or mainly false by circling the corresponding letter (T=True, F=False):

32.1 T F During partial ventilatory support, the patient is responsible for some or all of the minute ventilation.

32.2 T F The selection of a particular initial ventilatory support mode depends mainly upon the patient's underlying pathophysiologic problem.

32.3 T F When initiating mechanical ventilation, the initial $FIO_2$ setting should provide a $PaO_2$ of at least 60 mm Hg ($SaO_2 \geq 90\%$).

32.4 T F Permissive hypercapnia is a ventilating strategy in which the $PaCO_2$ is gradually allowed to be lowered by increasing tidal volume delivery.

32.5 T F During flow–limited, patient–triggered breaths, the inspiratory flow and trigger level can affect the patient's inspiratory work of breathing.

32.6 T F The routine use of sigh breaths during ventilatory support is highly recommended.

32.7 T F A disconnect alarm is mandatory on all ventilatory support apparatus.

32.8 T F A primary emphasis in the ventilatory support of patients with ARDS should be to keep plateau pressures elevated.

32.9 T F The main needs of patients with neuromuscular disorders who require ventilatory support include adequate lung inflation and aggressive airway management.

32.10 T F Independent lung ventilation (ILV) with LFPPV–ECCO$_2$R is the treatment of choice for ventilator management in patients with unilateral lung disease.

32.11 T F No single ventilatory support mode has proved best in treating patients with bronchopleural fistula.

32.12 T F Changing the minute ventilation in pressure–targeted modes is very much a trial and error process.

32.13 T F Oxygenation adjustments can be made by changing either the $FIO_2$ or PEEP/CPAP level.

32.14 T F a/A values below 0.15 indicate V/Q imbalances requiring simple oxygen therapy.

32.15 T F The smaller the endotracheal tube and the greater the minute ventilation, the lower the imposed work of breathing.

**Short Answer:** Complete each statement by filling in the correct information in the space(s) provided:

32.16 When used, sigh volumes normally are set at _____ times the tidal volume.

32.17 During machine–assisted, pressure–triggered breaths, the trigger level should be set _____ below the baseline pressure.

32.18 Most patients requiring uncomplicated or short–term ventilatory support can be adequately ventilated using a _____ or _____ flow pattern.

32.19 The plateau pressure should be kept below _____ cm $H_2O$ in acutely ill patients with obstructive disorders.

32.20 When mechanical hyperventilation is used to lower intracranial pressure, the target $PaCO_2$ level is typically _____ torr.

32.21 When positive pressure ventilation is applied to a patient with unilateral lung disease, most of the ventilation goes to the _____ lung.

32.22 The initial artificial airway cuff pressure should be set using either the _____ or _____ technique.

32.23 The adequacy of ventilation is assessed by measuring the patient's _____ level.

32.24 The difference between the peak and baseline or PEEP pressure is called the _____.

32.25 One of the most reliable indices of oxygenation is the _____ ratio.

32.26 Arterial hypoxemia that does not respond to high $F_{IO_2}$s is clinically known as _____.

32.27 Clinical studies have shown that decreasing the trigger level from –2 to –5 cm $H_2O$ can increase the patient's work of breathing by as much as _____.

32.28 The ideal PEEP/CPAP valve is a true _____ resistor.

**Multiple Choice:** Circle the letter corresponding to the single best answer from the available choices:

32.29 Which of the following are examples of full ventilatory support modes?
I.     PSVmax
II.    low–level PSV
III.   CMV
IV.    CPAP

a. I only                     c. I, III, and IV
b. I and III                  d. I, II, III, and IV

32.30 Partial ventilatory support modes that provide continuous distending pressure include:
I.     high rate SIMV with PEEP
II.    APRV
III.   BiPAP
IV.    CPAP

a. II and IV                  c. II, III, and IV
b. III and IV                 d. I, II, III, and IV

32.31 Patients with a combined hypercapnic and hypoxemic respiratory failure are candidates for:

a. CMV or normal rate IMV with PEEP
b. CPAP
c. low rate SIMV with PEEP
d. low level PSV with PEEP

32.32 A physician consults with an RCP regarding the use of pressure–targeted ventilation. All of the following statements are true *except:*

a. pressure–targeted ventilation guarantees a minimum minute volume
b. pressure–targeted ventilation limits and controls peak airway pressure
c. a decelerating inspiratory flow pattern is provided by most pressure–targeted modes
d. there is no firm evidence that the pressure–targeted approach results in better clinical outcomes

32.33 In order to avoid oxygen toxicity and absorption atelectasis following initiating of mechanical ventilation, the $F_{IO_2}$ should be decreased to below what level as soon as possible?

a. .70
b. .50
c. .40
d. .30

32.34 The goal in establishing a patient's minute ventilation during ventilatory support is to ensure adequate removal of $CO_2$, as judged by normalization of the:

a. mixed expired $P_{CO_2}$
b. bicarbonate
c. respiratory rate
d. arterial pH

32.35 A ventilator has separate rate and minute ventilation controls. A physician orders CMV mode ventilation with a tidal volume of 800 ml at a respiratory rate of 12/min in the CMV mode. What minute ventilation would you set on this ventilator?

a. 1700 ml/min (1.7 L/min)
b. 5800 ml/min (5.8 L/min)
c. 7500 ml/min (7.5 L/min)
d. 9600 ml/min (9.6 L/min)

32.36 A patient is receiving ventilatory support in the CMV control mode via a volume–cycled ventilator. Changes in which of the following parameters will alter this patient's $Pa_{CO_2}$?
I.     tidal volume
II.    $F_{IO_2}$
III.   rate
IV.    flow

a. II and IV                  c. I, II, and III
b. I and III                  d. I, II, III, and IV

32.37 For adolescents in the 8– to 16–year–old age range, which of the following ranges of ventilatory parameters is appropriate?

| Rate | Tidal Volume |
| --- | --- |
| a. 8–12/min | 12–15 ml/kg |
| b. 8–12/min | 8–10 ml/kg |
| c. 20–30/min | 12–15 ml/kg |
| d. 20–30/min | 8–10 ml/kg |

32.38 A physician orders intubation and mechanical ventilation in the IMV mode for a 70–kg adult male patient with a history of COPD. Which of the following parameters would be best for this patient?

| Rate | Tidal Volume |
| --- | --- |
| a. 8/min | 700 ml |
| b. 20/min | 700 ml |
| c. 12/min | 1100 ml |
| d. 16/min | 900 ml |

32.39 The inspiratory flow rate set during flow–limited ventilatory support in most adults should initially begin at:

a. equal to or greater than 20 L/min
b. equal to or greater than 40 L/min
c. equal to or greater than 60 L/min
d. equal to or greater than 90 L/min

32.40 A physician requests that the inspiratory flow be lowered on a patient with chronic airflow obstruction receiving ventilatory support in the assist–control mode, with a control rate of 16 breaths/min. What consequences might this action have?
I.    development of auto–PEEP
II.   worsening of gas exchange
III.  insufficient time for exhalation
IV.   decreased work of breathing

a. I and III
b. I, II, and IV
c. II, III, and IV
d. I, II, III, and IV

32.41 A patient suffering from postoperative complications has been receiving mechanical ventilation for 6 days via a volume–cycled ventilator. A heat and moisture exchanger (HME) is providing control over humidification and airway temperature. Over the past 24 hours, the patient's secretions have decreased in quantity but are thicker and more purulent. Which of the following actions would you suggest at this time?

a. add a second HME to the circuit
b. increase the frequency of tracheobronchial aspiration
c. switch over to a heated wick or cascade–type humidifier
d. replace the HME with a new one

32.42 Ventilatory support modes that have been reported to increase the survival of ARDS patients include all of the following except:

a. PCIRV
b. APRV
c. LFPPV–ECCO$_2$R
d. PSVmax

32.43 Guidelines for ventilatory support of ARDS patients include which of the following strategies?
I.    clinician should have experience with selected modes
II.   use empirical trials to determine minimum PEEP level
III.  increase tidal volume to 15 ml/kg
IV.   if high F$_{IO_2}$ required, accept Sa$_{O_2}$ slightly below 90%

a. I, II, and IV
b. I and IV
c. II, III, and IV
d. I, II, III, and IV

32.44 In managing patients in acute respiratory failure due to asthma, guidelines for ventilatory support include which of the following strategies?
I.    minimize plateau and peak airway pressures
II.   sedation or paralysis may be appropriate in some patients
III.  use lowest minute volume with acceptable gas exchange
IV.   monitor for and minimize auto–PEEP

a. I and IV
b. I, III, and IV
c. II, III, and IV
d. I, II, III, and IV

32.45 You are caring for a patient being ventilated in the CMV–control mode with a minute ventilation of 8.5 L/min and a Pa$_{CO_2}$ of 56 torr. If you wish to bring the Pa$_{CO_2}$ down to 40 torr, the new minute ventilation would be:

a. 13.0 L/min
b. 11.9 L/min
c. 10.0 L/min
d. 9.7 L/min

32.46 A patient receiving volume–targeted ventilation in the CMV assist–control mode has the following ABGs on an $FIO_2$ of 0.50: pH = 7.58; $Po_2$ = 70 torr; $Pco_2$ = 21 torr. The resident requests that you raise the patient's $Pco_2$. Which of the following actions would be appropriate?

a. increase the inspiratory flow
b. decrease the $O_2$ concentration
c. add mechanical deadspace
d. increase the set tidal volume

32.47 Which of the following statements is false regarding consequences of large bronchopleural fistulas (BPF)?

a. BPFs can cause atelectasis
b. BPFs can impair gas exchange
c. BPFs may prolong the need for mechanical ventilation
d. BPFs cannot be corrected surgically

32.48 During mechanical ventilatory support, the artificial airway cuff pressure at peak airway pressure should be maintained below:

a. 50 mm Hg
b. 40 mm Hg
c. 35 mm Hg
d. 25 mm Hg

32.49 You have just placed a COPD patient on ventilatory support in the IMV mode at a rate of 8/min, a tidal volume of 800 ml, and an $FIO_2$ of .40. In order to ensure proper equilibration between the alveolar and arterial gas tensions, how long should you wait before drawing a ABG?

a. 30 minutes
b. 20 minutes
c. 15 minutes
d. 10 minutes

32.50 In severe congestive heart failure, the effects of positive pressure ventilation may result in which of the following physiologic responses?
I.    decrease afterload
II.   increase left ventricular stroke volume
III.  decrease cardiac output

a. III only          c. II and III
b. I and II          d. I, II, and III

32.51 Ventilatory strategies used in the management of unilateral lung disease include which of the following?
I.    independent lung ventilation
II.   high inspiratory flows
III.  differential CPAP
IV.   bronchial blockers

a. I and II          c. I, III, and IV
b. I, II, and IV     d. I, II, III, and IV

32.52 A patient on a ventilator in the SIMV mode at a rate of 12/min has the following ABGs on an $FIO_2$ of 0.45: pH = 7.58; $Po_2$ = 88 torr; $Pco_2$ = 21 torr. The physician requests that you try to normalize the pH. Which of the following actions would be appropriate?

a. decrease the SIMV rate
b. decrease the inspiratory flow
c. increase the SIMV rate
d. increase the tidal volume

32.53 During airway pressure release ventilation, the clinician has control over which of the following parameters?
I.    baseline pressure
II.   release pressure
III.  release frequency
IV.   release time

a. I and II          c. II, III, and IV
b. II and IV         d. I, II, III, and IV

32.54 A patient has been set up to receive ventilatory assistance with BiPAP(c). The physician wants to know what the effects will be of an increased pressure differential on tidal volume delivery. Your response would be that:

a. tidal volume would tend to increase
b. tidal volume would tend to decrease
c. tidal volume would remain unchanged
d. tidal volume would initially increase, then decrease

32.55 A patient receiving pressure–targeted ventilation using APRV has the following ABGs on an $FIO_2$ of 0.40: pH = 7.25; $Pco_2$ = 55 mm Hg; $HCO_3$ = 27 mEq/L. The physician and RCP wish to increase $CO_2$ excretion. Which of the following strategies could be used?
I.    raise the baseline pressure
II.   increase the release frequency
III.  decrease the release time
IV.   lower the release pressure

a. I and III         c. II, III, and IV
b. I, II, and IV     d. I, II, III, and IV

32.56 Blood gases data for a 50–year–old man with COPD on ventilatory support at an $FIO_2$ of .40 are: pH = 7.35; $Paco_2$ = 60 mm Hg; $Pao_2$ = 50 mm Hg; barometric pressure = 760. Compute his or her a/A ratio:

a. .24
b. .30
c. .42
d. .51

32.57 The following data are gathered during a PEEP study ($FIO_2$ = 0.70):

| PEEP cm $H_2O$ | 0 | 5 | 10 | 15 | 20 | 25 |
|---|---|---|---|---|---|---|
| $Pao_2$ mm Hg | 42 | 55 | 63 | 72 | 84 | 91 |
| $Pvo_2$ mm Hg | 25 | 34 | 38 | 42 | 37 | 36 |
| $C(a-\bar{v})o_2$ Vol % | 6.2 | 6.1 | 5.7 | 4.9 | 5.6 | 6.3 |
| cardiac output L/min | 5.4 | 5.2 | 5.1 | 5.0 | 4.7 | 4.1 |
| oxygen delivery ml/min | 755 | 812 | 823 | 894 | 786 | 717 |

Based on these data, the optimum PEEP level is:

a. 5 cm $H_2O$
b. 10 cm $H_2O$
c. 15 cm $H_2O$
d. 20 cm $H_2O$

32.58 The following data are gathered during a PEEP study ($FIO_2$ = 0.60):

| PEEP cm $H_2O$ | 0 | 5 | 10 | 15 | 20 | 25 |
|---|---|---|---|---|---|---|
| $Pao_2$ mm Hg | 46 | 54 | 67 | 71 | 75 | 74 |
| compliance ml/cm $H_2O$ | 18 | 23 | 29 | 26 | 21 | 19 |
| systolic pressure | 125 | 123 | 114 | 108 | 104 | 94 |
| diastolic pressure | 90 | 88 | 83 | 75 | 76 | 68 |

Based on these data, the optimum PEEP level is:

a. 5 cm $H_2O$
b. 10 cm $H_2O$
c. 15 cm $H_2O$
d. 20 cm $H_2O$

32.59 Data for a 95–kg (209–lb) patient receiving ventilatory support are as follows:

| Ventilator Settings | | Blood Gases | |
|---|---|---|---|
| Mode | SIMV | pH | 7.43 |
| $V_T$ | 1000 ml | $Pco_2$ | 38 mm Hg |
| Rate | 8/min | $HCO_3$ | 23 mm Hg |
| $FIO2$ | 0.70 | $Pao_2$ | 43 mm Hg |

Which of the following changes would you recommend at this time?

a. raise the $V_T$ to 1200 ml
b. increase the rate to 12/min
c. apply 5 cm $H_2O$ PEEP
d. switch to assist–control

32.60 Data for a 78–kg (172–lb) patient receiving ventilatory support with 10 cm$H_2O$ PEEP are as follows:

| Ventilator Settings | | Blood Gases | |
|---|---|---|---|
| Mode | SIMV | pH | 7.34 |
| $V_T$ | 1000 ml | $Pco_2$ | 43 mm Hg |
| Rate | 8/min | $HCO_3$ | 22 mEq/L |
| $FIO2$ | 0.40 | $Pao_2$ | 145 mm Hg |

Which of the following changes would you recommend at this time?

a. lower the $V_T$ to 900 ml
b. increase the rate to 10/min
c. decrease the PEEP to 5 cm $H_2O$
d. switch to control mode

32.61 When utilizing partial ventilatory support, which of the following interventions may be useful in reducing imposed additional work on the patient?

I. using sufficient number of machine–assisted breaths
II. ensure adequate ventilator inspiratory flow rates
III. use PSV, when necessary, to augment spontaneous $V_T$

a. I only
b. I and II
c. II and III
d. I, II, and III

32.62 To determine the adequacy of machine flow, one assesses:

a. the end–tidal $CO_2$ waveform
b. the airway pressure waveform
c. the peak airway pressure
d. the exhaled minute ventilation

32.63 Factors that can prolong ventilator response time other than incorrect trigger sensitivity include which of the following?
I.    abdominal/rib cage paradox
II.   auto–PEEP
III.  low circuit deadspace
IV.   high tubing compliance

a. I and III
b. I, II, and III
c. I, II, and IV
d. I, II, III, and IV

32.64 The use of externally applied PEEP/CPAP to overcome auto–PEEP is most effective in patients with:

a. pure restrictive disorders
b. normal lungs
c. neuromuscular disorders
d. chronic airflow obstruction

## Management and Monitoring of the Patient in Respiratory Failure

## CONTENT EXERCISES

**True/False:** For each of the following statements, indicate whether it is mainly true or mainly false by circling the corresponding letter (T=True, F=False):

33.1   T   F   Changes in any variable that alter the total minute ventilation will affect the $Pa_{CO_2}$.

33.2   T   F   The Radford nomogram tends to overestimate the requirements of most patients requiring ventilatory support.

33.3   T   F   A low pressure or disconnect alarm should be incorporated into all ventilatory support systems.

33.4   T   F   Most ventilatory support systems increase insensible water loss through the lungs.

33.5   T   F   The less stable the patient, the greater the need for continuous data gathering.

33.6   T   F   The $P(A-a)O_2$ changes linearly with changes in inspired oxygen concentrations.

33.7   T   F   In order to measure the physiologic shunt, both an arterial and mixed venous blood sample must be obtained.

33.8   T   F   True end–capillary pulmonary blood cannot be sampled.

33.9   T   F   A normal mixed venous oxygen content indicates that tissue oxygenation is adequate for all body systems.

33.10   T   F   Fats produce the most $CO_2$ relative to oxygen consumption.

33.11   T   F   Ventilation must always be judged according to its effect on the pH.

33.12   T   F   Positive pressure ventilation tends to decrease physiologic deadspace.

**Short Answer:** Complete each statement by filling in the correct information in the space(s) provided:

33.13 In establishing initial ventilatory support settings, the primary aim is to stabilize the patient by providing adequate _____ and _____.

33.14 Both the patient and patient–ventilator system should be thoroughly assessed at least every _____ hours.

33.15 Patient heart rate can normally be observed continuously using the _____ monitor.

33.16 Oxygen exchange at the lung is adequate if the arterial $Po_2$ can be maintained between _____ and _____ mm Hg.

33.17 The most accurate and reliable measure of the efficiency of oxygen transfer between the lung and blood is measurement of the _____ _____.

33.18 A normal adult minute ventilation ranges between _____ and _____ liters/min.

33.19 The partial pressures gradient between the end–tidal and arterial $Pco_2$ levels is normally _____ mm Hg.

33.20 Normal individuals are able to generate a vital capacity of between _____ ml/kg.

33.21 At the bedside, the maximum voluntary ventilation (MVV) is measured over a time interval of between _____ and _____ seconds.

33.22 A reversible decrease in the force a muscle can develop during sustained or repeated contraction best defines _____.

33.23 Fatigued respiratory muscles may take anywhere from _____ to _____ hours to fully recover.

33.24 A Swan–Ganz catheter should not be maintained in the wedge position (balloon inflated) for longer than _____ seconds.

33.25 The pulmonary artery catheter is used to measure cardiac output by the _____ method.

**Matching:**

33.26 Below on the left are listed the results of several laboratory tests conducted on patients receiving respiratory care. On the right are listed possible interpretations of these results. Match each test result to the most likely interpretation:

| | Test | Result | Interpretation |
|---|---|---|---|
| ___ | a. Red blood cell count (male) | $7.4 \times 10^{-6}/mm^3$ | 1. within normal limits |
| ___ | b. Platelet count | $34,000/mm^3$ | 2. decreased $O_2$ transport |
| ___ | c. Serum chloride | 89 mEq/L | 3. hemodilution |
| ___ | d. Hemoglobin (female) | 7.8 g/dL | 4. decreased immunity |
| ___ | e. White blood cells | $22,000/mm^3$ | 5. chronic hypoxemia |
| ___ | f. Hematocrit (male) | 36% | 6. ketoacidosis |
| ___ | g. Prothrombin time (PT) | 13 seconds | 7. slow blood clotting |
| ___ | h. Serum sodium | 140 mEq/L | 8. metabolic acidosis |
| ___ | i. Creatinine | 3.9 mg/dL | 9. infection |
| ___ | j. Glucose | 212 mg/dL | 10. metabolic alkalosis |
| ___ | k. Serum potassium | 6.1 mEq/L | 11. renal failure |

**Multiple Choice:** Circle the letter corresponding to the single best answer from the available choices:

33.27 The most common medical complication of ventilatory support is:

a. hyper/hypoventilation
b. pneumothorax
c. hypotension
d. gastric distention

33.28 After intubating a patient in respiratory failure, a physician orders continuous mechanical ventilation. Before connecting the ventilator to the patient, you must:
I.   verify proper functioning of the device
II.  establish the initial ventilator settings
III. draw and analyze an arterial blood gas

a. I and II          c. I only
b. I and III         d. I, II, and III

33.29 Which of the following would you assess immediately after a patient is placed on a ventilatory support device?
I.   patient's airway
II.  patient's vital signs
III. patient's appearance
IV.  arterial blood gases

a. II and IV         c. III and IV
b. I, II, and III    d. I, II, III, and IV

33.30 Prior to drawing an arterial blood sample, you note that a patient has significantly elevated prothrombin and partial thromboplastin times (PT and PTT). Which of the following actions would be appropriate in this situation?

a. obtain a venous sample instead of an arterial one
b. allow extra time after the procedure to ensure hemostasis
c. use extra heparin in preparing the sampling syringe
d. switch to a larger bore (12 g) needle to obtain the sample

33.31 Which of the following clinical laboratory tests indicate potential renal failure?
I.   blood urea nitrogen of 58 mg/dL
II.  blood creatinine of 4.3 mg/dL
III. blood glucose of 100 mg/dL

a. I and II          c. I and III
b. II and III        d. I, II, and III

33.32 A patient receiving ventilatory support has a reported serum potassium of 2.1 mEq/L. Which of the following would you be on guard for with this patient?

I.    cardiac arrhythmias
II.   ketoacidosis
III.  metabolic alkalosis

a. I and II
b. II and III
c. I and III
d. I, II, and III

33.33 Which of the following methods may be used to monitor and guide a critically ill patient's fluid balance?

I.    pulmonary arterial pressure monitoring
II.   measurement of patient weight
III.  central venous pressure monitoring
IV.  fluid intake and output (I/O)

a. II and IV
b. I, II, and III
c. III and IV
d. I, II, III, and IV

33.34 Which of the following is *false* regarding nutrition and the respiratory care of patients receiving ventilatory support?

a. $O_2$ consumption/$CO_2$ production are unaffected by nutrient intake
b. malnutrition can occur commonly in critically ill patients
c. critically ill patients often have decreased nutrient intake
d. nutritional status can affect the ability to wean a patient

33.35 In which of the following patients would transcutaneous $Po_2$ ($Ptco_2$) monitoring most likely provide inaccurate or erroneous results?

a. a patient in hypovolemic shock
b. a newborn infant with RDS
c. a patient with hypoxemia
d. a patient with hyperpyrexia

33.36 You find that the Hb saturation readings for a patient being monitored by a bedside oximeter are consistently inaccurate when compared with an actual lab oximeter measurement on a blood sample. Which of the following would you check to determine the causes of this inconsistency?

I.    the lab oximeter report (for abnormal hemoglobins)
II.   the lighting conditions in the patient's room
III.  the alignment of the sensor's emitter/detector
IV.  the size of the sensor relative to its position

a. I and III
b. I, II, and III
c. III and IV
d. I, II, III, and IV

33.37 In evaluating the oxygenation status of a patient just placed on ventilatory support with an $F_{IO_2}$ of 1.0, you compute a $P(A - a)o_2$ of 400 mm Hg. Based on this data, this patient's percent physiologic shunt (Qs/Qt) is about:

a. 10%
b. 20%
c. 30%
d. 40%

33.38 Which of the following patients has the most serious problem with oxygenation?

| Patient | $F_{IO_2}$ | $Pao_2$ |
| --- | --- | --- |
| a. A | 1.00 | 85 |
| b. B | 0.70 | 90 |
| c. C | 0.40 | 95 |
| d. D | 0.28 | 65 |

33.39 With all else being equal, under which of the following conditions will the mixed venous oxygen content ($C\overline{v}o_2$) of a patient's blood decrease?

I.    when tissue oxygen uptake ($Vo_2$) increases
II.   when the arterial oxygen content ($Cao_2$) falls
III.  when cardiac output ($Q_T$) increases

a. I and II
b. II and III
c. I and III
d. I, II, and III

33.40 Which of the following are false regarding sampling of mixed venous blood for oxygen?

a. usually the $P\overline{v}o_2$ or $S\overline{v}o_2$ are used to assess tissue oxygenation
b. mixed venous blood indicates the adequacy of $O_2$ delivery and uptake
c. sampling is from the distal port of a pulmonary artery catheter
d. samples must be withdrawn slowly and with the balloon inflated

33.41 Tissue oxygenation is considered inadequate if the mixed venous hemoglobin saturation ($S\overline{v}o_2$) falls below:

a. 85%
b. 80%
c. 75%
d. 50%

33.42 In which of the following clinical circumstances can the use of mixed venous oxygen parameters to assess tissue oxygenation be misleading?

I. septic shock
II. cyanide poisoning
III. ARDS

a. I and II
b. II and III
c. I and III
d. I, II, and III

33.43 On analysis of the ABG reports for a patient receiving ventilatory support in the control mode, you note that her $Paco_2$ has been increasing over the last 8 hours, despite the fact that her minute ventilation has remained constant. Which of the following could explain this finding?

I. the patient has become febrile
II. physiologic deadspace has increased
III. lung compliance has increased

a. I and II
b. II and III
c. I and III
d. I, II, and III

33.44 The normal end–tidal $CO_2$ percentage as measured by capnography ranges between:

a. 4.6 and 5.6%
b. 8.6 and 9.8%
c. 35 and 45%
d. 0 and 4.5%

33.45 A patient being monitored by capnography has a measured arterial $Pco_2$ of 40 mm Hg but an end–tidal $Pco_2$ of 30 mm Hg. Which of the following best explains this difference?

a. the patient has an abnormal increase in pulmonary blood flow
b. the patient has an increase in physiologic deadspace (high V/Q)
c. there must be a leak somewhere in the sampling or analysis system
d. an arterial to end–tidal $CO_2$ gradient of this magnitude is normal

33.46 After gathering a concurrent mixed expired and arterial $Pco_2$ sample from a spontaneously breathing patient, you record the following: $PaPco_2$ = 48 mm Hg; $P_{\overline{E}}co_2$ = 20 mm Hg; average $V_T$ = 600 ml; and apparatus deadspace = 75 ml. What is this patient's physiologic deadspace ($V_{Dphy}$)?

a. 250 ml
b. 275 ml
c. 300 ml
d. 325 ml

33.47 Which of the following is *false* regarding analysis of the mixed expired $Pco_2$ ($P_{\overline{E}}co_2$) on patients receiving positive pressure ventilation?

a. a large–volume (greater than 10 L) collection bag is used
b. the deadspace of the collecting apparatus must be accounted for
c. the collected $P_{\overline{E}}co_2$ will be higher than the actual patient value
d. the ventilator's compressed volume contributes to the expired gas

33.48 Which of the following patients is least likely to be able to maintain adequate $CO_2$ removal at a tolerable level of ventilation?

| Patient | $V_D/V_T$ |
| --- | --- |
| a. A | 0.33 |
| b. B | 0.42 |
| c. C | 0.56 |
| d. D | 0.71 |

33.49 Assuming all else is equal, which of the following adult patients has the least efficient ventilation?

| Patient | $\dot{V}_E$ | $Paco_2$ |
| --- | --- | --- |
| a. A | 14.1 L/min | 42 mm Hg |
| b. B | 8.4 L/min | 35 mm Hg |
| c. C | 6.5 L/min | 29 mm Hg |
| d. D | 9.2 L/min | 45 mm Hg |

33.50 A patient receiving CMV with 8 cm $H_2O$ PEEP has a corrected $V_T$ of 740 ml, a peak pressure of 68 cm $H_2O$, and a plateau pressure during pause (EIP) of 53 cm $H_2O$. What is her effective compliance (Ceff)?

a. 5 ml/cm $H_2O$
b. 10 ml/cm $H_2O$
c. 12 ml/cm $H_2O$
d. 16 ml/cm $H_2O$

33.51 You measure the effective compliance (Ceff) of a patient receiving continuous mandatory ventilation at 11 AM to be 60 ml/cm $H_2O$. Two hours later, her Ceff is 30 ml/cm $H_2O$. Which of the following are possible causes of this change?
I.    developing atelectasis
II.   acute pulmonary edema
III.  a tension pneumothorax

a. I and II                c. I and III
b. II and III              d. I, II, and III

33.52 In patients receiving ventilatory support, the pressure necessary to overcome airway resistance is estimated by measuring the:

a. difference between the peak and atmospheric pressure
b. difference between the peak and the plateau pressure
c. difference between the peak and PEEP pressure
d. difference between the plateau pressure and PEEP pressure

33.53 At 8 AM you estimate the airway resistance ($R_{aw}$) of a patient receiving CMV to be 8 cm $H_2O$/L/sec. Two hours later, his estimated $R_{aw}$ is 20 cm $H_2O$/L/sec. Which of the following are possible causes of this change?
I.    pulmonary vascular congestion
II.   increased secretions
III.  bronchospasm
IV.   partial tube occlusion

a. II and IV              c. III and IV
b. I, II, and III         d. I, II, III, and IV

33.54 Over a two–hour period, you note that a patient's peak and plateau pressures have both been steadily increasing, but the difference between the two remains about the same. Which of the following is the best explanation for this observation?

a. the patient has increased secretions
b. the patient's compliance has decreased
c. the patient is developing bronchospasm
d. the patient's airway resistance has increased

33.55 Which of the following methods can be used at the bedside for assessing the respiratory muscle strength or endurance of a patient in respiratory failure?
I.    maximum voluntary ventilation (MVV)
II.   effective compliance (Ceff)
III.  forced vital capacity (VC)
IV.   maximum inspiratory force (MIF)

a. II and IV              c. I, III, and IV
b. I, II, and III         d. I, II, III, and IV

33.56 Which of the following is *false* regarding the bedside measurement of vital capacity (VC) when used to assess a patient's respiratory muscle strength or endurance?

a. results of the vital capacity maneuver are effort–independent
b. accurate results can be obtained only on cooperative patients
c. results are obtained using a mechanical or electronic spirometer
d. normal individuals can generate a VC of about 65 to 75 ml/kg

33.57 It is unlikely that a patient can support spontaneous ventilation for prolonged time periods when the vital capacity (VC) falls below:

a. 10–15 ml/kg
b. 25–35 ml/kg
c. 45–55 ml/kg
d. 55–65 ml/kg

33.58 In order to assure maximum stimulation when using the airway occlusion method to measure inspiratory force (MIF; NIF; $P_{Imax}$), you should occlude the airway for:

a. 5 seconds
b. 10 seconds
c. 20 seconds
d. 30 seconds

33.59 Which of the following maximum inspiratory force (MIF; NIF) measures taken on adult patients indicates that the respiratory muscle strength is not sufficient to support adequate spontaneous ventilation?

a. $-100$ cm $H_2O$
b. $-90$ cm $H_2O$
c. $-20$ cm $H_2O$
d. $-70$ cm $H_2O$

33.60 In observing a patient's pattern of breathing, you note that the abdomen moves outward while the lower rib cage moves inward during inspiration. Which of the following descriptions would you put in the respiratory notes?

a. "patient exhibits inspiratory retractions"
b. "patient exhibits asynchronous breathing"
c. "patient exhibits paradoxical breathing"
d. "patient exhibits normal breathing pattern"

33.61 Before performing puncture or cannulation of the radial artery, the practitioner should:

a. fix and tighten a tourniquet above the antecubital fossa
b. inject heparin into the adjoining subcutaneous tissues
c. apply firm pressure to the arterial site for 5 minutes
d. perform the Allen test to ensure collateral circulation

33.62 A physician requests that you obtain and set up an arterial line system for invasive monitoring of blood pressure. Which of the following equipment would you gather?
I.   a pressurized IV bag
II.  a continuous flush device
III. an arterial catheter
IV.  a pressure transducer
V.   an amplifier/monitor

a. I, III, and IV
b. II, III, IV, and V
c. I, II, IV, and V
d. I, II, III, IV, and V

33.63 In the arterial pressure waveform of a patient displayed on a bedside monitor, you observe a slight rebound or upward swing in pressure soon after the peak systolic level. Which of the following best explains this observation?

a. an upward swing after peak systole indicates aortic insufficiency
b. this rebound is abnormal, probably due to measurement artifact
c. this rebound is normal, marking opening of the AV valves
d. this rebound is normal, marking closure of the aortic valve

33.64 A patient has a systolic arterial pressure of 145 mm Hg and a diastolic pressure of 100 mm Hg. Her estimated mean arterial pressure (MAP) is:

a. 45 mm Hg
b. 122 mm Hg
c. 115 mm Hg
d. 245 mm Hg

33.65 In assessing the arterial line system of a patient in ICU, you note that blood has begun to flow back into the continuous flush device. Which of the following is the most likely cause of this problem?

a. the patient is developing hypotension or shock
b. the IV bag is not sufficiently pressurized
c. the catheter has become blocked by a blood clot
d. the pressure transducer is placed too high

33.66 In a patient with a brachial artery catheter in place, you note loss of a palpable radial pulse. Which of the following is the most likely cause of this problem?

a. arterial thrombosis distal to the cannula
b. blood loss into the subcutaneous tissues
c. blockage of the catheter by a blood clot
d. slippage of the catheter out of the artery

33.67 Complications of arterial cannulation include which of the following?
I.   infection
II.  embolization
III. hemorrhage
IV.  nerve damage

a. II and IV
b. I, II, and III
c. II and III
d. I, II, III, and IV

33.68 Through which of the following pulmonary artery catheter channels would you obtain a mixed venous blood sample?

a. the distal (catheter tip) channel
b. the proximal (right atrium) channel
c. the catheter thermistor connector
d. the accessory injection port

33.69 Failure to deflate the balloon on a pulmonary artery catheter after taking a wedge pressure reading can result in which of the following?

a. left ventricular failure
b. pulmonary infarction
c. tension pneumothorax
d. myocardial infarction

33.70 The normal range for the pulmonary artery wedge pressure (PAWP) as measured via the distal port of a Swan–Ganz catheter (with the balloon inflated) is:

a. 15–30 mm Hg
b. 5–16 mm Hg
c. 4–12 mm Hg
d. 10–22 mm Hg

33.71 Which of the following is not a potential cause of increased right atrial (RA) or CVP pressures?

a. cardiac tamponade
b. peripheral vasodilation
c. tricuspid stenosis
d. right ventricular failure

33.72 A patient has a mean pulmonary artery (PA) pressure of 34 mm Hg. Which of the following are possible causes of this finding?
I.      increased pulmonary vascular resistance
II.     decreased circulating blood volume
III.    left ventricular failure

a. II and III          c. I and III
b. I and II           d. I, II, and III

33.73 In order to obtain an accurate pulmonary artery wedge pressure (PAWP) from a patient receiving positive pressure ventilatory support, you should:

a. measure the PAWP at peak inspiration
b. remove the patient from the ventilator
c. advance the catheter at least 3–5 cm
d. measure the PAWP at the end of exhalation

33.74 A patient has an arterial $O_2$ content ($CaO_2$) of 18.5 ml/dL, a mixed venous $O_2$ content ($C\bar{v}O_2$) of 12.5 ml/dL, and an end–capillary $O_2$ content ($CcO_2$) of 20.5 ml/dL. What is his percent shunt?

a. 5%
b. 10%
c. 15%
d. 25%

33.75 An adult patient in ICU has bilateral infiltrates on chest x–ray and the following hemodynamic profile: systemic arterial pressure = decreased; systemic vascular resistance = increased; cardiac output = decreased; pulmonary artery pressure = increased; pulmonary artery wedge pressure = increased. What is the most likely cardiovascular problem?

a. left ventricular failure
b. adult respiratory distress syndrome
c. septic shock
d. dehydration

33.76 Complications associated with the use of pulmonary artery catheters include which of the following?
I.      thromboses
II.     cardiac arrhythmias
III.    pneumothorax
IV.     infection

a. II and IV          c. III and IV
b. I, II, and III      d. I, II, III, and IV

33.77 You are called by the coronary care charge nurse to check on a patient being supported by a volume–cycled ventilator. You note that both the low tidal volume and high pressure limit alarm are sounding on each inspiration. You first action should be to:

a. call the attending physician for further patient information
b. check the patient's chart for the original ventilator orders
c. increase the preset tidal volume to 1.5x the current setting
d. disconnect patient and provide manual ventilation with 100% $O_2$

33.78 When responding to an alarm on a patient receiving ventilatory support in the IMV mode, you note that the low exhaled minute volume indicator is flashing. Which of the following are possible causes for this condition?

I. a large leak in the patient–ventilator system
II. a decrease in the patient's spontaneous ventilation
III. a malfunctioning alarm/indicator system
IV. a change in the set frequency or tidal volume

a. II and IV
b. I, II, and III
c. III and IV
d. I, II, III, and IV

33.79 In assessing a patient receiving IMV on a Siemens Servo 900C ventilator, you note an increase in her spontaneous breathing rate and minute ventilation ($\dot{V}_E$). Which of the following are possible causes for this change?

I. agitation or irritation
II. increased metabolic demand
III. hypoxia
IV. CNS depression

a. II and IV
b. I, II, and III
c. III and IV
d. I, II, III, and IV

33.80 When performing a routine ventilator check, you note several potentially harmful discrepancies between the ventilator's current settings and those previously specified in the most recent physician's orders. The patient's attending physician is not available. Which of the following actions would be appropriate in this case?

a. ask the patient's nurse to write a new order to update the changes
b. record the new changes on the flowsheet and note "awaiting update"
c. ask the pulmonary resident to write an order to update the changes
d. restore the parameters back to their previously documented values

33.81 When performing a routine ventilator check, you note that the airway temperature indicator reads 26°C. The flowsheet indicates a prior temperature of 35°C. Which of the following could explain this discrepancy?

I. addition of cool water to the humidifier
II. alteration in the thermostat setting
III. failure of the thermostat mechanism

a. II only
b. II and III
c. I and III
d. I, II, and III

33.82 Which of the following will decrease the likelihood of successful weaning of a patient from ventilatory support?

I. poor muscle strength
II. use of sedatives
III. high–protein diet
IV. excessive secretions

a. II and IV
b. I, II, and IV
c. III and IV
d. I, II, III, and IV

33.83 Which of the following five adult patients receiving ventilatory support is the best candidate for weaning?

| Patient | $V_C$ | $\dot{V}_E$ | MVV | NIF | $V_D/V_T$ | % Shunt |
|---|---|---|---|---|---|---|
| a. | 0.5 L | 4.1 L | 6.3 L | –21 cm $H_2O$ | 0.49 | 16% |
| b. | 1.5 L | 4.6 L | 9.7 L | –33 cm $H_2O$ | 0.45 | 17% |
| c. | 0.9 L | 12.1 L | 14.3 L | –28 cm $H_2O$ | 0.76 | 12% |
| d. | 1.3 L | 6.3 L | 16.7 L | –42 cm $H_2O$ | 0.39 | 28% |

33.84 Which of the following statements regarding auto–PEEP are true:

I. auto–PEEP cannot be identified by standard observation of airway pressure
II. detection is aided by visualizing expiratory flow tracings
III. measurement is made by performing an end–expiratory hold maneuver
IV. the incidence of auto–PEEP in mechanically ventilated patients is low

a. II and IV
b. I, II, and III
c. I and II
d. I, II, III, and IV

## Labeling:

33.85 Below is a low–speed capnograph tracing for a patent receiving mechanical ventilation.

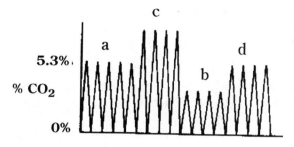

**Figure 33–1** Low–speed capnograph tracing for a patent receiving mechanical ventilation

For each of the four labeled stages of the tracing (a – d), specify whether the patient's alveolar ventilation is normal, excessive (hyperventilation), or insufficient (hypoventilation):

a. _____

b. _____

c. _____

d. _____

33.86 Below are three pressure–volume curves obtained from a patient receiving mechanical ventilatory support.

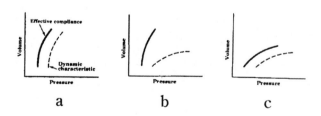

**Figure 33–2** Pressure volume curves

Assuming that Figure 33–3a is normal, indicate for b and c (1) whether the primary problem is a change in resistance or compliance; (2) the direction of the change (increased/decreased); and (3) at least two possible causes for the change identified:

b.
1. _____

2. _____

3. _____

c.
1. _____

2. _____

3. _____

33.87 Below are pictured three plethysmographic tracings of rib cage (RC) and abdominal (Ab) motion plotted against tidal volume ($V_T$).

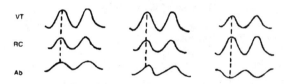

**Figure 33–3** Motion of rib cage and abdomen

Match each tracing label (a – c) on the left (Figure 33–3) to the proper breathing pattern description on the right below:

a. _____    paradoxical breathing

b. _____    normal pattern

c. _____    asynchronous breathing

33.88 Below on the left are arterial line pressure tracings obtained from six patients in an ICU. Label each tracing by the cardiovascular disorder most likely present for that patient:

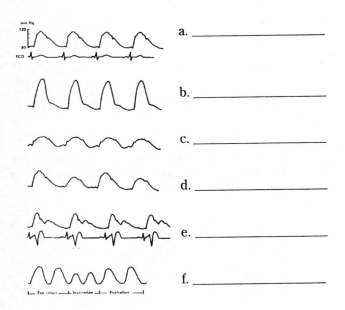

a. _____

b. _____

c. _____

d. _____

e. _____

f. _____

33.89 Below is a pressure tracing obtained while a physician was inserting a Swan–Ganz pulmonary artery catheter in a patient in ICU:

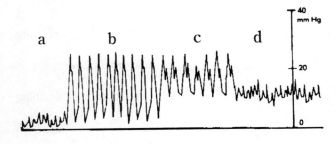

**Figure 33–5** Pressure tracing with Swan–Ganz catheter

Match each pressure tracing component (a – d) to the location from which that pressure was obtained:

a. _____     PA wedge pressure

b. _____     pulmonary artery

c. _____     right atrium

d. _____     right ventricle

# CHAPTER
## 34

# Discontinuing Ventilatory Support

## CONTENT EXERCISES

**True/False:** For each of the following statements, indicate whether it is mainly true or mainly false by circling the corresponding letter (T=True, F=False):

34.1 T F Removing most patients from ventilatory support is a relatively quick and easy process.

34.2 T F The primary reason why patients cannot be removed from ventilatory support is an imbalance between ventilatory demand and ventilatory capacity.

34.3 T F Neurologically, most patients undergoing withdrawal of ventilatory support have a normal or decreased drive to breathe.

34.4 T F A muscle's endurance is best described as its ability to sustain work load over time.

34.5 T F Too high a carbohydrate load can decrease the respiratory quotient and lower $CO_2$ production.

34.6 T F The airway occlusion pressure is the inspiratory pressure measured 100 milliseconds after airway occlusion.

34.7 T F Oxygen cost of breathing represents the sum of oxygen consumption during both spontaneous and controlled ventilation.

34.8 T F Patients who fail spontaneous breathing trials tend to exhibit significantly greater asynchrony and paradox than those having a successful outcome.

34.9 T F Psychologic factors are a minor determinant of outcome in patients requiring prolonged ventilatory support.

34.10 T F Patients who exhibit anxiousness and psychotic behavior from sleep deprivation are poor candidates for withdrawal from ventilatory support.

34.11 T F Use of rapid weaning protocols are not common among postoperative cardiac surgery patients receiving ventilatory support.

34.12 T F The use of flow–triggered spontaneous ventilation is a reasonable alternative to traditional T–tube trials.

34.13 T F Mandatory minute ventilation, or MMV, guarantees a constant minute volume and is adjusted automatically by end–tidal $CO_2$ monitors.

34.14 T F Changes in end–tidal $P_{CO_2}$ do not always reflect changes in arterial $P_{CO_2}$ during weaning.

**Short Answer:** Complete each statement by filling in the correct information in the space(s) provided:

34.15 The process of slowly reducing ventilatory support is commonly referred to as _____.

34.16 Two aspects of muscle performance affecting ventilatory capacity are _____ and _____.

34.17 In terms of respiratory muscle endurance, normal individuals can sustain about _____ % of their maximum voluntary ventilation for extended periods of time.

34.18 Regarding feeding strategies, most patients should receive a daily caloric intake between _____ and _____ times their resting energy expenditure.

34.19 The most widely used weaning technique and most common primary mode of ventilation is _____ _____.

34.20 During weaning from mechanical ventilation, changes in $Pa_{CO_2}$ levels are common in the range of _____ mm Hg or torr.

34.21 The single most important cause of ventilator dependency is _____.

**Multiple Choice:** Circle the letter corresponding to the single best answer from the available choices:

34.22 Key factors which hinder the "science" of weaning include:

I. limited ability to accurately predict who will wean
II. no one superior technique for weaning identified
III. majority of clinicians do not understand ventilators

a. I only
b. I and II
c. I and III
d. I, II, and III

34.23 Several studies of general medical and surgical patients undergoing ventilatory support have shown that weaning success occurs in better than:

a. 60% or 6 out of 10
b. 70% or 7 out of 10
c. 80% or 8 out of 10
d. 90% or 9 out of 10

34.24 Which of the following contributing factors may contribute to ventilator dependence?

I. arterial hypoxemia
II. malnutrition
III. psychologic dependence
IV. cardiovascular instability

a. I and IV
b. II and III
c. I, II, and III
d. I, II, III, and IV

34.25 A patient's ventilatory demand is primarily determined by which of the following factors?

I. metabolic rate
II. CNS drive
III. internal locus of control
IV. ventilatory deadspace

a. I and II
b. II, III, and IV
c. I, II, and IV
d. I, II, III, and IV

34.26 Factors which may decrease ventilatory drive include all of the following *except:*

a. hypothyroidism
b. metabolic acidosis
c. sleep deprivation
d. starvation

34.27 Prolonging the decision to begin the ventilator withdrawal process has the potential to:

I. result in lower morbidity
II. result in psychologic stress
III. result in increased cost of care
IV. result in improved patient satisfaction

a. II only
b. I, III, and IV
c. II and III
d. I, II, III, and IV

34.28 Which of the following questions should clinicians ask in order to identify patients who are clearly not ready to be weaned?

I. is the patient getting better?
II. is the initial reason for providing support being resolved?
III. is the patient clinically stable?
IV. is the patient's insurance company requesting intervention?

a. I and III
b. II and IV
c. I, II, and III
d. I, II, III, and IV

34.29 Patients exhibiting which of the following physical signs are considered clinically unstable and require further ventilatory support?

I. pulse rate over 120 or under 70/min
II. presence of palpable scalene muscle during inspiration
III. presence of palpable abdominal tensing during expiration
IV. presence of an irregular breathing pattern

a. I and IV
b. I, II, and III
c. II, III, and IV
d. I, II, III, and IV

34.30 Which of the following measures are included in the CROP score?

I. dynamic compliance
II. respiratory frequency (spontaneous)
III. arterial–to–alveolar oxygen tension ratio
IV. maximum inspiratory pressure

a. II and IV
b. I and III
c. I, III, and IV
d. I, II, III, and IV

34.31 Physical signs associated with stress and anxiety in the ventilated patient include:

I. increased heart rate
II. diaphoresis
III. constricted and fixed pupils
IV. hypertension

a. I, II, and III
b. I, II, and IV
c. II, III, and IV
d. I, II, III, and IV

34.32 All of the following are the primary methods available for withdrawing patients from ventilatory support *except:*

a. T–tube trials
b. pressure support ventilation
c. assist–control ventilation
d. intermittent mandatory ventilation

34.33 While monitoring a patient during a traditional T–tube weaning trial, you note the following: increased patient agitation; increased heart rate (from 85 to 110/min); and increased respiratory rate (from 15 to 34/min with some paradoxical motion). Which of the following actions would be appropriate at this time?

a. encourage the patient to relax and continue careful monitoring
b. reconnect the patient to the ventilator with prior settings
c. request that the patient be given a strong sedative/hypnotic
d. conduct a full bedside assessment of ventilatory mechanics

34.34 Indications for the use of rapid weaning protocols in clinical practice include:
I.   following surgery where heavy anesthesia was used
II.  neuromuscular disorders resulting in respiratory failure
III. uncomplicated cases of narcotic drug overdose
IV.  acute exacerbations of COPD lasting a week or longer

a. I and III        c. II, III, and IV
b. I and II         d. I, II, III, and IV

34.35 All of the following statements are reasons for applying CPAP during T–tube weaning *except:*

a. CPAP may support oxygenation during transition from mechanical support to spontaneous breathing
b. CPAP replaces the glottic closure mechanism during expiration, helping to prevent airway collapse
c. CPAP improves phrenic nerve function and strengthens nerve impulse conduction
d. CPAP reduces the inspiratory work of breathing without increasing end–expiratory lung volume

34.36 Which are poor candidates for weaning via IMV?
I.   patients with chronic obstructive pulmonary disease
II.  patients who are unstable and cannot be monitored closely
III. patients with CNS depression or impaired respiratory drive

a. I and II         c. I and III
b. II and III       d. I, II, and III

34.37 An alert patient receiving ventilatory support in the IMV mode at a rate of 10/min and a tidal volume of 800 ml has stable vital signs and satisfactory blood gases on an $F_{IO_2}$ of 0.40. In order to initiate weaning for this patient, you would:

a. switch to the assist–control mode
b. decrease the tidal volume to 600 ml
c. decrease the mandatory rate to 6–8/min
d. increase the oxygen concentration to 50%

34.38 Proponents of IMV as a weaning tool argue which of the following clinical advantages?
I.   maintains respiratory muscle function
II.  lowers mean airway pressure
III. helps prevent asynchronous breathing
IV.  prevents respiratory alkalosis

a. I and IV         c. I, III, and IV
b. I, II, and IV    d. I, II, III, and IV

34.39 When using pressure support ventilation for weaning, the amount of work performed by the patient is adjusted by altering:

a. inspiratory flow
b. breathing frequency
c. level of inspiratory pressure
d. level of tidal volume

34.40 Examples of mechanical ventilators capable of providing mandatory minute ventilation include:
I.   Engstrom Erica
II.  Bear 1000
III. Hamilton Veolar
IV.  Siemens Servo 900C

a. I and IV         c. I, III, and IV
b. I, II, and III   d. I, II, III, and IV

34.41 Potential disadvantages of computer–based weaning include which of the following?
I. algorithm may induce nonphysiologic breathing patterns
II. adequate target value can be difficult to adjust
III. target variable may give false information if other data not examined

a. I only
b. I and II
c. II and III
d. I, II, and III

34.42 A failed weaning attempt is usually indicated when the $PaO_2$ increases:

a. greater than 30 torr above baseline
b. greater than 10 torr above baseline
c. greater than 40 torr above baseline
d. greater than 20 torr above baseline

34.43 Indicators of adequate upper airway function in postoperative patients include which of the following?
I. MIP > –40 cm $H_2O$
II. MEP > 60 cm $H_2O$
III. FRC > 15 ml/kg
IV. deep cough on suctioning

a. I and II
b. II, III, and IV
c. I, II, and IV
d. I, II, III, and IV

34.44 Common clinical conditions that can hinder weaning include:
I. anemia
II. pain
III. infection/sepsis
IV. bronchospasm

a. I, II, and IV
b. II and III
c. II, III, and IV
d. I, II, III, and IV

34.45 Basic criteria used for confirming cardiovascular stability include all of the following *except:*

a. systolic blood pressure 80–180 mm Hg
b. no major arrhythmias present
c. hemoglobin 12–15 mg/dL
d. radial artery pulse equal bilaterally

34.46 A patient is undergoing clinical evaluation of hemodynamic performance prior to ventilator weaning. In the presence of poor ventricular reserve, an abrupt transition to spontaneous breathing can actually worsen cardiac function due to:

a. decreased right heart preload
b. vasodilation of systemic arteries
c. increased left ventricular afterload
d. decreased right ventricular end–diastolic pressure

34.47 Metabolic imbalances can impair weaning by:

a. increasing ventilatory demand in the presence of metabolic acidosis
b. decreasing muscle load in the presence of metabolic acidosis
c. increasing ventilatory drive in the presence of metabolic alkalosis
d. increasing muscle load in the presence of normal blood pH

34.48 A patient being evaluated for withdrawal of ventilatory support has the following electrolyte values: $Mg^{++}$ = 1.2 mg/dL; $Po_4^{++}$ = 1.3 mg/dL; $K^+$ = 2.5 mEq/dL. The physician asks what your recommendation would be. Which of the following actions would you recommend?

a. correct only the $K^+$ level since it is too high
b. all of the electrolyte values are abnormal and require correction
c. increase the $Mg^{++}$ level to normal range
d. decrease the $Po_4^+$ to 1.0 mg/dL since it is too high

34.49 Which of the following statements regarding airway occlusion pressure or $P_{0.1}$ are true?
I. $P_{0.1}$ correlates with central respiratory drive
II. Patients with COPD who fail weaning have $P_{0.1} \geq$ 6 cm $H_2O$
III. $P_{0.1}$ measurement requires patient cooperation
IV. $P_{0.1}$ is effort–independent

a. I and II
b. II, III, and IV
c. I, II, and IV
d. I, II, III, and IV

34.50 All of the following statements regarding the ratio of spontaneous breathing frequency to tidal volume ($f/V_T$) are true *except:*

a. predictive power is less for patients on ventilator > 8 days
b. may not be useful in predicting weaning success among elderly
c. the threshold criterion is 100 breaths/min/L
d. values greater than 110 indicate successful weaning

34.51 Which of the following five adult patients receiving ventilatory support is the best candidate for weaning?

| Patient | VC | $\dot{V}_E$ | MVV | MIF | $V_D/V_T$ | % Shunt |
|---------|------|--------|--------|----------------|-----------|---------|
| a. A | 0.7 L | 5.4 L | 7.1 L | −18 cm $H_2O$ | 0.65 | 11% |
| b. B | 1.5 L | 4.6 L | 9.7 L | −33 cm $H_2O$ | 0.45 | 17% |
| c. C | 0.9 L | 12.1 L | 14.3 L | −28 cm $H_2O$ | 0.76 | 12% |
| d. D | 1.3 L | 6.3 L | 16.7 L | −42 cm $H_2O$ | 0.39 | 28% |

34.52 Newer measured indices used to predict weaning success include all of the following *except:*

a. airway occlusion pressure ($P_{0.1}$)
b. the rapid–shallow breathing index ($f/V_T$ ratio)
c. oxygen cost of breathing (OCB)
d. static compliance

34.53 Studies of the mechanical work of breathing in patients receiving ventilatory support indicate successful weaning is unlikely unless spontaneous work levels are below:

a. 1.6 kg m/min
b. 2.0 kg m/min
c. 3.2 kg m/min
d. 4.0 kg m/min

34.54 Examples of multivariate indices used to identify factors affecting patient's responses to withdrawal from ventilatory support include:
I.     CROP index
II.    WINNER score
III.   adverse/ventilator score
IV.   WI or weaning index

a. I and II
b. I, II, and III
c. I, III, and IV
d. I, II, III, and IV

# 35

# Neonatal and Pediatric Intensive Care

## CONTENT EXERCISES

**True/False:** For each of the following statements, indicate whether it is mainly true or mainly false by circling the corresponding letter (T=True, F=False):

35.1 (T) F  Maternal blood and fetal blood never physically mix.

35.2 T (F)  Fetal hemoglobin is normally completely replaced by adult hemoglobin within the first four to six days of life.

35.3 (T) F  The fetal lung is normally filled with liquid to a volume equivalent to the FRC.

35.4 (T) F  The normal newborn infant achieves normal gas exchange within the first 12 to 24 hours of life.

35.5 T (F)  In proportion to the body as a whole, the head of the infant is smaller than the adult head.

35.6 T (F)  The anatomic deadspace of the newborn is proportionately larger than the adult's.

35.7 (T) F  When exposed to severe hypoxemia, a newborn responds with either a decrease in ventilation or apnea.

35.8 T (F)  LGA infants (those weighing over 4000 g at birth) have lower mortality rates than normal term babies.

35.9 T (F)  Most conditions leading to respiratory distress are immediately apparent at birth.

35.10 T (F)  Grunting is the most common of all signs of respiratory distress in infants.

35.11 T (F)  Fetal capillary samples provide useful information on blood oxygenation.

35.12 (T) F  Critically ill newborn infants tend to be more susceptible to developing nosocomial infections than adults.

35.13 (T) F  In some critically ill neonates it is impossible to maintain an acceptable level of arterial oxygenation without dangerously high $FIO_2$s.

35.14 (T) F  Ideally, $FIO_2$s delivered to newborn infants should be analyzed continuously.

35.15 (T) F  CPAP can decrease lung compliance in some infants, especially in those with hyaline membrane disease.

35.16 (T) F  Leaving an endotracheal tube in place without CPAP is contraindicated in infants being treated for respiratory distress syndrome.

35.17 T (F)  Too high a level of PEEP can increase right–to–left shunting in some infants.

35.18 (T) F  Infants with severe meconium aspiration syndrome are among the most difficult to ventilate.

35.19 (T) F  Definitive diagnosis of hyaline membrane disease is usually made by chest x–ray.

35.20 (T) F  High mean airway pressures do not usually affect blood pressure and cardiac output in infants with hyaline membrane disease.

35.21 T (F)  Apnea of prematurity is usually of the obstructive type.

35.22 T (F)  Bronchopulmonary dysplasia develops over a much shorter course than hyaline membrane disease.

35.23 (T) F  The best treatment of bronchopulmonary dysplasia is prevention.

35.24 (T) F  SIDS is the leading cause of death in infants less than one year old in the United States.

35.25 (T) F  The role of the RCP during transport is to assist in pulmonary stabilization and airway management.

**Short Answer:** Complete each statement by filling in the correct information in the space(s) provided:

35.26 Fetal blood which is freshly oxygenated in the placenta returns to the fetus via the _umbilical Vein_.

35.27 The major factor aiding $O_2$ uptake by fetal blood at the placenta is _HBf_.

35.28 Most of the blood entering the fetal pulmonary circulation is shunted from the main pulmonary artery to the descending aorta via the _Ductus Arteriosus_.

35.29 The length of the normal newborn trachea averages _3_ centimeters. _5–6_

35.30 The newborn infant must generate a transpulmonary pressure gradient of about _40 cm H2o_ cm $H_2O$ before inflation with air can begin.

35.31 Normal tidal volumes (adjusted for body weight) in newborn infants are approximately ___3___ ml per kilogram. 6~7

35.32 The average frequency of breathing in the normal full–term newborn is __20~40__ per minute. 40-60

35.33 Fetal lung maturity (the existence of a stable pathway for surfactant production) is indicated when the lethicin to sphingomyelin (L/S) ratio first rises above __2:1__ .

35.34 A "term" infant is born between __38__ and __42__ weeks' gestation.

35.35 The maximum time limit for application of suction to a small infant is ____5____ seconds.

35.36 The minimum flow through an infant oxyhood system should be no less than __6-10__ liters per minute. 7

35.37 A vacuum setting of __80-100__ mm Hg should be used for nasopharyngeal or nasotracheal suctioning of a neonate. -60 - -80

35.38 The most common cause of hypercapnic respiratory failure in newborn infants is a __depressed__ resp. Drive correct .

35.39 The initial inspiratory time range recommended for newborn infants being placed on time–cycled, pressure–limited ventilation is between __.4__ and __.5__ seconds. -.2. - -.5

35.40 A condition in which the fetus inhales amniotic fluid containing bowel contents best describes ____ __Meconium aspiration__ .

35.41 Most cases of bronchiolitis are caused by ____ __RSV__ .

35.42 ____ECmo____ is a form of cardiopulmonary bypass used to provide gas exchange.

35.43 __Surfactant Replacement__ is recommended for small infants (<1350 g) and for larger infants who show signs of pulmonary immaturity.

**Labeling:**

35.44 Match the structures listed on the right to the letter labels corresponding to the components of the fetal circulation in the following diagram:

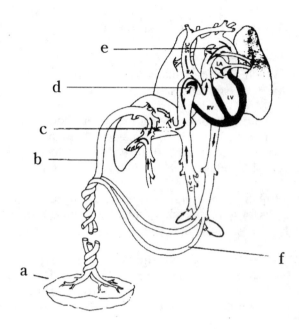

| | | |
|---|---|---|
| a. | __placenta__ | ductus venosus |
| b. | __UV__ | foramen ovale |
| c. | __DV__ | ductus arteriosus |
| d. | __FO__ | placenta |
| e. | __DA__ | umbilical arteries |
| f. | __UA__ | umbilical vein |

**Multiple Choice:** Circle the letter corresponding to the single best answer from the available choices:

35.45 The umbilical cord of the fetus contains:

a. one umbilical vein and one umbilical artery
b. one umbilical vein and two umbilical arteries
c. two umbilical veins and two umbilical arteries
d. two umbilical veins and one umbilical artery

35.46 Abnormalities of the placenta which may cause intrauterine growth retardation or fetal asphyxia include which of the following?

I.    uteroplacental insufficiency
II.   placenta previa
III.  abruptio placenta

a. I and II
b. II and III
c. I and III
d. I, II, and III

35.47 Which of the following is *false* regarding maternal–fetal exchange at the placenta?

a. maternal drugs may move across intervillous space
b. certain bacteria and viruses may cross the placenta
c. maternal oxygen readily diffuses to fetal blood
d. maternal blood and fetal blood mix with each other

35.48 Which of the following represent normal blood gas values for a sample taken from the umbilical vein of a term fetus?

a. pH = 7.35; $P_{CO_2}$ = 42 mm Hg; $P_{O_2}$ = 30 mm Hg
b. pH = 7.33; $P_{CO_2}$ = 46 mm Hg; $P_{O_2}$ = 16 mm Hg
c. pH = 7.35; $P_{CO_2}$ = 46 mm Hg; $P_{O_2}$ = 16 mm Hg
d. pH = 7.33; $P_{CO_2}$ = 42 mm Hg; $P_{O_2}$ = 75 mm Hg

35.49 In the fetal heart, the foramen ovale allows blood to flow from the:

a. right atrium to right ventricle
b. right atrium to left atrium
c. right atrium to left ventricle
d. pulmonary artery to aortic arch

35.50 Which of the following is *false* regarding the fetal pulmonary circulation?

a. less than 10% of the pulmonary flow perfuses the lungs
b. mean pulmonary artery pressure exceeds mean aortic pressure
c. most of the pulmonary flow is shunted into the aorta
d. due to low $P_{O_2}$s, pulmonary vascular resistance is low

35.51 Which of the following factors stimulate a newborn infant to breathe?

I.    tactile stimulus
II.   acidosis
III.  hypoxia
IV.  thermal stimulus

a. II and IV
b. I, II, and III
c. III and IV
d. I, II, III, and IV

35.52 With initiation of breathing and proper lung expansion, the newborn infant's $Pa_{O_2}$ increases, while the $Pa_{CO_2}$ decreases and the pH rises back toward normal. In combination, these changes cause which of the following?

I.    a decrease in pulmonary vascular resistance
II.   an increase in pulmonary vascular blood flow
III.  constriction of the ductus arteriosus

a. I and II
b. II only
c. I and III
d. I, II, and III

35.53 Compared with an adult's, which of the following is *false* regarding the upper airway of infants?

a. the epiglottis is longer and less flexible
b. the tongue is larger relative to the oral cavity
c. the nasal passages are proportionately smaller
d. the larynx is positioned lower in the neck

35.54 Which of the following are true regarding lung development after birth?

I.    respiratory units increase in number as an infant ages
II.   the number of alveoli at 8–10 years is similar to an adult's
III.  airways increase in size as the infant develops and ages
IV.  after 8–10 years alveoli grow mainly in size, not number

a. I, II, and III
b. II and IV
c. II, III, and IV
d. I, II, III, and IV

35.55 Which of the following are true regarding the pattern of breathing commonly observed among premature or preterm infants?

I.    frequent periods of short duration apnea are common
II.   periodic breathing is common during sleep or feeding
III.  apneic spells are often accompanied by tachycardia
IV.  apneic spells are due to a decreased response to $CO_2$

a. II and IV
b. II and III
c. I, II, and IV
d. I, II, III, and IV

35.56 The specific compliance of a neonate's lung is:

a. one–tenth that of an adult
b. one–fifth that of an adult
c. about the same as an adult
d. one–half that of an adult

35.57 Fetal ultrasonography can provide information useful in assessing all of the following *except:*

a. the presence of major anatomic anomalies
b. the qualitative status of the amniotic fluid
c. fetal growth and gestational age
d. the state of pulmonary maturation

35.58 While observing the fetal heart rate monitor of a woman in labor, you note that the heart rate tends to drop well after the onset of uterine contractions. Which of the following is the most likely cause of this observation?

a. failure of the lung to complete maturation
b. vagal stimulation due to head compression
c. short periods of umbilical cord compression
d. impaired maternal blood flow to the placenta

35.59 A scalp capillary blood sample obtained from a fetus during the later stages of labor has a pH of 7.17. Which of the following conclusions can you draw from this information?
I. a combined respiratory and metabolic acidosis is present
II. anerobic metabolism is causing lactic acidosis buildup
III. the probability of fetal tissue hypoxia is high

a. I and II
b. II and III
c. I and III
d. I, II, and III

35.60 At 1 minute after birth, a newborn infant exhibits the following: heart rate of 65; a slow and irregular respiratory rate; some muscle flexion; a grimace when nasally suctioned; and a pink body with blue extremities. What is this infant's 1 minute Apgar score?

a. 2
b. 3
c. 4
d. 5

35.61 Which problems are common to small preterm babies?
I. their high body surface area/weight ratio promotes heat loss
II. their immature vasculature is more prone to hemorrhage
III. their lungs are not yet fully prepared for gas exchange
IV. their immune system is not fully able to fight infection

a. II and IV
b. I, II, and III
c. III and IV
d. I, II, III, and IV

35.62 Which of the following is *false* regarding infant "grunting"?

a. grunting increases airway pressure during expiration
b. grunting occurs only in hyaline membrane disease
c. grunting prevents airway closure and alveolar collapse
d. grunting is exhalation against a partially closed glottis

35.63 While observing a newborn infant breathe, you note indrawing of chest wall between the ribs and below the sternum during inspiration. Which of the following conclusions is most consistent with this observation?

a. airway resistance is less than normal
b. pulmonary (lung) compliance is increased
c. total impedance to breathing is increased
d. the infant has hyaline membrane disease

35.64 Which of the following arterial blood gas results would be considered within normal limits for a normal preterm infant 1 hour after birth?

a. pH = 7.29; $P_{CO_2}$ = 51 mm Hg; $HCO_3$ = 22 mEq/L; BE = –4; $P_{O_2}$ = 57 mm Hg
b. pH = 7.33; $P_{CO_2}$ = 35 mm Hg; $HCO_3$ = 20 mEq/L; BE = –5; $P_{O_2}$ = 69 mm Hg
c. pH = 7.35; $P_{CO_2}$ = 36 mm Hg; $HCO_3$ = 20 mEq/L; BE = –3; $P_{O_2}$ = 79 mm Hg
d. pH = 7.38; $P_{CO_2}$ = 43 mm Hg; $HCO_3$ = 23 mEq/L; BE = –1; $P_{O_2}$ = 83 mm Hg

35.65 A right radial arterial blood sample in a newborn infant has a $P_{O_2}$ of 69 mm Hg, while the umbilical artery $P_{O_2}$ is 56 mm Hg. Which of the following best explains this difference?

a. the higher temperature of the umbilical artery sample
b. a left–to–right shunt through a patent foramen ovale
c. a right–to–left shunt through a patent ductus arteriosus
d. the lower partial pressure of $CO_2$ of the radial sample

35.66 A newborn infant will require a precise and stable $F_{IO_2}$ for at least 5 to 7 days. Which of the following devices would you recommend to provide $O_2$ to this infant?

a. mask
b. catheter
c. isolette
d. oxyhood

35.67 In setting up an oxyhood system using an oxygen blender and a heated "all–purpose" nebulizer to deliver an $F_{IO_2}$ of 0.40, you would set the nebulizer entrainment port to:

a. 28%
b. 40%
c. 60%
d. 100%

35.68 Potential hazards of high partial pressures of oxygen administered to infants include which of the following?
I.   bronchopulmonary dysplasia
II.  retrolental fibroplasia
III. oxygen toxicity

a. I and II              c. I and III
b. II and III            d. I, II, and III

35.69 Adjunctive methods to clear secretions mobilized with chest physical therapy are always needed in infants and small children because:

a. infants and small children do not have a cough reflex
b. their airways are too small to allow effective coughing
c. infants and small children cannot generate a cough on command
d. their expiratory muscles are too weak for effective coughing

35.70 Which of the following size (internal diameter) endotracheal tubes would you select to intubate a 2300–gram newborn infant?

a. 2.5 mm
b. 3.5 mm
c. 4.5 mm
d. 5.5 mm

35.71 Which of the following French size catheters would you use to suction an infant with a 3.5 mm ID endotracheal tube in place?

a. 5 Fr
b. 6 Fr
c. 8 Fr
d. 10 Fr

35.72 When using a mask to ventilate a small infant, which of the following should the practitioner avoid?
I.   keeping the mouth open under the mask
II.  forcefully raising the mandible (jaw)
III. overextending the head and neck

a. I and II              c. I and III
b. II and III            d. I, II, and III

35.73 Which of the following is *false* regarding infant endotracheal tubes?

a. malpositioning of the head can cause tube obstruction
b. infant endotracheal tube diameters are very small
c. infant endotracheal tubes normally come with cuffs
d. infant tubes can be easily kinked or obstructed

35.74 Which of the following are true regarding infant intubation?
I.   the MacIntosh (curved) laryngoscope blade is normally used
II.  small tube movements can result in endo-bronchial intubation
III. the distance between the cords and carina is very small
IV.  tube stabilization is essential to prevent extubation

a. II and IV             c. II, III, and IV
b. I, II, and III        d. I, II, III, and IV

35.75 Signs of infant respiratory distress indicating a potential need for CPAP include which of the following?
I.   cyanosis on 50% or more $O_2$
II.  an x–ray indicating RDS
III. grunting on expiration
IV.  severe inspiratory retractions

a. III and IV            c. II, III, and IV
b. I, II, and III        d. I, II, III, and IV

35.76 The oximetry saturation readings of an infant receiving CPAP via nasal prongs with an $F_{IO_2}$ of 0.40 drop substantially during frequent episodes of crying. Which of the following actions would you recommend in this situation?

a. switch to CPAP via an endotracheal tube
b. increase the CPAP level by 2–4 cm $H_2O$
c. place the infant in an oxyhood with 40% $O_2$
d. increase the oxygen concentration to 50%

35.77 An infant with respiratory distress syndrome is placed on 5 cm $H_2O$ nasal CPAP at an $F_{IO_2}$ of 0.50. After five minutes, grunting, retractions, and cyanosis are still present. A peripheral ABG cannot be obtained, and blood gas analysis will have to await umbilical artery catheterization. Which of the following actions would you recommend at this time?

a. increase the CPAP pressure to 7 cm $H_2O$
b. increase the oxygen concentration to 60%
c. decrease the CPAP pressure to 3 cm $H_2O$
d. decrease the oxygen concentration to 40%

35.78 Hazards and complications of infant CPAP include which of the following?
I. overdistention/decreased compliance
II. impedance to venous return
III. increased intracranial pressures
IV. increased physiologic deadspace
V. increased risk of barotrauma

a. II, III, IV, and V
b. I, III, and IV
c. III, IV, and V
d. I, II, III, IV, and V

35.79 All of the following are true regarding time–cycled, pressure–limited ventilation in infants *except:*

a. when the exhalation valve is open, spontaneous breathing can occur
b. pressure stays constant as long as gas flows out the relief valve
c. with the pressure relief open, gas continues to flow into the lungs
d. system pressure rises until the preset pressure limit is reached

35.80 Which of the following would you expect to occur if the endotracheal tube of an infant receiving time–cycled, pressure–limited ventilation became kinked or plugged?

a. the pressure limit alarm–indicator would actuate
b. cycling would continue, no volume would be delivered
c. the ventilator inoperative alarm–indicator would actuate
d. the apnea alarm would actuate, opening the relief valve

35.81 A time–cycled, pressure–limited ventilator is set as follows on a 3.5–kg infant: inspiratory time = 0.4 sec; flow = 8 L/min. If you were to set the pressure limit above that required to deliver this flow over the duration of inspiration, what tidal volume would this device deliver?

a. 32 ml
b. 41 ml
c. 53 ml
d. 77 ml

35.82 By setting the rate and I:E ratio on an infant ventilator with separate controls for these values, which of the following parameters will result?
I. inspiratory flow
II. inspiratory time
III. expiratory time

a. I and II
b. II and III
c. I and III
d. I, II, and III

35.83 In order to ensure adequate alveolar ventilation and elimination of $CO_2$ in a newborn infant receiving time–cycled, pressure–limited ventilation, what initial breathing frequency or rate would you recommend?

a. 10–20/min
b. 20–30/min
c. 30–40/min
d. 40–50/min

35.84 An infant receiving time–cycled, pressure–limited ventilation at a rate of 40/min has a $P_{CO_2}$ of 58 mm Hg and a pH of 7.21. Which of the following changes in ventilatory support parameters would you recommend at this time?

a. increase the preset rate of breathing
b. increase the inspiratory pressure limit
c. decrease the preset inspiratory time
d. apply 6–8 cm $H_2O$ PEEP to the system

35.85 What initial range of peak inspiratory pressure (PIP) would you suggest for a newborn infant being placed on time–cycled, pressure–limited ventilation?

a. 5–10 cm $H_2O$
b. 10–15 cm $H_2O$
c. 15–20 cm $H_2O$
d. 20–25 cm $H_2O$

35.86 If you were to increase the flow setting during time–cycled, pressure–limited ventilation of an infant, which of the following would occur?

a. the duration of the pressure plateau would increase
b. the tidal volumes delivered to the infant would increase
c. the infant's spontaneous ventilatory demands would not be met
d. the rate at which inspiratory pressure rises would decrease

35.87 In observing the airway pressure manometer of a ventilator providing continuous flow IMV support to an infant, you note negative deflections of –2 to –4 cm $H_2O$ during spontaneous breathing efforts. Which of the following actions would you recommend at this time?

a. increase the flow
b. increase the pressure limit
c. increase the inspiratory time
d. decrease the pressure limit

35.88 All of the following ventilatory support components pose high risk to infants *except:*

a. peak pressures above 30 cm $H_2O$
b. PEEP levels greater than 8 cm $H_2O$
c. $F_{IO_2}$s greater than 0.7
d. breathing rates above 30/min

35.89 Ventilatory support parameters for an infant being weaned include: an $F_{IO_2}$ of 0.45; a peak pressure (PIP) of 38 cm $H_2O$; a PEEP level of 6 cm $H_2O$; a rate of 30/min; and an inspiratory time (ti) of 0.5 sec. Which of these parameters would you recommend trying to reduce first?

a. the $F_{IO_2}$
b. the PIP
c. the PEEP level
d. the rate

35.90 Ventilatory support parameters for an infant being weaned include: an $F_{IO_2}$ of 0.40; a peak pressure of 20 cm $H_2O$; a PEEP level of 5 cm $H_2O$; a rate of 15/min; and an inspiratory time of 0.4 sec. Assuming that blood gases are acceptable on these settings, which of the following actions would you now recommend?

a. switch the infant to 5 cm $H_2O$ CPAP
b. decrease the PEEP level to 2 cm $H_2O$
c. decrease the breathing rate to 5/min
d. increase the peak pressure to 25 cm $H_2O$

35.91 Arterial blood gas analysis of the infant with meconium aspiration syndrome (MAS) will usually show which of the following?

a. hypoxemia with an acute respiratory acidosis only
b. hypoxemia with a mixed respiratory and metabolic acidosis
c. hypoxemia with an acute metabolic acidosis only
d. hypoxemia with a mixed respiratory and metabolic alkalosis

35.92 When meconium–stained amniotic fluid is present at birth, the likelihood of the infant progressing to true meconium aspiration syndrome (MAS) can be minimized by:

a. immediate administration of supplemental oxygen
b. vigorous chest physical therapy/suctioning after birth
c. vigorous oropharyngeal suctioning before the first breath
d. immediate administration of corticosteroids

35.93 Despite CPAP at 10 cm $H_2O$ with an $FIO_2$ of 0.45, an infant with meconium aspiration syndrome (MAS) develops a progressively worsening hypoxemia and respiratory acidosis. Which of the following actions would you recommend at this time?

a. increase the CPAP system pressure to 12 cm $H_2O$ and $FIO_2$ to 0.50
b. ventilate with short expiratory times and high peak pressures
c. administer an organic buffer like THAM to restore the pH
d. ventilate with short inspiratory times and low peak pressures

35.94 The severe hypoxemia seen in hyaline membrane disease (HMD) or respiratory distress syndrome (RDS) can lead to which of the following additional problems?
I.    increased pulmonary vascular resistance
II.   increased cardiac right–to–left shunting
III.  impaired pulmonary surfactant production

a. II and III          c. I and III
b. I and II            d. I, II, and III

35.95 Findings characteristic of the chest x–ray in infants with respiratory distress syndrome (RDS) or newborn respiratory distress syndrome include which of the following?
I.    reticulogranular densities
II.   hyperlucency at the bases
III.  air bronchograms

a. I and II          c. I and III
b. II and III        d. I, II, and III

35.96 Despite nasal CPAP at 10 cm $H_2O$ with an $FIO_2$ of 0.50, an infant with respiratory distress syndrome (RDS) still has unsatisfactory arterial oxygenation. Which of the following actions would you recommend at this time?

a. increase CPAP system pressure to 12 cm $H_2O$ and $FIO_2$ to 0.55
b. intubate, provide mechanical ventilatory support with PEEP
c. intubate, provide endotracheal CPAP at 10 cm $H_2O$ and 50% $O_2$
d. intubate and provide pressure support ventilation at 10 cm $H_2O$

35.97 An adjunctive therapy for hyaline membrane disease (neonatal respiratory distress syndrome) which appears to show promise as a rescue treatment is:

a. parenteral high carbohydrate nutrition
b. vitamin E replacement therapy
c. mechanical ventilation at low frequencies
d. surfactant replacement therapy

35.98 A few hours after birth, a term infant develops tachypnea and mild hypoxemia but has a normal pH and $Paco_2$. The chest x–ray shows some hyperinflation with perihilar streaking. The infant responds well to low $FIO_2$s by hood. Which of the following is the most likely problem?

a. transient tachypnea of the newborn
b. apnea of prematurity
c. hyaline membrane disease
d. bronchopulmonary dysplasia

35.99 Which of the following statements is *false* regarding treatment of apnea of prematurity?

a. apnea of prematurity responds well to the methyl-xanthines
b. severe or recurrent apnea may require mechanical ventilation
c. continuous respiratory and heart rate monitoring is essential
d. CPAP is contraindicated for apnea of prematurity

35.100 Factors implicated in the pathogenesis of bronchopulmonary dysplasia (BPD) include which of the following?
I.    positive pressure ventilation
II.   oxygen toxicity
III.  pulmonary immaturity

a. I and II          c. I and III
b. II and III        d. I, II, and III

35.101 According to the National Institutes of Health (NIH), home cardiopulmonary monitoring of infants is medically indicated for all of the following groups *except:*

a. infants with a history of prior severe life–threatening events
b. preterm infants with apnea of prematurity ready for discharge
c. infants with conditions such as central hypoventilation
d. preterm infants with no major cardiopulmonary symptoms

35.102 exhibits persistent respiratory distress despite good systemic hydration and oxygen therapy, the next step is usually:

a. administration of aerosolized ribavirin (Virazole)
c. intubation and mechanical ventilatory support
d. nasal continuous positive airway pressure
b. administration of an adrenergic bronchodilator

35.103 The normal regimen for administration of aerosolized ribavirin (Virazole) to an infant with bronchiolitis is:

a. 4–6 hours of aerosolization per day via oxyhood for 3–7 days
b. 12–18 hours of aerosolization per day via oxyhood for 3–7 days
c. 4–6 hours of aerosolization per day via face mask for 3–7 days
d. 6–8 hours of aerosolization per day via oxyhood for 1–2 days

35.104 Administration of aerosolized ribavirin (Virazole) to ventilator–dependent children must be done with caution because:

a. precipitation of the aerosol often plugs the endotracheal tube
b. drug aerosolization via ventilator circuits causes bronchospasm
c. ventilator–dependent children poorly tolerate aerosolized drugs
d. precipitation of the aerosol can clog the expiratory valve

35.105 Management of the child with mild to moderate croup may involve all of the following *except:*

a. cool mist therapy
b. supplemental oxygen administration
c. intubation and mechanical ventilation
d. corticosteroid administration

35.106 The primary etiologic agent causing epiglottitis is:

a. *Streptococcus pyogenes*
b. *Staphylococcus aureus*
c. *Klebsiella pneumoniae*
d. *Haemophilus influenzae*

35.107 Clinical manifestations of epiglottitis include which of the following?
I.      high fever
II.     cyanosis
III.    labored breathing
IV.     "barky" cough
V.      dysphagia

a. I, II, IV, and V          c. III and IV
b. I, II, III, and V         d. I, II, III, IV, and V

35.108 Immediate management of the child with diagnosed epiglottitis involves:

a. placement in the prone position, with neck hyperextended
b. intubation under general anesthesia by a skilled practitioner
c. immediate bacterial culture and sensitivity testing
d. initiation of cool mist therapy with supplemental oxygen

35.109 Late complications of cystic fibrosis include which of the following?
I.      cor pulmonale
II.     bronchiectasis
III.    tracheomalacia

a. I and II                  c. I and III
b. II and III                d. I, II, and III

35.110 All of the following are inclusion criteria for neonatal ECMO *except:*

a. irreversible lung disease
b. gestational age >35 weeks
c. no preexisting cerebral hemorrhage
d. significant shunting

35.111 All of the following are considered congenital cardiac defects *except:*

a. tetrology of Fallot
b. ventricular septal defect
c. Wilson–Mikity syndrome
d. patent ductus arteriosus

# 36

## Health Education and Health Promotion

### CONTENT EXERCISES

**True/False:** For each of the following statements, indicate whether it is mainly true or mainly false by circling the corresponding letter (T=True, F=False):

36.1  T  F  Most of the infectious diseases that ravaged Americans in the early 1900s have been eradicated.

36.2  T  F  Peak Performance USA is an AARC program designed to bring better asthma care to the nation's children.

36.3  T  F  Diseases related to the environment are now the leading cause of death in the United States.

36.4  T  F  The public is generally unaware of the impact of poor health habits on health and quality of life.

36.5  T  F  Many consumers tend to view the health care delivery system as the solution for all matters pertaining to health.

36.6  T  F  The most effective means for reducing premature mortality and morbidity is greater attention to acute care.

36.7  T  F  Achievement of a "healthy people" requires collaborative effort among multiple health–related disciplines.

36.8  T  F  Health promotion assumes that health status depends mainly on external factors beyond an individual's control.

36.9  T  F  The value individuals place on health determines the extent to which they follow a recommended health regimen.

36.10 T  F  For health education to be successful, participants must be actively engaged in the learning process.

36.11 T  F  Health education activities must not attempt to influence the values and health beliefs of the learners.

36.12 T  F  An individual's self–esteem can inhibit the ability to make sound health behavior decisions.

36.13 T  F  The development of unhealthy behaviors never begins until adulthood.

36.14 T  F  The family plays a crucial role in developing and maintaining the well–being of its members.

**Short Answer:** Complete each statement by filling in the correct information in the space(s) provided:

36.15  At least _____ of American adults smoke cigarettes, are overweight, and/or do not exercise regularly.

36.16  Throughout this century, the organization and delivery of health care has been based mainly on the _____ model.

36.17  The medical model asserts that disease and disability arise _____ of the individual.

36.18  _____ includes measures which can be used by the government and other agencies, as well as by industry, to protect people from harm.

36.19  When individuals experience _____ , they have achieved and are maintaining a balance in integrating all six dimensions.

**Listing:** Complete each list as directed in its statement.

36.20  List six (6) simple behaviors that can significantly increase individual life expectancy:

1. _____

2. _____

3. _____

4. _____

5. _____

6. _____

36.21 List the six (6) dimensions of health recognized by supporters of holistic health care:

1. _____

2. _____

3. _____

4. _____

5. _____

6. _____

**Multiple Choice:** Circle the letter corresponding to the single best answer among the available choices:

36.22 Major causes of disease and disability include:
I.     human biological factors
II.    inadequate health care
III.   unhealthy lifestyles
IV.    environmental hazards

a. II and IV                 c. I and III
b. I, II, and III            d. I, II, III, and IV

36.23 Which of the following is *false* regarding lifestyle behaviors and health?

a. much heart disease and cancer is related to lifestyle patterns
b. only a small percentage of Americans have unhealthy lifestyles
c. life expectancy can be increased by following simple behaviors
d. over half of all deaths are related to unhealthy lifestyles

36.24 Under the medical model of health care, primary responsibility for preserving, maintaining, and restoring health rests with:

a. the individual consumer
b. insurance companies
c. the health care system
d. one's family members

36.25 Which of the following assumptions underlie the medical model of health care?
I.     sick people should be treated by the medical care system
II.    disease and disability arise outside of the individual
III.   sick people are not responsible for their conditions
IV.    unhealthy lifestyles are a major factor in disease

a. II and IV                 c. I and III
b. I, II, and III            d. I, II, III, and IV

36.26 Based on the medical model, the U.S. health care delivery system has become increasingly characterized by which of the following?
I.     specialization of health care providers
II.    treatment that focuses on curing disease
III.   a high reliance on medical technology

a. I and II                  c. II only
b. II and III                d. I, II, and III

36.27 Primary health services provided to individuals by health care professionals best describes which of the following components of health promotion and disease prevention?

a. health protection
b. preventive services
c. health promotion
d. public health

36.28 Measures used by the government and other agencies, as well as industry, to safeguard people from harm best describes which of the following components of health promotion and disease prevention?

a. health promotion
b. diagnostic services
c. health protection
d. preventive services

36.29 Activities designed to foster healthy lifestyles among individuals or communities best describes which of the following?

a. health promotion
b. preventive services
c. health protection
d. public health services

36.30 Which of the following activities are included with the concept of health promotion?
I. high–level wellness
II. holistic health care
III. disease prevention

a. I and II
b. II and III
c. II only
d. I, II, and III

36.31 That dimension of health consisting of one's level of fitness and biological functioning (including the existence of disease or predisposing risk factors) best describes:

a. physical health
b. social health
c. spiritual health
d. mental health

36.32 That dimension of health concerned with the quality of interaction and level of satisfaction with interpersonal relationships best describes:

a. spiritual health
b. emotional health
c. vocational health
d. social health

36.33 That dimension of health consisting of one's ability to express appropriate feelings best describes:

a. vocational health
b. mental health
c. emotional health
d. social health

36.34 Which of the following dimensions of health is generally difficult to define or understand?

a. physical health
b. spiritual health
c. social health
d. vocational health

36.35 Vocational health includes all of the following *except*:

a. sharing of work experience with others
b. gaining recognition for one's contributions
c. believing in some unifying source
d. achieving financial success and advancement

36.36 The chief responsibility for primary disease prevention rests with:

a. the individual (oneself)
b. the health professional
c. one's family members
d. one's employer

36.37 Activities designed to enhance or ensure the well–being of healthy individuals best describes:

a. primary disease prevention
b. high–level wellness programs
c. tertiary disease prevention
d. health behavior assessment

36.38 Which of the following are good examples of primary disease prevention activities?
I. choosing not to smoke
II. eating a balanced diet
III. breast self–examination
IV. wearing seat belts

a. II and IV
b. I, II, and III
c. I, II, and IV
d. I, II, III, and IV

36.39 Early diagnosis and periodic disease screening are components of:

a. primary disease prevention
b. high–level wellness programs
c. tertiary disease prevention
d. secondary disease prevention

36.40 Major responsibility for secondary prevention activities (such as early diagnosis and disease screening) rests with:
I. the health care consumer
II. the immediate family
III. the health care provider
IV. the employing agency

a. II and IV
b. I, II, and III
c. I and III
d. I, II, III, and IV

36.41 Which of the following is *not* an example of secondary disease prevention?

a. pulmonary function screening
b. periodic pap smears
c. breast self–examination
d. pulmonary rehabilitation

36.42 Good examples of tertiary disease prevention include:
I.   pulmonary rehabilitation
II.  cardiac rehabilitation
III. periodic eye examinations

a. I and II                 c. II only
b. II and III               d. I, II, and III

36.43 Efforts to rehabilitate and restore functioning to an individual and to minimize any further consequences of disease or disability best describes:
a. health behavior assessment
b. primary disease prevention
c. high–level wellness programs
d. tertiary disease prevention

36.44 A process of planned learning opportunities designed to enable individuals to make decisions and act on information affecting their health best describes:

a. health education
b. vocational counseling
c. health promotion
d. disease prevention

36.45 Which of the following factors must be assessed in planning a health education program?
I.   factors that reinforce healthy behaviors
II.  factors that predispose healthy behaviors
III. factors that enable healthy behaviors

a. I and II                 c. II only
b. II and III               d. I, II, and III

36.46 Which of the following is *false* regarding health education?

a. health education activities are directed toward individuals
b. health education aims to make healthy behaviors involuntary
c. health education programs use multiple methods and strategies
d. health education programs require careful preliminary assessment

36.47 Which of the following is *not* a specific social indicator useful in assessing the quality of life in a population targeted for health education?

a. unemployment rates
b. welfare data
c. sex distribution
d. population statistics

36.48 Nonhealth factors contributing to an individual or group's quality of life include which of the following?
I.   employment
II.  transportation
III. race/ethnicity
IV.  education

a. I, II, and III           c. II and III
b. II and IV                d. I, II, III, and IV

36.49 Nonbehavioral causes of chronic lung disease include all of the following *except:*

a. family history
b. air pollution
c. smoking
d. genetic defect

36.50 Variables such as an individual's knowledge, attitudes, values, and perceptions regarding health best describe which major category of factors impacting on health education programming?

a. enabling factors
b. self–esteem factors
c. reinforcing factors
d. predisposing factors

36.51 Variables such as the availability of resources, accessibility of resources, and requisite skills and knowledge best describe which major category of factors impacting on health education programming?

a. economic factors
b. reinforcing factors
c. predisposing factors
d. enabling factors

36.52 Variables such as the attitudes and behavior of health personnel or significant others (peers, parents, and employers) best describe which major category of factors impacting on health education programming?

a. economic factors
b. self–esteem factors
c. enabling factors
d. reinforcing factors

36.53 The ultimate test of the effectiveness of a health education program is whether it:

a. increases participants' knowledge of healthy behaviors
b. results in participants' satisfaction with the program
c. affects behaviors causally related to health outcomes
d. attends to participants' individual values and beliefs

36.54 A good example of respiratory care professionals aiding in the primary prevention of lung disease is:

a. providing pulmonary rehabilitation programs
b. providing pulmonary function screening
c. participating in assessing work site hazards
d. providing smoking awareness/cessation programs

36.55 A good example of respiratory care professionals aiding in the secondary prevention of lung disease is:

a. participating in exercise stress testing
b. providing pulmonary function screening
c. participating in assessing work site hazards
d. providing pulmonary rehabilitation programs

36.56 A good example of respiratory care professionals aiding in the tertiary prevention of lung disease or disability is:

a. providing pulmonary rehabilitation programs
b. participating in exercise stress testing
c. participating in assessing work site hazards
d. providing smoking awareness/cessation programs

36.57 Which of the following benefits can health promotion at the work site help achieve?
I.    reduced employee absenteeism
II.   increased productivity
III.  lower insurance costs
IV.   increased job satisfaction

a. II and IV            c. I and III
b. I, II, and III       d. I, II, III, and IV

36.58 In order to develop effective health education programs involving the family, the respiratory care practitioner must be sensitive to which of the following?
I.    socioeconomic status
II.   level of education
III.  race/ethnicity
IV.   cultural background

a. II and IV            c. I and III
b. I, II, and III       d. I, II, III, and IV

36.59 Which of the following statements are true regarding the DHHS Administration on Aging (AoA)?
I.    AoA supports state and local efforts to address health care
II.   AoA addresses economic and social concerns of older Americans
III.  AoA programs fall outside the scope of health promotion involvement for RCPs

a. I and II             c. II and III
b. II only              d. I, II, and III

## PROBLEMS FOR THOUGHT AND DISCUSSION

The AARC believes that respiratory care practitioners, in addition to striving to render the highest quality of care, should assume leadership and advocacy roles in public respiratory health. Describe some practical ways in which you could assume either a leadership or advocacy role in health promotion or disease prevention.

A local middle school has asked you to develop a smoking awareness/cessation program for its 7th graders. Specify how you would go about planning this program to meet the needs of the participants. (Hint: Apply a program development process like that described in the chapter.)

# 37

# Pulmonary Rehabilitation

## CONTENT EXERCISES

**True/False:** For each of the following statements, indicate whether it is mainly true or mainly false by circling the corresponding letter (T=True, F=False):

37.1   T   F   As more survive the acute phases of various illnesses, there are increasing numbers of individuals with chronic disorders.

37.2   T   F   Patients with various chronic cardiopulmonary disorders have little in common.

37.3   T   F   Sufficient trained personnel and physical facilities exist to meet the needs for pulmonary rehabilitation.

37.4   T   F   Comprehensive home care cannot succeed without complementary pulmonary rehabilitation efforts.

37.5   T   F   Pulmonary rehabilitation benefits include significant changes in pulmonary function.

37.6   T   F   Long–term results of pulmonary rehabilitation are contradictory and often difficult to interpret.

37.7   T   F   Rehabilitation must focus on the patient as a whole.

37.8   T   F   Traditional pulmonary function measures are the best predictors of the likelihood of a COPD patient being rehospitalized.

37.9   T   F   When the anaerobic threshold is exceeded, energy production increases.

37.10  T   F   The muscles of a COPD patient consume less oxygen per work unit than normal.

37.11  T   F   The most successful rehabilitation programs focus solely on physical reconditioning.

37.12  T   F   Depression and hostility are common correlates of many chronic diseases.

37.13  T   F   COPD patients lacking a strong social support structure are at higher risk for rehospitalization than those with such networks in place.

37.14  T   F   The physiological impairment of chronic lung disease can severely restrict a patient's ability to perform even the most routine tasks.

37.15  T   F   Many disabled pulmonary patients are in their economically productive years.

37.16  T   F   The psychosocial outcomes of rehabilitation are easier to substantiate than physiologic measures.

37.17  T   F   Cardiopulmonary stress tests can help differentiate between primary respiratory or cardiac causes of exercise limitation.

37.18  T   F   Reconditioning and rehabilitation will have little or no value if the patient still smokes.

37.19  T   F   Effective pulmonary rehabilitation can eliminate the occurrence of dyspnea in chronic disease patients.

37.20  T   F   Cardiovascular rehabilitation outcomes tend to have greater validity and acceptance than pulmonary rehabilitation.

**Short Answer:** Complete each statement by filling in the correct information in the space(s) provided:

37.21 The restoration of an individual to the fullest medical, mental, emotional, social, and vocational potential best describes _____.

37.22 Patients with chronic cardiopulmonary disorders all share an inability to _____ with their disease process.

37.23 Rehabilitation programs should address both the physiological impairment and its _____ consequences.

37.24 In the broadest sense, pulmonary rehabilitation is any method designed to improve the _____ _____ experienced by patients with disabling pulmonary disease.

37.25 _____ may be a contributing factor in rehabilitation efforts where no improvements in pertinent physical or psychosocial measures are obtained.

37.26 If the body is unable to deliver adequate $O_2$ for the demands of energy metabolism during exercise, blood _____ levels increase.

37.27 The _____ is that point during exercise at which increased lactic acid production results in an increased $\dot{V}CO_2$ and $\dot{V}_E$.

37.28 At the anaerobic threshold, the RQ is approximately _____.

37.29 Normally, an individual can achieve _____ of their MVV value on maximum exercise.

37.30 A normal resting $CO_2$ consumption for a 70–kilogram adult is about _____ ml/min.

37.31 The educational content of any pulmonary rehabilitation effort should be based on the _____ _____ _____.

37.32 In order to help ensure compliance with the reconditioning goals of a rehabilitation program, patients should maintain a _____ of home exercise activities.

37.33 The _____ is a convenient way for a patient to carry out a well–defined amount of activity without equipment.

37.34 By following the guidelines for a comprehensive outpatient rehab facility (CORF), Medicare will reimburse up to _____ % of the allowable charge for a rehabilitation program.

37.35 CORF regulations allow reimbursement for services provided by a respiratory care practitioner on an _____ basis.

**Listing:** Complete each list as directed in its statement.

37.36 List at least seven (7) goals common to most pulmonary rehabilitation programs:

1. _____

2. _____

3. _____

4. _____

5. _____

6. _____

7. _____

37.37 List the minimum equipment needed for a pulmonary rehabilitation class of 6–10 participants:

1. _____

2. _____

3. _____

4. _____

5. _____

6. _____

7. _____

8. _____

**Compare and Contrast:**

37.38 Compare and contrast the accepted benefits of pulmonary rehabilitation exercise reconditioning with those benefits considered unlikely:

Accepted Benefits:

_____

_____

_____

_____

_____

_____

Unlikely Benefits:

_____

_____

_____

_____

_____

**Multiple Choice:** Circle the letter corresponding to the single best answer from the available choices:

37.39 The principal objectives of pulmonary rehabilitation include which of the following?
I.    to control the symptoms/complications of respiratory impairment
II.   to reverse the course or progression of the disease process
III.  to help patients achieve optimal capability for daily living

a. I and III          c. II only
b. I and II           d. I, II, and III

37.40 Which of the following would you not expect to observe after a COPD patient completes a sound pulmonary rehabilitation program?

a. a reduced pulse rate during exercise
b. a permanent increase in $FEV_1$ and $FEF_{25-75}$
c. a decreased breathing rate during exercise
d. a reduction in $CO_2$ production during exercise

37.41 Which of the following have been implicated as reasons for pulmonary rehabilitation programs failing to produce the desired physical or psychosocial benefits for participants?
I.    inadequate training in rehabilitation methods
II.   a lack of uniformity in rehabilitation teams
III.  treatment courses that are too short

a. I and II           c. II only
b. II and III         d. I, II, and III

37.42 Knowledge from the social sciences is used in pulmonary rehabilitation programming mainly to:
I.    determine the impact of the disability on the patient/family
II.   quantify the extent of physiologic impairment due to disease
III.  establish ways to improve the patient's quality of life

a. II and III         c. II only
b. I and III          d. I, II, and III

37.43 Which of the following occur when the anaerobic threshold is exceeded during exercise?
I.    metabolism becomes anaerobic
II.   energy production decreases
III.  fatigue increases

a. I and II           c. I only
b. II and III         d. I, II, and III

37.44 Which of the following formulas can be used to estimate a patient's maximum voluntary ventilation (MVV)?

a. FVC x 35
b. $\dot{V}_{CO_2}/\dot{V}_{O_2}$
c. $FEV_1$ x 35
d. IRV/FRC

37.45 A normal resting respiratory quotient (mixed diet) is about:

a. 0.2
b. 0.4
c. 0.6
d. 0.8

37.46 Which of the following diets would result in the highest respiratory quotients (RQ)?

a. pure carbohydrate
b. pure fat
c. 50% carbohydrate/50% fat
d. pure protein

37.47 Which of the following factors are responsible for the high degree of intolerance COPD patients exhibit for increased levels of physical activity?
I.    proportionately high $\dot{V}_{CO_2}$
II.   development of dyspnea
III.  respiratory acidosis
IV.   proportionately high $\dot{V}_{O_2}$

a. II and IV          c. I and III
b. I, II, and III     d. I, II, III, and IV

37.48 In order to physically recondition a patient and increase his or her exercise tolerance, which of the following need to be accomplished?
I.    the body's overall oxygen utilization must be improved
II.   the patient's essential muscle groups must be strengthened
III.  the cardiovascular response to exercise must be enhanced

a. I and II           c. II only
b. II and III         d. I, II, and III

37.49 Attrition in pulmonary rehabilitation programs is best associated with which of the following?

a. the success of the physical reconditioning component
b. the scope and depth of the group educational activities
c. the comprehensiveness of the preliminary patient evaluation
d. the degree to which patients' psychosocial needs are met

37.50 Which of the following is *false* regarding the social needs of patients with chronic lung disease participating in a rehabilitation program?

a. social support should be provided only after program completion
b. social support helps determine how well one adapts to disability
c. lack of social support increases the risk of rehospitalization
d. patients derive support by informal association with each other

37.51 Accepted benefits of physical reconditioning in patients with chronic lung disease include all of the following *except:*

a. increased maximum oxygen consumption
b. increased activity with decreased heart rate
c. improved resting arterial blood gas values
d. increased overall physical endurance
e. increased activity with decreased ventilation

37.52 Which of the following blood gas abnormalities should the practitioner be on guard for when conducting physical reconditioning for patients with chronic lung disease?
I.    arterial $O_2$ desaturation
II.   metabolic alkalosis
III.  elevated $CO_2$ (hypercapnia)

a. I and II          c. I and III
b. II and III        d. I, II, and III

37.53 Which of the following is *not* a potential hazard of physical reconditioning for patients with chronic lung disease?

a. dehydration
b. cardiac arrhythmias
c. hyperglycemia
d. $O_2$ desaturation

37.54 A patient is being considered for participation in a pulmonary rehabilitation program. Which of the following pulmonary function tests would you recommend be performed as a component of the preliminary evaluation?
I.    lung volumes (including FRC)
II.   diffusing capacity ($D_{Lco}$)
III.  lung and thoracic compliance
IV.   pre/post bronchodilator flows

a. II and IV         c. I and II
b. I, II, and IV     d. I, II, III, and IV

37.55 Which of the following stress test findings (compared with normal) is most consistent with exercise intolerance due primarily to a ventilatory impairment?

a. increased max $O_2$ consumption
b. normal arterial $Pao_2$
c. increased arterial $Paco_2$
d. low anaerobic threshold

37.56 Which of the following blood gases obtained from a patient breathing room air during the later stages of a cardiopulmonary stress test is most consistent with exercise intolerance due primarily to a ventilatory impairment?

a. pH = 7.53; $Paco_2$ = 33 mm Hg; $Pao_2$ = 59 mm Hg
b. pH = 7.55; $Paco_2$ = 31 mm Hg; $Pao_2$ = 87 mm Hg
c. pH = 7.29; $Paco_2$ = 55 mm Hg; $Pao_2$ = 53 mm Hg
d. pH = 7.38; $Paco_2$ = 42 mm Hg; $Pao_2$ = 55 mm Hg

37.57 In order to maximize patient safety during cardiopulmonary stress testing, which of the following precautions would you recommend?
I.    immediate availability of a "crash cart"
II.   staff training in emergency life support
III.  presence of a physician throughout testing
IV.   patient physical exam/ECG before testing

a. II and IV         c. I and III
b. I, II, and III    d. I, II, III, and IV

37.58 While you are assisting in a treadmill cardiopulmonary stress test procedure, the patient complains to you that she is developing severe shortness of breath and some chest pain. Which of the following actions would you recommend at this time?

a. increase the $O_2$ flow rate
b. decrease the treadmill speed
c. terminate the procedure at once
d. encourage her to try harder

37.59 In preparing an outpatient for a cardiopulmonary stress test to be conducted the next day, which of the following instructions would you provide?

I. the patient should fast for at least 8 hours before testing
II. the patient should wear loose–fitting clothing/sneakers
III. the patient should review his or her drugs with the physician
IV. the patient should stop all medications at once

a. I, II, and III
b. II and IV
c. I and III
d. I, II, III, and IV

37.60 Which of the following patients is *not* a good candidate for pulmonary rehabilitation?

a. a patient with exercise limitations due to severe dyspnea
b. a patient with a chronic mucociliary clearance problem
c. a patient with moderate to severe obstructive lung disease
d. a patient with a severe neuromuscular abnormality

37.61 Which of the following patients would benefit least from pulmonary rehabilitation?

a. a patient with chronic bronchitis
b. a patient with pulmonary emphysema
c. a patient with malignant lung cancer
d. a patient with pulmonary fibrosis

37.62 Which of the following patients are good candidates for pulmonary rehabilitation?

I. patients with exercise limitations due to severe dyspnea
II. patients with severe arthritis or neuromuscular abnormalities
III. patients with malignant neoplasms involving the lungs
IV. patient with moderate to severe obstructive lung disease

a. I, II, and III
b. II and IV
c. I and IV
d. I, II, III, and IV

37.63 The maximum oxygen consumption ($Vo_2max$) at termination of exercise (as a percent of predicted) for four patients appears below. Which of these patients is the best candidate for pulmonary rehabilitation?

| Patient | $Vo_2max$ (%predicted) |
|---|---|
| a. A | 120% |
| b. B | 95% |
| c. C | 85% |
| d. D | 65% |

37.64 Below what level of the predicted $FEV_1$% ($FEV_1$/FVC) are patients with irreversible airway obstruction considered good candidates for pulmonary rehabilitation?

a. 60%
b. 70%
c. 75%
d. 80%

37.65 Which of the following pulmonary function tests are most useful in determining whether a patient with restrictive lung disease should be considered for pulmonary rehabilitation?

I. $FEV_1$% ($FEV_1$/FVC)
II. total lung capacity (TLC)
III. diffusing capacity ($D_{Lco}$)

a. I and II
b. II and III
c. II only
d. I, II, and III

37.66 For which of the following patients would you recommend an "open–ended" format for a pulmonary rehabilitation program?

I. patients with scheduling difficulties
II. patients who require individual attention
III. patients who are self–directed

a. I and II
b. II and III
c. II only
d. I, II, and III

37.67 An absolute prerequisite for participation in any formal pulmonary rehabilitation program is that patients be:

a. wealthy
b. lonely
c. destitute
d. nonsmokers
e. healthy

37.68 The physical reconditioning component of a pulmonary rehabilitation program usually includes which of the following?
I.   aerobic exercises for the upper extremities
II.   aerobic exercises for the lower extremities
III.   inspiratory resistive breathing exercises

a. I and II        c. II only
b. II and III     d. I, II, and III

37.69 Reconditioning the inspiratory muscles of patients undergoing pulmonary rehabilitation is accomplished via:

a. walking aerobically for a specified time period
b. performing inspiratory resistive breathing exercises
c. using a rowing machine for a specified time period
d. pedaling a stationary bicycle for a specified distance

37.70 Which of the following educational topics covered in a typical pulmonary rehabilitation program are most suitable for presentation by a respiratory care practitioner?
I.   diaphragmatic and pursed–lip breathing techniques
II.   respiratory structure, function, and disease
III.   methods of relaxation and stress management
IV.   recreation and vocational counseling

a. II and IV     c. I and II
b. I, II, and III   d. I, II, III, and IV

37.71 Which of the following health professionals would be best for conducting a pulmonary rehabilitation session on methods of relaxation and stress management?

a. a physical therapist
b. a clinical nutritionist
c. a respiratory therapist
d. a clinical psychologist

37.72 Which of the following topics should be covered in a rehabilitation education session covering respiratory home care?
I.   self–administration of therapy
II.   safety and equipment cleaning
III.   home care equipment use

a. II and III    c. II only
b. I and II     d. I, II, and III

37.73 Appropriate topical areas to be covered in a rehabilitation education session on nutrition include which of the following?
I.   elements of a good diet
II.   proper eating habits
III.   foods to avoid
IV.   daily menu planning

a. II and IV     c. I and III
b. I, II, and III   d. I, II, III, and IV

37.74 In order to deal with incidents of hypoxemia, dyspnea, or airway hyperreactivity during physical reconditioning activities, which of the following should be available in the rehabilitation area?
I.   bronchodilator agents
II.   an intubation tray
III.   emergency oxygen

a. I and II        c. I and III
b. II and III     d. I, II, and III

37.75 Which Medicare provision allows for reimbursement for outpatient services provided by a respiratory care practitioner?

a. Diagnosis Related Groups/prospective payment regulations
b. Certificate–of–Need statutes (Health Planning Facilities Act)
c. Comprehensive Outpatient Rehabilitative Facilities (CORFs)
d. Clinical Laboratory Improvement Act (CLIA)

37.76 In comparing pulmonary and cardiac rehabilitation, which of the following statements is *false*?

a. both incorporate education and physical exercise
b. both monitor the same parameters during exercise
c. both use a stress test for preliminary evaluation
d. both employ a multidisciplinary team approach

# Respiratory Home Care

## CONTENT EXERCISES

**True/False:** For each of the following statements, indicate whether it is mainly true or mainly false by circling the corresponding letter (T=True, F=False):

38.1  T  F  Most home care currently is initiated after an acute–care hospitalization.

38.2  T  F  Before 1970, respiratory therapy was almost exclusively administered within the hospital.

38.3  T  F  The number of organizations providing respiratory home care is decreasing.

38.4  T  F  Most patients for whom respiratory home care is considered are those with acute disease.

38.5  T  F  Home oxygen therapy can improve survival in patient groups.

38.6  T  F  Home oxygen therapy has been the most improperly prescribed and abused form of respiratory home care.

38.7  T  F  Safety measures for home cylinder oxygen are the same as those applied in the hospital.

38.8  T  F  Home gaseous cylinder systems continually lose gas due to venting.

38.9  T  F  Membrane oxygen concentrators provide a lower $F_{IO_2}$ than that provided by molecular sieve concentrators.

38.10  T  F  The oxygen mixture delivered by a membrane concentrator must be humidified.

38.11  T  F  Most ventilators used within the home environment are positive pressure devices.

38.12  T  F  Home care fraud or abuse can result in criminal prosecution.

**Short Answer:** Complete each statement by filling in the correct information in the space(s) provided:

38.13  Oxygen and related equipment became reimbursable under Part B of _____ in 1967.

38.14  An equipment management company should offer its services _____ hour a day, _____ days a week.

38.15  National uniform medical criteria for the coverage of home oxygen therapy are published by the _____.

38.16  The accepted maximum duration of need for home oxygen therapy without recertification is _____.

38.17  The oxygen in the inner reservoir of a home liquid oxygen system is maintained at a temperature of about _____°F.

38.18  Small home liquid oxygen cylinders hold about _____ liters of liquid oxygen.

38.19  One cubic foot of liquid oxygen is equivalent to _____ cubic feet of gaseous oxygen.

38.20  When not in use, pressure in a home liquid oxygen system is maintained between _____ and _____ psig.

38.21  At normal operating pressures, one pound of liquid oxygen equals approximately _____ liters of gaseous oxygen.

38.22  Most portable liquid oxygen units can provide _____ hours of $O_2$ at flows of 2 L/min.

38.23  At flows between 1 and 2 L/min, a molecular sieve $O_2$ concentrator provides oxygen concentrations of _____ %.

38.24  In some patients, adequate oxygenation can be achieved with transtracheal catheter flows as low as _____ L/min.

38.25  Transtracheal catheters and their tubing should be replaced every _____ to avoid product failure.

38.26  Routine removing and cleaning of the transtracheal oxygen catheter should be performed by the _____.

38.27 A reservoir cannula set at _____ L/min can provide $SaO_2$s equivalent to that available with a regular cannula set at 2 L/min.

38.28 The recommended vacuum pressure when using a home portable suction unit for airway clearance in adults is _____.

38.29 The American Respiratory Care Foundation (ACRF) recommends an _____ for home disinfection of respiratory equipment.

**Listing:** Complete each list as directed in its statement.

38.30 List ten (10) criteria used to assess the clinical stability of patients under consideration for home mechanical ventilation (as recommended by the ACCP):

1. _____

_____

2. _____

_____

3. _____

_____

4. _____

_____

5. _____

_____

6. _____

_____

7. _____

_____

8. _____

_____

9. _____

_____

10. _____

_____

38.31 List the essential equipment and supplies that a DME company should normally provide for a ventilator–dependent home care patient:

1. _____

_____

2. _____

_____

3. _____

_____

4. _____

_____

5. _____

_____

6. _____

_____

7. _____

_____

8. _____

_____

9. _____

_____

38.32 List at least five (5) common areas of potential ethical or legal impropriety in the delivery of respiratory home care:

1. _____

   _____

2. _____

   _____

3. _____

   _____

4. _____

   _____

5. _____

   _____

**Multiple Choice:** Circle the letter corresponding to the single best answer from the available choices:

38.33 For which of the following categories of disorders is respiratory home care not considered appropriate?

a. cystic fibrosis
b. acute restrictive disorders
c. chronic obstructive pulmonary disease
d. chronic neuromuscular disorders

38.34 The American Association for Respiratory Care (AARC) standards for respiratory home care include which of the following provisions?
I.    the need for therapy must be clearly established
II.   a medical record must be established and maintained
III.  proper maintenance of equipment must be ensured
IV.   patients must receive periodic follow–up evaluations

a. I and III             c. II and IV
b. I, II, and III        d. I, II, III, and IV

38.35 Which of the following areas is not addressed in the Joint Commission for Accreditation of Healthcare Organizations (JCAHO) generic standards for home care?

a. infection control
b. patient/client care
c. the home care record
d. patient age

38.36 Criteria for considering patient discharge to the home care environment include which of the following?
I.    patient status
II.   education and training
III.  home conditions
IV.   family support

a. II and IV             c. I and IV
b. I and III             d. I, II, III, and IV

38.37 Establishing therapeutic objectives for home care normally is the responsibility of which member of the respiratory home care team?

a. physical therapy
b. attending physician
c. respiratory care
d. nursing services

38.38 Providing necessary home care equipment and supplies and handling any emergency situations involving delivery or equipment operation is the responsibility of which member of the respiratory home care team?

a. social services
b. discharge planning
c. DME company
d. nursing services

38.39 A patient discharge plan should include at least which of the following key points?
I.    therapeutic goals for home care
II.   equipment needed for implementation
III.  patient instruction and set–up
IV.   plans for follow–up and evaluation

a. II and IV             c. I and III
b. I, II, and III        d. I, II, III, and IV

38.40 Patients being discharged from a hospital and requiring home care services may be referred to which of the following?

I.    skilled nursing facility
II.   home health agency (HHA)
III.  visiting nurse service (VNA)
IV.   durable medical equipment (DME) supplier

a. II and IV            c. I and III
b. II, III, and IV      d. I, II, III, and IV

38.41 Factors to consider when advising a patient on selection of a home care equipment management company (DME) include all of the following *except:*

a. finder's fees
b. dependability
c. cost/charges
d. availability

38.42 DME companies usually provide which of the following respiratory home care services?

I.    acceptance of insurance coverage
II.   most respiratory care modalities
III.  24–hour, 7–day–a–week service
IV.   home instruction and follow–up

a. II and IV            c. I and IV
b. I, II, and III       d. I, II, III, and IV

38.43 Sources of home care equipment other than durable medical equipment (DME) companies include which of the following?

I.    home health agencies (HHA)
II.   private concerns
III.  charitable organizations
IV.   hospitals

a. II and IV            c. I and III
b. I, II, and III       d. I, II, III, and IV

38.44 Under HCFA regulations, which of the following is *false* regarding home oxygen therapy?

a. hypoxemia can be confirmed by blood gas analysis
b. a $PaO_2$ at or below 55 mm Hg documents need
c. an $SaO_2$ 88% or less during exercise documents need
d. "prn" prescriptions for oxygen are acceptable

38.45 Conditions or symptoms that can help justify reimbursement coverage for home oxygen include all of the following *except:*

a. erythrocytosis
b. impaired cognitive processes
c. pulmonary hypertension
d. peripheral vascular disease

38.46 In addition to specifying the liter flow or concentration, which of the following must a doctor include in a home oxygen prescription?

I.    duration of need for oxygen
II.   appropriate medical diagnosis
III.  laboratory evidence of hypoxemia
IV.   frequency of use of oxygen

a. II, III, and IV      c. III and IV
b. I, III, and IV       d. I, II, III, and IV

38.47 Disadvantages of using compressed oxygen cylinders in the home include all of the following *except:*

a. high pressure hazards
b. limited volume of oxygen
c. gas wastage when not used
d. need for frequent deliveries

38.48 A home care patient will be receiving low–flow nasal oxygen using a large compressed gas cylinder. Which of the following additional equipment would you specify for this patient?

I.    a pressure–reducing valve with flowmeter
II.   a cylinder safety stand or "donut" base
III.  an adjustable humidifier heating element

a. I and III            c. II and III
b. I and II             d. I, II, and III

38.49 On visiting a home care patient receiving nasal $O_2$ via cylinder, you note that the humidifier diffusing element is producing only large bubbles, and its pressure relief is sounding. When asked, the patient indicates that tap water is used in the humidifier. Which of the following is the likely cause of this problem?

a. the nasal cannula has become obstructed with secretions
b. the diffusing element is occluded by mineral deposits
c. the cylinder gas is contaminated with particulate matter
d. the humidifier pressure relief valve is defective

38.50 The gauge reading of a 50–pound home liquid oxygen system indicates that the cylinder is 2/3 full. What is the duration of flow of this system at 2 L/min?

a. 24 hours
b. 48 hours
c. 72 hours
d. 94 hours

38.51 The purpose of the small refillable liquid oxygen tank that comes with many stationary home liquid oxygen reservoirs is:

a. to serve as a backup should the primary reservoir fail
b. to collect and save gas vented by the primary reservoir
c. to provide oxygen to ambulatory patients outside the home
d. to allow transfilling from the LOX delivery truck

38.52 A home care patient who uses $O_2$ only during ambulatory rehabilitation activities calls you and complains that her large liquid oxygen reservoir tank is "hissing." You would:

a. immediately call her oxygen service company for a repair visit
b. explain that the hissing is due to an abnormal system leak
c. tell her to immediately turn off all home electrical devices
d. explain that the hissing is due to normal reservoir venting

38.53 When visiting a home care patient receiving nasal oxygen at 3 L/min via a molecular sieve–type oxygen concentrator, you measure the $O_2$ concentration of the outlet gas as 41%. Which of the following actions would be appropriate at this time?

a. none–this $F_{IO_2}$ is normal at this flow
b. replace the zeolite pellet canisters
c. replace the internal/external filters
d. replace the gas diffusion membrane

38.54 At flows between 3 and 5 L/min, the molecular sieve oxygen concentrator provides oxygen concentrations of:

a. 95%
b. 85–93%
c. 70–80%
d. 60–70%

38.55 At flows of 10 L/min, the membrane oxygen concentrator can provide oxygen concentrations of about:

a. 80%
b. 70%
c. 60%
d. 40%

38.56 In setting up a home care patient with COPD for continuous low–flow oxygen therapy via an oxygen concentrator, which of the following additional equipment must you provide?

a. a pressure–reducing valve
b. an emergency generator
c. a bag–mask resuscitator
d. a backup gas cylinder

38.57 Routine in–home monthly maintenance of an oxygen concentrator should include which of the following?
I.    cleaning and replacing of internal and external filters
II.   confirming the $F_{IO_2}$ with a calibrated oxygen analyzer
III.  flushing the system for 20 minutes with an inert gas

a. I and II          c. I and III
b. II and III        d. I, II, and III

38.58 Compared with a nasal cannula, a transtracheal catheter can provide comparable $Pa_{O_2}$s with how much less flow?

a. 10–20% less flow
b. 20–30% less flow
c. 30–50% less flow
d. 50–70% less flow

38.59 While visiting a patient who has been receiving transtracheal oxygen therapy for 6 months, you note marked cracking of the catheter. Which of the following actions would be appropriate at this time?

a. question the patient/family regarding their cleaning methods
b. liberally apply tape to the catheter
c. promptly report your observations to the prescribing physician
d. immediately replace the catheter and discard the old one

38.60 Compared with a typical continuous flow nasal cannula delivery system, the flow requirements of a reservoir cannula are about:

a. 1/3 to 2/5 as much
b. 1/4 to 1/2 as much
c. 1/7 to 1/3 as much
d. 1/2 to 2/3 as much

38.61 For achieving comparable oxygenation, which of the following delivery devices uses the least oxygen?

a. reservoir cannula
b. transtracheal catheter
c. demand flow system
d. simple cannula

38.62 Which of the following patients are good candidates for mechanical ventilation in the home?
I.    a patient who cannot maintain adequate ventilation at night
II.   a patient who requires continuous ventilation to survive
III.  a terminally ill patient who requires ventilatory support

a. I and II                    c. II only
b. II and III                  d. I, II, and III

38.63 Which of the following criteria are prerequisite to considering long–term mechanical ventilation in the home setting?
I.    presence of adequate professional support
II.   willingness of family to accept responsibility
III.  patient's condition, especially stability
IV.   overall viability of the home care plan

a. I, II, and III              c. III and IV
b. II and IV                   d. I, II, III, and IV

38.64 You have been asked to organize a patient/family education program as part of a discharge plan for a patient requiring home ventilatory support. Which of the following methods would be best for training the family in operation of the ventilator chosen?

a. set up and review the ventilator after the patient gets home
b. take the family into a back room and show them a ventilator
c. give the family a lecture on principles of ventilatory support
d. apply the device to the patient while still hospitalized

38.65 Legitimate goals for mechanical ventilatory support in the home setting include which of the following?
I.    to enhance the quality of life
II.   to reduce morbidity
III.  to extend life
IV.   to provide cost benefits

a. I, II, and III              c. I and III
b. II and IV                   d. I, II, III, and IV

38.66 According to the AARC, which of the following standards should be met when considering ventilatory support outside the acute care hospital?
I.    services must be based on the attending doctor's prescription
II.   those providing the support should be appropriately trained
III.  appropriate recording and reporting mechanisms should exist
IV.   safe, effective, and appropriate equipment must be provided

a. II and IV                   c. I and III
b. I, II, and III              d. I, II, III, and IV

38.67 For which of the following patients requiring home ventilatory support would you consider noninvasive positive pressure ventilation (NIPPV)?
I.    patients with chronic neuromuscular or neurologic disorders
II.   patients with COPD requiring only periodic support
III.  patients with idiopathic hypoventilation syndrome

a. I and II                    c. I only
b. II and III                  d. I, II, and III

38.68 You are conducting a routine visit to a ventilator–dependent patient in a home care setting. Which of the following would you be sure to perform while on this visit?
I.    carefully assess patient's status
II.   administer prescribed respiratory therapy
III.  check and clean equipment (as needed)
IV.   complete all appropriate documentation

a. II and IV                   c. I and III
b. I, II, and III              d. I, II, III, and IV

38.69 A home care patient with a tracheostomy requires continuous aerosol therapy but no supplemental oxygen. Which of the following systems would be appropriate for these circumstances?
I.    electrically powered (ultrasonic) nebulizer
II.   jet nebulizer with 50 psig air compressor
III.  jet nebulizer with large air cylinder/regulator

a. I only                 c. I and III
b. II and III             d. I, II, and III

38.70 Legitimate home care applications for intermittent positive pressure breathing (IPPB) include which of the following?
I.    treating restrictive lung diseases such as kyphoscoliosis
II.   overcoming airway obstruction in patients with tumors
III.  administering bronchodilators to certain COPD patients

a. I and II               c. I and III
b. II and III             d. I, II, and III

38.71 In order to control the cost of suction supplies for a home care patient, which of the following is an acceptable strategy?

a. save used catheters for resterilization with ethylene oxide
b. wash catheters in detergent and hot water between uses
c. save used catheters for resterilization via autoclave
d. use 1 catheter per day, place in disinfectant between uses

38.72 After fitting a home care patient with a CPAP nasal mask, you set the prescribed pressure and turn the flow generator on. At this point the mask pressure reading is 0 cm $H_2O$. The most likely cause of this problem is:

a. electrical failure
b. a large system leak
c. patient asynchrony
d. too high a flow

38.73 Common problems encountered when using adult nasal CPAP to treat sleep apnea include all of the following except:

a. sinusitis
b. conjunctivitis
c. barotrauma
d. rhinitis

38.74 Which of the following would you recommend to a home care patient as a source of water for an oxygen humidification device?

a. boiled tap water kept refrigerated, discarded after 24 hours
b. sterile water supplied by a DME company
c. USP water obtained from a local pharmacy
d. only water that has undergone electrolysis
e. plain tap water (as long as it is "soft")

38.75 Which of the following factors would you consider in determining the frequency of follow–up visits needed by a home care patient?
I.    level of self–care the patient is able to provide
II.   type and complexity of home care equipment used
III.  patient's condition and therapeutic objectives
IV.   level of family or caregiver support available

a. I, II, and III         c. I and III
b. II and IV              d. I, II, III, and IV

38.76 As a full–time hospital staff member, you take a part–time job with a home care company that has taken patient referrals from your employer. Which of the following should you do?

a. quit the hospital job to avoid a conflict of interest
b. inform the home care company about your hospital job
c. inform Medicare Part B carriers about this relationship
d. inform both parties about this new job relationship

## PROBLEMS FOR THOUGHT AND DISCUSSION

A 76–year–old ventilator–dependent male patient with end–stage COPD is being discharged to the home care setting. Both his wife (69 years old and in good health) and daughter (a 45–year–old college graduate) will assume primary caregiver responsibilities. Develop an outline for an educational program designed to prepare this patient and his family for home care.

# Suggested Readings

# Chapter 1

Burner ST, Waldo DR, McKusic DR: National health expenditure projections through 2030, *Health Care Financing Review* 14(1):1–29, 1992.

O'Neil EH: *Health professions education for the future: schools in service to the nation*, San Francisco, 1993, Pew Health Professions Commission.

Cummings KC, Abell RM: Loosing sight of the shore: how a future integrated American health care organization might look, *Health Care Management Review* 18(2):41–42, 1993.

Joint Review Committee for Respiratory Therapy Education: *Essentials and guidelines of an accredited educational program for the respiratory therapy technician and respiratory therapist,* Euless, TX, 1986, Joint Review Committee for Respiratory Therapy Education.

Angell M: How much will health care reform cost? *N Engl J Med* 328(24):1778–1779, 1993.

# Chapter 2

American Association for Respiratory Therapy, Administrative standards for respiratory care services and personnel (official statement), *Respir Care* 28(8):1033–1038, 1983.

Bunch D: Restructuring hospitals for the future, *AARC Times* 16(3):29–36, 1992.

Elliott CG: Quality assurance for respiratory care services: a computer–assisted program, *Respir Care* 38(1):54–59, 1993.

Greenway L, Jeffs M, Turner K: Computerized management of respiratory care. *Respir Care* 38(1):42–53, 1993.

Scanlan CL: The prospective payment system: What you see is what you get, *Pul Med Tech* 1(5): 19–34, 1984.

Snyder GM: Patient–focused hospitals: an opportunity for respiratory care practitioners, *Respir Care* 37(5):448–454, 1992.

# Chapter 3

Bruner J: Hazards of electrical apparatus, *Anesthesiology*, 28:945–957, 1967.

Scanlan, CL: *Electrical safety in respiratory therapy,* Part I. Dallas, 1978, American Association for Respiratory Therapy.

Scanlan, CL: *Electrical safety in respiratory therapy,* Part II. Dallas, 1978, American Association for Respiratory Therapy.

DiMatteo MP: A social–psychological analysis of physician–patient rapport: toward a science of the art of medicine, *J Soc Issues* 35:17–31, 1979.

Bray KA: Managing conflict, *Crit Care Nurs,* 3(2):77–78, 1983.

# Chapter 4

Hooton TM: Protecting ourselves and our patients from nosocomial infections, *Respir Care,* 34(2):111–115, 1989.

Chatburn RL: Decontamination of respiratory care equipment: What can be done, what should be done, *Respir Care,* 34(2):98–110, 1989.

Tobin MJ: Diagnosis of pneumonia: techniques and problems, *Clin Chest Med* 8(3):513–527, 1987.

Grim PS, Gottlieb LJ, Boddie A, Batson E: Hyperbaric oxygen therapy, *JAMA* 263(16):2216–2220, 1990.

Horsburgh CR Jr: Mycobacterium avium complex infection in the acquired immunodeficiency syndrome, *N Engl J Med* 324:1332–1338, 1991.

Greenberg SB: Viral pneumonia, *Infect Dis Clin North Am* 5(3):603–621, 1991.

Bjornson HS: Diagnosis and treatment of bacterial pneumonia in the intensive care unit: an overview, *Respir Care* 32(9):773–780, 1987.

American Respiratory Care Foundation: Guidelines for disinfection of respiratory care equipment used in the home, *Respir Care,* 33:801–808, 1988.

Weber DJ, Wilson MB, Rutala WA, et al.: Manual ventilation bags as a source for bacterial colonization of intubated patients, *Am Rev Respir Dis* 142(4):892–894, 1990.

Crutcher JM, Lamm SH, Hall TA: Procedures to protect health–care workers from HIV infection: category I (health–care) workers, *Am Ind Hyg Assoc J* 52(2):A100–103, 1991.

# Chapter 5

Edge R, Groves R: *The ethics of health care: a guide for practice,* Albany, NY, 1994, DelMar.

Francoeur RT: *Biomedical ethics, a guide to decision making,* New York, 1983, Wiley Medical Publications.

Evans RE: Health care technology and the inevitability of resource allocation and rationing decisions, *JAMA* 249:2208–2219, 1983.

Larson K: DME referrals: what's legal and what's not, *AAR Times* 10(8):28–31, 1986.

Blendon RJ.: Health policy choices for the 1990s, *Issues in Science and Technology* 2:65, 1986.

The President's Commission for the Study of Ethical Problems in Medicine and Biomedical and Behavioral Research. Washington: U. S. Government Printing Office, 1983. (10 reports)

# Chapter 6

Chatburn RL: Measurement, physical quantities and le systeme international d'unites (SI units), *Respir Care* 33(10):861–873, 1988.

McQueen MJ: Conversion to SI units, *JAMA* 256:3001–3002, 1986.

Pulmonary terms and symbols: A report of the ACCP–ATS Joint Committee on Pulmonary Nomenclature, *Chest* 67:583, 1975.

Young DS: Standardized reporting of laboratory data, *N Engl J Med* 290:368, 1974.

# Chapter 7

Flitter HH: *An introduction to physics in nursing,* ed 7, St Louis, 1976, Mosby–Year Book.

Green JF: *Mechanical concepts in cardiovascular and pulmonary physiology,* Philadelphia, 1977, Lea & Febeger.

Kacmarek RM: Chemical and physical background. In Pierson DJ and Kacmarek RM, editors: *Foundations of Respiratory Care,* New York, 1992, Churchill Livingston.

Kimball WR: Fluid mechanics. In Kacmarek RM, Hess D and Stoller JK, editors: *Monitoring in Respiratory Care,* St. Louis, 1993, Mosby–Year Book.

Rau JL: An evaluation of fluidic control in ventilators. *Respir Ther,* 6:29–32, 1976.

# Chapter 8

Demers RR: Some potential pitfalls associated with the use of computers and microprocessors, *Respir Care,* 27:842845, 1982.

East TD: Microcomputer data acquisition and control. *Int J Clin Monit Comput* 3:225–238, 1986.

Lampotang S: Microprocessor–controlled ventilation systems and concepts. In: Kirby RR, Banner MJ, Downs JB (eds), *Clinical Application of Ventilatory Support.* New York, Churchill Livingston, 1990.

Meehan PA: Hemodynamic assessment using the automated physiologic profile, *Crit Care Nurse,* 6(1):2946, 1986.

Morozoff PE, Evans RW: Closed–loop control of $SaO_2$ in the neonate. *Biomed Instrum Technol,* 26:117–123, 1992.

Schwartz WB, Patil RS, and Szolovits. P.: Artificial intelligence in medicine: where do we stand? *N Engl J Med,* 316:685688, 1987.

# Chapter 9

Lai Fook SJ: Mechanics of the pleural space: fundamental concepts. *Lung* 165(5):249, 1987.

Celli BR: Clinical and physiologic evaluation of respiratory muscle function, *Clin Chest Med* 10(2): 199, 1989.

Barnes PJ: Neural control of human airways in health and disease, *Am Rev Respir Dis* 134(6): 1289, 1986.

Charan B: The bronchial circulatory system: structure, function and importance, *Respir Care* 29: 1226, 1984.

Johanson WG: Lung defense mechanisms, *Basics Respir Disease,* 6(2):7, 1977.

Fels AO, Cohn ZA: The alveolar macrophage, *J Appl Physiol* 60(2): 353, 1986.

# Chapter 10

Berne RM, Levy MN: *Cardiovascular physiology,* ed 4, St Louis, 1981, Mosby–Year Book.

Johnson PL: *The microcirculation and local and humoral control of the circulation.* In Guyton AC, Jones CE, editors: *Cardiovascular physiology,* Baltimore, 1974, University Park Press.

Guyton AC, Jones CE, Coleman TC: *Circulatory physiology: cardiac output and its regulation,* Philadelphia, 1973, WB Saunders.

Downing SE: *Baroreceptor regulation of the heart.* In Berne SR, Sperelakis N, Geiger SR, editor: Handbook of physiology, Sect 2, *The cardiovascular system,* Vol I, The heart, Bethesda, MD, 1979, American Physiological Society.

Phillips RE, Feeney MK: *The cardaic rhythms: a systematic approach to interpretation.* Philadelphia, 1973, WB Saunders.

# Chapter 11

Report of the ACCP–ATS Joint Committee on Pulmonary Nomenclature, *Chest* 67: 583, 1975.

Wright JR, Hagwood S: Pulmonary surfactant metabolism, *Clin Chest Med,* 10(1):83, 1989

Robinson DR, Chaudhary BA, Speir WS: Expiratory flow limitation in large and small airways, *Arch Intern Med* 144:1457, 1984.

Otis AB: The work of breathing, *Physiol Rev* 34: 449–458, 1954.

Celli BR: Clinical and physiologic evaluation of respiratory muscle function, *Clin Chest Med* 10(2): 199–214, 1989.

# Chapter 12

West JB: Ventilation–perfusion relationships, *Am Rev Resp Dis* 116:919, 1977.

Dantzker DR; Guiterrez G. The assessment of tissue oxygenation. *Respir Care* 1985; 30(6)456–462.

Thomas HM III; Lefrak SS, Irwin RS, Fritts HW Jr, Caldwell PR. The oxyhemoglobin dissociation curve in health and disease: role of 2,3–diphosphoglycerate, *Am J Med* 57(3)331–348, 1974.

Gregory IC: The oxygen and carbon dioxide capacities of fetal and adult hemoglobin, *J Physiol* 236:625, 1974.

Winter PM. Miller JN. Carbon monoxide poisoning, *JAMA* 236(13):1502, 1976.

Kacmarek RM: Carbon dioxide production, carriage and transport. In Pierson DJ, Kacmarek RM, editors: *Foundations of respiratory care,* New York, 1992, Churchill–Livingstone.

# Chapter 13

Metheny NM: *Fluid and electrolyte balance.* Nursing considerations, ed. 3, Philadelphia, 1987, JB Lippincott.

Tietz NW, editor: *Clinical guide to laboratory tests.* ed 2, Philadelphia, 1990, WB Saunders.

Webster PO: Electrolyte balance in heart failure and the role for magnesium ions. *Am J Cardiol,* 70:44s–49s, 1992.

York K: The lung and fluid electrolyte and acid base imbalances, *Nurs Clin N Am*, 22:805 814, 1987.

# Chapter 14

Martin L: *Pulmonary physiology in clinical practice: the essentials for patient care and evaluation*, St. Louis, 1987, Mosby–Year Book.

Siggaard Andersen O: *The acid–base status of the blood*, ed 4, Baltimore, 1974, Williams & Wilkins.

Shapiro BA, Harrison RA, Walton JR: *Clinical application of blood gases*, ed 3, Chicago, 1982, Mosby–Year Book.

Malley WJ: *Clinical blood gases: application and noninvasive alternatives*, Philadelphia 1990, WB Saunders.

Jovaheri S, Kazemi H: Metabolic alkalosis and hypoventilation in humans, *Am Rev Respir Dis* 136:1011–1016, 1987.

# Chapter 15

Dantzker DR: Oxygen transport and utilization, *Respir Care* 33(10):874–880, 1988.

Hudson LD, Pierson DJ: Hypoxemia. In: Pierson DJ, Kacmarek RM, editors: *Foundations of respiratory care*, New York, 1992, Churchill Livingston.

Pierson DJ: Normal and abnormal oxygenation: physiology and clinical syndromes, *Respir Care* 38(6):587–599, 1993.

Phang PT, Russell JA: When does $Vo_2$ depend on $Do_2$? *Respir Care* 38(6):618–626, 1993.

Higgins TL, Yared J: Clinical effects of hypoxemia and tissue hypoxia, *Respir Care* 38(6):603–615, 1993.

Johnson NT, Pierson DJ: Restrictive disorders. In Pierson DJ, Kacmarek RM, editors: *Foundations of Respiratory Care*, New York: 1992, Churchill Livingston.

# Chapter 16

Gravelyn TR and Weg JG: Respiratory rate as an indicator of acute respiratory dysfunction, *JAMA* 244:1123, 1980.

Mier–Jedrzejowicz A, et al: Assessment of diaphragm weakness, *Am Rev of Respir Dis* 137:877, 1988.

Wilkins RL, Dexter JR: Comparing RCPs to physicians for the description of lung sounds: are we accurate and can we communicate: *Respir Care* 35:969–976, 1990.

Nicholson D: Cyanosis: five grams of history, *Respir Care*, 32:113–114, 1987.

Wilkins RL, Sheldon RL, Krider SJ: *Clinical assessment in respiratory care*, ed 2, St Louis, 1990, Mosby–Year Book.

# Chapter 17

Hess D, Kacmarek RM: Techniques and devices for monitoring oxygenation, *Respir Care* 38:646–671, 1993.

American Association for Respiratory Care: AARC clinical practice guideline: In–vitro pH and blood gas analysis and hemoximetry, *Respir Care* 38:505–510, 1993.

Chernow B: The bedside laboratory: a critical step forward in ICU care, *Chest* 97:183s–184s, 1990.

Tobin MJ: Respiratory monitoring, *JAMA* 264:244–251, 1990.

American Association for Respiratory Care: Clinical practice guideline: pulse oximetry, *Respir Care* 36(12): 1406–1409, 1991.

Graybeal JM, Russel GB: Capmometry in the surgical ICU: an analysis of the arterial–to–end–tidal carbon dioxide difference, *Respir Care* 38:923–928, 1993.

Hess D, et al: An evaluation of the usefulness of end–tidal $Pco_2$ to aid weaning from mechaincal ventilation following cardiac surgery, *Respir Care* 36:837–843, 1991.

# Chapter 18

Zibrak JD, O'Donnell CR, Marton K: Idications for pulmonary function testing. *Ann Intern Med* 112:793–794, 1990.

American Association for Respiratory Care Clinical Practice Guideline: Spirometry, *Respir Care* 36: 1414–1417, 1991.

ATS Statement: Standardization of spirometry 1987 update. *Am Rev Respir* 136:1285–1998, 1987. Reprinted in *Respir Care* 32:1039–1060, 1987.

Knudson RJ, Kaltenborn WT, Burrows B: The effects of cigarette smoking and smoking cessation on the carbon dioxide diffusing capacity of the lung in asymptomatic subjects. *Am Rev Respir Dis* 140:645–51, 1989.

Crapo RO, Morris AM: Standardized single breath normal values for carbon monoxide diffusing capacity. *Am Rev Respir Dis* 123:185–189, 1981.

Clausen JL: Prediction of normal values in pulmonary function testing. *Clin Chest Med* 10:135–43, 1989.

Glindmeyer HW, Jones RN, Barkman HW, Weill H: Spirometry: quantitative test criteria and test acceptability. *Am Rev Respir Dis* 136:449–52, 1987.

# Chapter 19

Felson B: *Chest roentgenology.* Philadelphia, 1973, WB Saunders.

Nadich DP, Zeritowin EA, Speelman SS: *Computed Tomography and Magnetic Resonance of the Thorax,* ed 2: New York, 1991, Raven Press.

Freundlich IM, Bragg D: *A Radiologic Approach to Diseases of the Chest,* 1992, Williams & Wilkins.

# Chapter 20

American Thoracic Society: Standards for the diagnosis and care of patients with chronic obstructive pulmonary disease (COPD) and asthma. *Am Rev Resp Dis* 136:225, 1987.

American Thoracic Society: Indications and standards for cardiopulmonary sleep studies. *Am Rev Resp Dis* 139:559, 1989.

Buist AS: Asthma mortality: what have we learned? *J Allery Clin Immunol* 84:275, 1989.

Collins FS: Cystic fibrosis: molecular biology and therapeutic implications. *Science* 256:774, 1992.

Hudgel DW: Mechanisms of obstructive sleep apnea, *Chest* 101:541, 1992.

Seale DD, Beaver BM: Pathophysiology of lung cancer, *Nurs Clin North Am* 27:603, 1992.

Snider GL: Emphysema: the first two centuries–and beyond. *Am Rev Resp Dis* 146:1615, 1992.

US Department of Health and Human Services, Public Health Service: Prevention and control of influenza: Recommendations of the immunization practices advisory committee, *MMWR,* 41(RR–9):1–17, 1992.

Volosky RL, Rubin FL: The re–emergence of tuberculosis: a previously forgotten disease becomes a problem for caregivers [editorial], *Respir Care* 38:880–883, 1993.

# Chapter 21

Busse, W. Asthma in the 1990s. A new approach to therapy, *Postgrad Med* 92(6):177, 1992.

Pinnas JL, et al: Multicenter study of bitolterol and isoproterenol nebulizer solutions in nonsteroid using patients, *J Allergy Clin Immunol* 79:768, 1987.

Simons FE, Soni NR, Watson WT, and Becker AB: Bronchodilator and bronchoprotective effects of salmeterol in young patients with asthma [see comments], *J Allergy Clin Immunol* 90(5):840, 1992.

Jobe A: Pulmonary Surfactant Therapy, *NEJM* 328(12):861, 1993.

Selcow JE, Mendelson LM, Rosen JP: Clinical benefits of cromolyn sodium aerosol (MDI) in the treatment of asthma in children, *Ann Allergy* 62(3):195, 1989.

Aylward RB, Burdge DR: Ribavirin therapy of adult respiratory syncytial virus pneumonitis, *Arch Intern Med* 151(11):2303, 1991.

Kacmarek RM: Care–giver protection from exposure to aerosolized pharmacologic agents. Is it necessary? *Chest* 100(4):1104, 1991.

Haverkos HW, Assessment of therapy for pneumocystis carinii pneumonia, *Am J Med* 76:501, 1984.

Montgomery AB, Debs RJ, Luce JM: Selective delivery of pentamidine to the lung by aerosol, *Am Rev Respir Dis* 137:477, 1988.

# Chapter 22

AARC clinical practice guideline: Endotracheal suctioning of mechanically ventilated adults and children with artificial airway, *Respir Care* 38(5) 500–504, 1993.

AARC clinical practice guidelines: Nasotracheal suctioning, *Respir Care* 37(8):898–901, 1992.

Ackerman MH: The use of bolus normal saline instillations in artificial airways Is it useful or necessary, *Heart Lung* 14(5) 505–506, 1985.

Chulay M: Arterial blood gas changes with a hyperinflation and hyperoxygenation suctioning intervention in critically ill patients, *Heart Lung* 17(6) 654–61, 1988.

Day SL, Wooton L, MacIntrye N: Rapid analysis of exhaled $CO_2$ to assess endotracheal tube placement, *Respir Care* 37(10) 1161–1165, 1992.

Godwin JE and Heffner JE: Special critical care considerations in tracheostomy management, *Clin Chest Med* 12(3) 573–583, 1991.

Guyton D, Banner MJ, Kirby RR: High–volume, low pressure cuffs. Are they always low pressure, *Chest* 100(4): 1076–1081, 1991.

Heffner JE: Airway management in the critically ill patient, *Crit Care Clin* 6(3) 533–550, 1990.

Kacmarek RM: The role of the respiratory therapist in emergency care, *Respir Care* 37(6) 523–32, 1992.

Rudy EB, et al: The relationship between endotracheal suctioning and changes in intra–cranial pressure: A review of the literature, *Heart Lung* 15(5) 488–494, 1986.

Stauffer JL: Medical management of the airway, *Clin Chest Med* vol 12(3) 449–482, 1991.

Stone KS, Preusser BA, Groch KF, Karl JI, Gonyon DS: The effect of lung hyperinflation and endotracheal suctioning on cardiopulmonary hemodynamics, *Nurs Res* 40(2): 76–80, 1991.

Wood DE, Mathesen DJ: Late complications of tracheostomy, *Clin Chest Med* Sept 12(3): 597–609, 1991.

# Chapter 23

Kacmarek RM: The role of the respiratory therapist in emergency care, *Respir Care,* 37(6):523–530, 1992.

American Heart Association: Guidelines for cardiopulmonary resuscitation and emergency cardiac care: Recommendations of the 1992 National Conference, *JAMA* (Suppl. ), 268:16, 2135–2302, 1992.

Council on Ethical and Judicial Affairs, American Medical Association: Guidelines for the appropriate use of do–not–resuscitate orders, *JAMA* 265:1868–1871, 1991.

Brenner BE, Kauffman J: Reluctance of internists and medical nurses to perform mouth–to–mouth resuscitation, *Arch Intern Med* 153(15):1763–1769, 1993.

Reines, HD: Airway management options, *Respir Care* 37(7):695–705, 1992.

Barnes TA: Emergency ventilation techniques and related equipment, *Respir Care* (7):673–90, 1992.

Barnes TA, McGarry W: Evaluation of ten disposable manual resuscitators, *Respir Care* 35:960–968, 1990.

Branson RD: Intrahospital transport of critically ill, mechanical ventilated patients, *Respir Care* 37(7):775–803, 1992.

Mathewson HS, Conyers, D: Advanced cardiac life support update: Uses of drugs, *Respir Care* 38(9):1020–1023, 1993.

# Chapter 24

Bancroft ML, Steen JA: Health device legislation: an overview of the law and its impact on respiratory care, *Respir Care* 23:1179, 1978.

National Fire Protection Association: Fire hazards in oxygen–enriched atmospheres (NFPA 53M). Quincy, MA, 1990, National Fire Protection Association.

Roberts JD, Polaner DM, Lang P, Zapol WM: Inhaled nitric oxide in persistent pulmonary hypertension of the newborn, *Lancet* 340(8823): 818–9, 1992.

Anderson WR: Oxygen pipeline supply failure: a coping strategy, *J Clin Monit* 7(1):39–41, 1991.

Oxygen regulator fire caused by use of two yoke washers, *Health Devices* 19(11 Spec No):426–427, 1990.

West GA, Primeau P: Nonmedical hazards of longterm oxygen therapy, *Respir Care* 28(7):906–12, 1983.

# Chapter 25

Scanlan C: Humidity and Aerosol Therapy. In Scanlan CL, Spearman CB, Sheldon RL, editors: *Egan's Fundamentals of Respiratory Care,* ed 5, St Louis, 1990, Mosby–Year Book.

American College of Chest Physicians—NHLBI: National Conference on oxygen therapy, *Respir Care* 29:922, 1984.

AARC Clinical Practice Guidelines: Humidification during mechanical ventilation, *Respir Care* 37(8):887–890, 1992.

Dreyfuss D, Djedaini K, Weber P, Brun P, Lanore J, Rahmani J, Boussougant Y, Coste F: Prospective study of nosocomial pneumonia and of patient and circuit colonization during mechanical ventilation with circuit changes every 48 hours versus no change, *Am Rev Resp Dis* 143:738–743, 1991.

Hess D, Horney D, Snyder T: Medication–delivery performance of eight small–volume, hand–held nebulizers: Effects of diluent volume, gas flowrate and nebulizer model, *Respir Care* 34:717–723, 1989.

Kacmarek RM, Kratohvil J: Evaluation of a double–enclosure double–vacuum unit scavenging system for ribavirin administration, *Respir Care* 37:37–45, 1992.

AARC Clinical Practice Guidelines: Selection of aerosol delivery device, *Respir Care* 37(8):891–7, 1992.

Ebert J, Adams AB, Green–Eide B: An evaluation of MDI spacers and adapters: Their effect on the respirable volume of medications, *Respir Care* 37:862–868, 1992.

# Chapter 26

American Association for Respiratory Care: Clinical Practice Guideline—Oxygen Therapy in the Acute Care Hospital, *Respir Care,* 36(12):1410–1413, 1991.

American Association for Respiratory Care: Clinical Practice Guideline—Oxygen Therapy in the home or extended care facility, *Respir Care,* 37(8):918–922, 1991.

Ryerson EG, Block AJ: Oxygen as a drug: clinical properties, benefits, modes, and hazards of administration, In Burton GG, Hodgkin JE, Ward JJ: *Respiratory Care: A Guide to Clinical Practice,* ed 3, Philadelphia, 1991, JB Lippincott.

Jackson RM. Molecular, pharmacologic, and clinical aspects of oxygen–induced lung injury, *Clin Chest Med* 11(1):73–86, 1990.

Aubier M; Murciano D; Milic–Emili J; Touaty E; Daghfous J; Pariente R; Derenne JP. Effects of the administration of $O_2$ on ventilation and blood gases in patients with chronic obstructive pulmonary disease during acute respiratory failure, *Am Rev Respir Dis* 122(5):747–754, 1980.

George DS, et al.: The latest on retinopathy of prematurity, *MCN* 13:254–258, 1988.

Branson RD: The nuts and bolts of increasing arterial oxygenation: devices and techniques, *Respir Care* 38(6):672–686, 1993.

Dunlevy CL, Tyl SE: The effect of oral versus nasal breathing on oxygen concentrations received from nasal cannulas, *Respir Care* 37:357–360, 1992.

Woolner DF, Larkin J: An analysis of the performance of a variable venturi–type oxygen mask, *Anaesth Intensive Care* 8(1):44–51, 1980.

Fracchia G, Torda TA: Performance of venturi oxygen delivery devices, *Anaesth Intensive Care* 8(4):426–430, 1980.

Klaus MH, Fanaroff AA, editors: *Care of the high risk neonate*, ed 3, Philadelphia, 1986, Saunders.

Tiep BL: Long–term home oxygen therapy, *Clin Chest Med* 11(3):505–521, 1990.

NHLBI workshop summary. Hyperbaric oxygenation therapy, *Am Rev Respir Dis* 144(6):1414–21, 1991.

# Chapter 27

Marini JJ: Postoperative atelectasis: pathophysiology, clinical importance, and principles of management, *Respir Care* 29(5):516–528, 1984.

Celli BR, Rodriguez KS, Snider GL: A controlled trial of intermittent positive pressure breathing, incentive spirometry, and deep breathing exercises in preventing pulmonary complication after abdominal surgery, *Am Rev Respir Dis* 130:12–15, 1984.

American Association for Respiratory Care: Clinical practice guideline: incentive spirometry, *Respir Care* 36(12):1402–1405, 1991.

American Association for Respiratory Care: Clinical practice guideline. Intermittent positive pressure breathing, *Respir Care* 38(11):1189–1195, 1993.

American Association for Respiratory Care: Clinical practice guideline. Selection of aerosol delivery device, *Respir Care* 37(8):891–897, 1992.

American Association for Respiratory Care: Clinical practice guideline: Use of positive airway pressure adjuncts to bronchial hygiene therapy, *Respir Care* 38(5):516–521, 1993.

Malmeister MJ, Fink JB, Hoffman GL: Positive expiratory pressure mask therapy: theoretical and practical considerations and a review of the literature, *Respir Care*, 36:1218–1229, 1991.

Paul WL, Downs JB: Postoperative atelectasis: intermittent positive pressure breathing, incentive spirometry, and face–mask positive end–expiratory pressure, *Arch Surg* 116:861–863, 1981.

# Chapter 28

Murray J: The ketchup–bottle method, *N Eng J Med* 300:1155–1157, 1979.

Tyler ML: Complications of positioning and chest physiotherapy, *Respir Care* 27:458–466, 1982.

Kirilloff LH, Owens GR, et al.: Does chest physical therapy work?, Chest 88:436–444, 1985.

American Association for Respiratory Care: Clinical practice guideline: postural drainage therapy, *Respir Care* 36(12):1418–1426, 1991.

American Association for Respiratory Care: Clinical practice guideline: directed cough, *Respir Care* 38(5):495–499, 1993.

American Association for Respiratory Care: Clinical practice guideline: use of positive airway pressure adjuncts to bronchial hygiene therapy, *Respir Care* 38(5):516–521, 1993.

Marini JJ: Postoperative atelectasis: Pathophysiology, clinical importance, and principles of management, *Respir Care* 29:515–522, 1984.

Hess D, Agarwal NN, Myers CL: Positioning, lung function, and kinetic bed therapy, *Respir Care* 37(2):181–197, 1992.

Anderson JB, Falk M: Chest physiotherapy in the pediatric age group, *Respir Care* 36(6):546–552, 1991.

Bach JR: Mechanical insufflation–exsufflation, *Chest* 104:1553–1562, 1993.

Larson JL, Kim MJ, Sharp JT: Inspiratory muscle training with a threshold resistive breathing device in patients with chronic obstructive pulmonary disease, *Am Rev Respir Dis* 133:A100, 1986.

# Chapter 29

Demers RR, Irwin RS: Management of hypercapnic respiratory failure: a systemic approach, *Respir Care*, 24:328–335, 1979.

Brandstetter RD: The adult respiratory distress syndrome—1986, *Heart & Lung* 15:155–164, 1986.

Fein A, Wiener–Kronish JP, Niederman M, Matthay MA: Pathophysiology of the adult respiratory distress syndrome. What have we learned from human studies? *Crit Care Clin* 2(3):429–453, 1986.

Schuster DP: A physiologic approach to initiating, maintaining, and withdrawing mechanical ventilatory support during acute respiratory failure, *Am J Med* 88(3):268–78, 1990.

Husdon LD: Pharmacologic approaches to respiratory failure, *Respir Care* 38(7):754–764, 1993.

Lewis JF, Jobe AH: Surfactant and the adult respiratory distress syndrome, *Am Rev Respir Dis* 147:218–233, 1993.

American Association for Respiratory Care: Consensus conference on the essentials of mechanical ventilators, *Respir Care* 37:999–1130, 1992.

# Chapter 30

Chatburn RL: Classification of mechanical ventilators, *Respir Care* 37:1009–1025, 1992.

Branson RD: Flow–triggering systems, *Respir Care* 39: 138–144, 1994.

Marini JJ, Rodriguez RM, Lamb V: The inspiratory workload of patient–initiated mechanical ventilation, *Am Rev Respir Dis* 134:902–909, 1986.

Blanch PB, Jones M, et al: Pressure–preset ventilation (part 1): pysiologic and mechanical considerations, *Chest* 104:590–599, 1993.

Blanch PB, Jones M, et al: Pressure–preset ventilation (part 2): mechanics and safety, *Chest* 104(3):904–912, 1993.

Kacmarek RM, Hess D: Pressure–controlled inverse–ratio ventilation: Panacea or auto–PEEP? [editorial], *Respir Care* 35(10):945–948, 1990.

Quan SF, Parides GC, Knoper SR: Mandatory minute volume (MMV) ventilation: an overview, *Respir Care* 35(9):898–904, 1990.

Hurst JM, DeHaven CB Jr, Branson RD: Comparison of conventional mechanical ventilation and synchronous independent lung ventilation (SILV) in the treatment of unilateral lung injury, *J Trauma* 25(8):766–770, 1985.

Waldhorn RE: Nocturnal nasal intermittent positive pressure ventilation with bi–level positive airway pressure (BiPAP) in respiratory failure, *Chest* 101(2):516–521, 1992.

Garner W, Downs JB, Stock MC, et al: Airway pressure release ventilation (APRV). A human trial, *Chest* 94:779–781, 1988.

Pierson DJ. Complications associated with mechanical ventilation, *Crit Care Clin,* 6(3):711–24 1990.

Marini JJ, Ravenscraft SA: Mean airway pressure: physiologic determinants and clinical importance—Part 1: Physiologic determinants and measurements, *Crit Care Med* 20(10):1461–1472, 1992.

# Chapter 31

Chatburn RL: Classification of mechanical ventilators, *Respir Care* 37:1009–1025, 1992.

Branson RD, Chatburn RL: Technical description and classification of modes of ventilator operation, *Respir Care* 37:1026–1044, 1992.

Rau JL: Inspiratory flow patterns: the 'shape' of ventilation, *Respir Care* 38(1):132–140, 1993.

Chatburn RL, Lough MD, Primiano FP Jr.: Mechanical ventilation, In: Chatburn RL, Lough MD. *Handbook of respiratory care,* 2nd ed, Chicago, 1990, Mosby–Year Book.

MacIntyre NR, Day S: Essentials for ventilator–alarm systems, *Respir Care* 37:1108–1112, 1992.

American Association for Respiratory Care: Consensus Statement on the Essentials of Mechanical Ventilators—1992, *Respir Care* 37(9):1000–1008, 1992.

# Chapter 32

Kacmarek RM: Essential gas delivery features of mechanical ventilators, *Respir Care* 37(9):1045–1055, 1992.

MacIntyre NR: Clinically available new strategies for mechanical ventilatory support, *Chest* 104(2):560–565, 1993.

Slutsky AS (Chair): ACCP Consensus Conference: mechanical ventilation, *Chest* 104:1833–1859, 1993.

American Association for Respiratory Care. Clinical practice guideline. Humidification during mechanical ventilation, *Respir Care* 37(8):887–890, 1992.

American Association for Respiratory Care. Clinical practice guideline. Patient–ventilator system checks, *Respir Care* 37(8):882–886, 1992.

Campbell RS: Managing the patient–ventilator system: system checks and circuit changes, *Respir Care* 39(3):227–236, 1994.

Marcy TW, Marini JJ: Inverse ratio ventilation in ARDS, Rationale and implementation, *Chest* 100(2):494–504, 1991.

Adoumie R, Shennib H, Brown R, et al.: Differential lung ventilation. Applications beyond the operating room, *J Thorac Cardiovasc Surg* 105:229–233, 1993.

Wright J, Gong H Jr: "Auto–PEEP": incidence, magnitude, and contributing factors, *Heart Lung* 19(4):352–357, 1990.

# Chapter 33

Vaz Fragoso CA: Monitoring in adult critical care, in Kacmarek RM, Hess D, Stoller JK, editors: *Monitoring in Respiratory Care,* St. Louis, 1993, Mosby–Year Book.

Tobin MJ: Respiratory monitoring in the intensive care unit, *Am Rev Respir Dis* 138(6):1625–1642, 1988.

Kacmarek RM, Hess D, Stoller JK: Perspectives on monitoring in respiratory care, in Kacmarek RM, Hess D, Stoller JK, editors: *Monitoring in Respiratory Care,* St. Louis, 1993, Mosby–Year Book.

Hess D: Noninvasive monitoring in respiratory care—present, past and future: An overview, *Respir Care* 35(6):482–496, 1990.

Martin RJ: Transcutaneous monitoring: instrumentation and clinical applications, *Respir Care* 35(6):577–583, 1990.

Nelson LD: Assessment of oxygenation: oxygenation indices, *Respir Care* 38(6):631–640, 1993.

Pierson DJ: Normal and abnormal oxygenation: physiology and clinical syndromes, *Respir Care* 38(6):587–599, 1993.

Hess D: Capnometry and capnography: Technical aspects, physiologic aspects, and clinical applications, *Respir Care* 35(6):557–573, 1990.

Marini JJ: Lung mechanics determinations at the bedside: Instrumentations and clinical application, *Respir Care* 35(7):669–693, 1990.

Marini JJ: Obtaining meaningful data from the Swan–Ganz catheter, *Respir Care* 30:572–581, 1987.

Tobin MJ: What should the clinician do when a patient "fights the ventilator"? *Respir Care* 36(5):395–406, 1991.

# Chapter 34

American College of Chest Physicians: ACCP Consensus Conference: mechanical ventilation, *Chest* 104:1833–1859, 1993.

Geisman LK, Ahrens T: Auto–PEEP: an impediment to weaning in the chronically ventilated patient, *AACN Clin Issues Crit Care Nurs* 2(3):391–397, 1991.

Knebel AR: Weaning from mechanical ventilation: current controversies, *Heart Lung* 20(4):321–31, 1991.

Yang KL, Tobin MJ: A prospective study of indexes predicting the outcome of trials of weaning from mechanical ventilation, *N Engl J Med* 324(21):1445–1450, 1991.

Yang KL: Reproducibility of weaning parameters. A need for standardization, *Chest* 102(6):1829–32, 1992.

Kacmarek RM. The role of pressure support in reducing the work of breathing, *Respir Care* 33:99–120, 1988.

Banner MJ, Kirby RR, et al.: Decreasing imposed work of the breathing apparatus to zero using pressure support ventilation, *Crit Care Med* 21(9):1333–1338, 1993.

Quan SF, Parides GC, Knoper SR: Mandatory minute volume (MMV) ventilation: an overview, *Respir Care* 35(9):898–904, 1990.

Tomlinson JR, Miller KS, et al.: A prospective comparison of IMV and T–piece weaning from mechanical ventilation, *Chest* 96(2):348–352, 1989.

Knebel AR, Janson–Bjerklie SL, et al.: Comparison of breathing comfort during weaning with two ventilatory modes, *Am J Respir Crit Care Med* 149(1):14–18, 1994.

Boysen PG: Weaning from mechanical ventilation: Does technique make a difference? *Respir Care* 36(5):407–416, 1991.

Shekleton ME: Respiratory muscle conditioning and the work of breathing: a critical balance in the weaning patient, *AACN Clin Issues Crit Care Nurs* 2(3):405–414, 1991.

Holliday JE, Hyers TM: The reduction of weaning time from mechanical ventilation usiug tidal volume and relaxation biofeedback, *Am Rev Respir Dis* 141:1214–1220, 1990.

Nochomovitz ML, Montenegro HD, et al.: Placement alternatives for ventilator–dependent patients outside the intensive care unit, *Respir Care* 36(3):199–204, 1991.

# Chapter 35

Koff PB: Development of cardiopulmonary system, in Koff PB, Eitzman DV, Neu J: *Neonatal and pediatric respiratory care,* ed 2, St. Louis, 1993, Mosby–Year Book.

Muller N, Bryan AC: Chest wall mechanics and respiratory muscles in infants, *Ped Clin N Am* 26:503–516, 1979.

Carlo WA, Martin RJ: Principles of neonatal assisted ventilation, *Ped Clin N Am* 33:221–237, 1985.

Behnke M: Patient assessment, in Koff PB, Eitzman DV, Neu J: *Neonatal and pediatric respiratory care,* ed 2, St. Louis, 1993, Mosby–Yearbook.

American Thoracic Society: Respiratory mechanics in infants: physiologic evaluation in health and disease, *Am Rev Respir Dis* 147:474–496, 1993.

Salyer JW: Respiratory monitoring in the neonatal intensive care unit, In Kacmarek RM, Hess D, Stoller JK, editors.: *Monitoring in respiratory care.* St. Louis, 1993, Mosby–Year Book.

Rau JL: Delivery of aerosolized drugs to neonatal and pediatric patients, *Respir Care* 36(6):514–542, 1991.

Chatburn RL: Principles and practice of neonatal and pediatric mechanical ventilation, *Respir Care* 36(6):569–593, 1991.

Bernstein G: Synchronous and patient–triggered ventilation in newborns, *Neonatal Respir Dis,* 3(2):1–4, 9–11, 1993.

Coghill CH, Haywood JL, Chatburn RL, Carlo WA: Neonatal and pediatric high–frequency ventilation: principles and practice, *Respir Care,* 36(6): 596–609, 1991.

Clark RH, Gerstmann DR, et al.: Prospective randomized comparison of high–frequency oscillatory and conventional ventilation in respiratory distress syndrome, *Pediatrics* 89(1):5–12, 1992.

O'Rourke PP: ECMO: Where have we been? Where are we going? *Respir Care* 36(7):683–692, 1991.

Sayler JW: Transport of the critically ill and injured, *Respir Care* 36(7):720–733, 1991.

Katz VL, Bowes WA Jr: Meconium aspiration syndrome: reflections on a murky subject, *Am J Obstet Gynecol,* 166(1 Pt 1):171–83, 1992.

Jobe AH: Pulmonary surfactant therapy, *N Engl J Med* 328(12): 861–868, 1993.

Guntheroth WG, Spiers PS: Sleeping prone and the risk of sudden infant death syndrome, *JAMA* 267(17):2359–2362, 1992.

Orenstein DM: Cystic fibrosis, *Respir Care* 36(7):746–752, 1991.

## Chapter 36

Martin–Peterson J, Cottrell RR: Self–concept, values, and health behavior, *Health Educ* 18:6–9, 1987.

Mason JO, McGinnis JM: *"Healthy People 2000":* an overview of the national health promotion and disease prevention objectives, Public Health Reports 105:441–446.

Public Health Service, Office of Disease Prevention and Health Promotion: *Healthy people 2000,* Washington, DC: US Government Printing Office, 1990. PHS Publication No. (PHS) 90–50212.

Breslow L: Health status measurement in the evaluation of health promotion, *Med Care* 27(3 suppl):S205–216, 1989.

Crooks CE, Iammarino NK, Weinberg AD: The family's role in health promotion, *Health Values* 11(2):7–12, 1987.

American Public Health Association, Healthy Communities 2000: Model Standards (Guidelines for community attainment of the year 2000 national health objectives), ed 3, Washington, DC: The American Public Health Association, 1991.

## Chapter 37

American Thoracic Society Executive Committee: Pulmonary rehabilitation—an official statement of the American Thoracic Society, *Am Rev Respir Dis* 124:663–666, 1981.

Ries AL: Scientific basis of pulmonary rehabilitation: position paper of the American Association of Cardiovascular and Pulmonary Rehabilitation, *J Cardiopulmonary Rehabil,* 10:418, 1990.

Niederman MS, Clemente PH, Fein AM, Feinsilver SH, Robinson DA, Ilowit JS, and Berstein MG: Benefits of a multidisciplinary pulmonary rehabilitation program. Improvements are independent of lung function, *Chest,* 1991, 99(4):798–804.

Zu Wallack RL, Patel K, Reardon JZ, Clark BA 3d, and Normandin EA: Predictors of improvement in the 12–minute walking distance following a six–week outpatient pulmonary rehabilitation program, *Chest,* 99(4):805–808, 1991.

Reisman–Beytas LJ, Connors GL: Organization and management of a pulmonary rehabilitation program, in Hodgkin JE, Connors GL, Bell JE, editors, *Pulmonary Rehabilitation: Guidelines to Success,* ed 2, Philadelphia, JB Lippincott, 1993.

Wasserman, K. , Sue DY, Casaburi R, and Moricca RB: Selection criteria for exercise training in pulmonary rehabilitation, *Eur Respir J Suppl,* 7:604s–610s, 1989.

Gilmartin ME: Pulmonary rehabilitation–patient and family education, *Clin Chest Med* 7:619–627, 1986.

## Chapter 38

American Association for Respiratory Care: Standards for respiratory therapy home care—An official statement by the American Association for Respiratory Care, *Respir Care* 24:1080–1082, 1979.

Fields AI, Rosenblatt A, Pollack MM, Kaufman J: Home care cost–effectiveness for respiratory technology–dependent children, *Am J Dis Child* 145(7):729–733, 1991.

American Association for Respiratory Care: Clinical practice guideline: Oxygen therapy in the home or extended care facility, *Respir Care* 37(8):918–922, 1992.

Petty TL: Home oxygen—a revolution in the care of advanced COPD, *Med Clin North Am* 74(3):715–729, 1990.

Christopher KL: Travel for patients with chronic respiratory disease, in Pierson DJ and Kacmarek RM (eds): *Foundations of respiratory care,* New York, 1992, Churchill Livingstone.

O'Donohue WJ: Oxygen conserving devices, *Respir Care* 32(1):37–42, 1987.

Shigeoka JW: Oxygen conservers, home oxygen prescriptions and the role of the respiratory care practitioner, *Respir Care* 36(3): 178–183, 1991.

Gilmartin ME: Long–term mechanical ventilation: patient selection and discharge planning, *Respir Care* 36(3):205–216, 1991.

Gilmartin ME: Monitoring in the home and outpatient setting, in Kacmarek RM, Hess D, Stoller JK, editors: *Monitoring in Respiratory Care,* St. Louis, 1993, Mosby–Year Book.

Bach JR, Alba AS, Saporito LR: Intermittent positive pressure ventilation via the mouth as an alternative to tracheostomy for 257 ventilator users. *Chest* Jan;103(1):174–82, 1993. Jan; 103(1): 174–82, 1993; ISSN: 0012–3692.

Piper AJ, Parker S, Torzillo PJ, et al.: Nocturnal nasal IPPV stabilizes patients with cystic fibrosis and hypercapnic respiratory failure, *Chest* 102(3):846–850, 1992.

# Answer Key

# Chapter 1

1.1 T
1.2 F
1.3 F
1.4 T
1.5 F
1.6 T
1.7 F
1.8 F
1.9 F
1.10 T
1.11 personal health services
1.12 18
1.13 public
1.14 credentialing
1.15 licensure
1.16 Certification
1.17 National Board for Respiratory Care (NBRC)
1.18 skilled nursing facility (SNF)
1.19 diagnosis related group (DRG)
1.20 places hospitals at risk financially
1.21 Joint Commission on Accreditation of Healthcare Organizations (JCAHO)
1.22 American Association for Respiratory Care (AARC)
1.23
   1. human biology
   2. environment
   3. lifestyle behavior
   4. health care system
1.24
   1. direct, or "out-of-pocket," payments
   2. private insurance
   3. government programs, principally Medicare
   4. charitable contributions
1.25
   1. Blue Cross/Blue Shield
   2. Medicare/Medicaid
   3. private insurers
1.26
   1. hospitals
   2. nursing homes
   3. physicians' offices
   4. health maintenance organizations
   5. home care programs
   6. local health departments
1.27
   1. HMOs provide comprehensive health care services to a voluntarily enrolled consumer population
   2. enrollment in an HMO is an alternative to other forms of health insurance
   3. HMO enrollees are guaranteed a defined set of benefits for a fixed fee
   4. HMO fees are the same for all like members, regardless of extent of services utilized
   5. HMO enrollment is primarily on a year–to–year (contractual) basis
1.28
   1. the growing cost of health care in the United States
   2. inequities in access to health care (entitlement)
   3. new technology—safety, efficacy, ethical, and moral consequences
   4. consumers' lack of information and involvement in decision making regarding allocation, distribution, and use of health services
   5. the need for more efficient, effective, and economical structure in the system

# Chapter 2

2.1 T
2.2 T
2.3 T
2.4 F
2.5 T
2.6 T
2.7 F
2.8 F
2.9 T
2.10 T
2.11 T
2.12 T
2.13 F
2.14 Joint Commission on the Accreditation of Healthcare Organizations (JCAHO)
2.15 governing board of directors
2.16 technical director
2.17 Preventive maintenance
2.18 policy and procedure manual
2.19
   1. therapeutic gas administration
   2. aerosol and humidity therapy
   3. intermittent positive pressure breathing (IPPB)
   4. hyperinflation therapy (incentive spirometry)
   5. bronchial hygiene/chest physiotherapy
   6. aerosol drug administration
2.20
   1. pulmonary function testing
   2. blood gas evaluation
2.21
   1. electrocardiography
   2. echocardiography
   3. cardiovascular catheterization

4. pulmonary function and stress testing
5. sleep disorders
6. hemodynamic monitoring

2.22
1. home care
2. outpatient rehabilitation
3. health education

2.23
1. broaden skills of providers
2. move services closer to patient
3. simplify processes
4. streamline paperwork and eliminate duplication
5. focus patient population

2.24
1. clearly stated objectives
2. outline of protocol including decision tree
3. description of alternate choices at decision and action points
4. description of potential complications and corrections
5. description of end–points and decision points where doctor must be contacted

2.25
1. identify problem
2. determine problem cause(s)
3. rank problems
4. develop strategies for problem resolution
5. develop measurement techniques
6. implement problem resolution strategies
7. analyze intervention results
8. report results
9. evaluate intervention outcomes

2.26 d.
2.27 d.
2.28 c.
2.29 c.
2.30 c.
2.31 d.
2.32 d.
2.33 d.
2.34 d.

# Chapter 3

3.1  T
3.2  F
3.3  T
3.4  T
3.5  T
3.6  T
3.7  F
3.8  T
3.9  F
3.10 F
3.11 T
3.12 health communication
3.13 physical
3.14 shared
3.15 symbols
3.16 attention
3.17 Tolerance
3.18 empathetic
3.19 intrapersonal communication
3.20 Current
3.21
1. personal feelings
2. attitudes
3. dispositions
4. values
5. motivations

3.22
1. attitudes of sender/receiver
2. knowledge of sender/receiver
3. social background of sender/receiver
4. cultural background of sender/receiver

3.23
1. Flammable material present
2. Flammable material heated to or above ignition temperature

3.24 b; c; a; d; e
3.25 b; a; e; c; d
3.26 d.
3.27 c.
3.28 d.
3.29 c.
3.30 d.
3.31 d.
3.32 b.
3.33 d.
3.34 d.

# Chapter 4

4.1  T
4.2  F
4.3  T
4.4  F
4.5  F
4.6  T
4.7  T
4.8  T
4.9  F
4.10 F
4.11 F
4.12 F
4.13 F

4.14  T
4.15  F
4.16  T
4.17  F
4.18  T
4.19  F
4.20  T
4.21  T
4.22  F
4.23  T
4.24  T
4.25  F
4.26  T
4.27  T
4.28  F
4.29  F
4.30  F
4.31  T
4.32  F
4.33  F
4.34  F
4.35  T
4.36  T
4.37  F
4.38  T
4.39  T
4.40  F
4.41  T
4.42  F
4.43  T
4.44  T
4.45  F
4.46  T
4.47  Gram stain
4.48  acid–fast stain
4.49  *Neisseria meningitidis*
4.50  *Bordetella pertussis*
4.51  *Corynebacterium diphtheriae*
4.52  parainfluenza
4.53  respiratory syncytial
4.54  *Chlamydia trachomatis*
4.55  droplet contact
4.56  vehicle
4.57  Airborne transmission
4.58  sterilization
4.59  disinfection
4.60  spores
4.61  moist heat (steam under pressure)
4.62  high–level disinfection
4.63  24
4.64  impervious bag
4.65  cohorting
4.66  their own (endogenous) flora
4.67  48–72 hours

4.68  open skin lesions (exudative lesions or weeping dermatitis)
4.69  biological
4.70  removed from use and reprocessed
4.71
   1. the genus *Bacillus*
   2. the genus *Clostridium*
4.72
   1.  diabetes mellitus
   2.  lymphoma
   3.  leukemia
   4.  neoplasia
   5.  uremia
   6.  treatment with certain antimicrobials
   7.  treatment with corticosteroids
   8.  treatment with irradiation
   9.  treatment with immunosuppressive agents
   10. old age
   11. chronic debilitating disease
   12. shock
   13. coma
   14. traumatic injury
   15. surgical procedures
   16. burn injuries
4.73
   a. Gloves should be worn for touching blood and body fluids, mucous membranes, or non–intact skin of all patients; for handling items or surfaces soiled with blood or body fluids; and for performing venipuncture and other vascular access procedures.
      Gloves should be changed after contact with each patient.
   b. Masks and protective eyewear or face shields should be worn during procedures that are likely to generate droplets of blood or other body fluids to prevent exposure of mucous membranes of the mouth, nose, and eyes.
   c. Gowns or aprons should be worn during procedures that are likely to generate splashes of blood or other body fluids.
   d. To prevent needlestick injuries, needles should not be recapped; purposely bent or broken by hand; removed from disposable syringes; or otherwise manipulated by hand. After they are used, disposable syringes and needles, scalpel blades, and other sharp items should be placed in puncture–resistant containers for disposal; the puncture–resistant containers should be located as close as practical to the use area. Large–bore reusable needles should be placed in a puncture–resistant container for transport to the reprocessing area.

e. Pregnant health care workers are not known to be at greater risk of contracting HIV infection than others, but if a health care worker develops HIV infection during pregnancy, the infant is at risk of infection resulting from perinatal transmission. Because of this risk, pregnant health care workers should be especially familiar with and strictly adhere to precautions to minimize the risk of HIV transmission.

4.74

| | |
|---|---|
| *Staphylococcus aureus* | d |
| *Haemophilus influenzae* | c |
| *Clostridium botulinum* | f |
| *Mycobacterium tuberculosis* | e |
| *Leptospirae* | b |
| *Pseudomonas aeruginosa* | a |
| *Clostridium tetani* | f |
| *Bordetella pertussis* | c |
| *Streptococcus pneumoniae* | d |
| *M. avium–intracellulare* | e |
| *Clostridium perfringens* | f |
| *Neisseria meningitidis* | g |
| *Legionella pneumophila* | a |
| *Serratia marcescens* | a |
| *Corynebacterium diphtheriae* | h |
| *Escherichia coli* | a |
| *Treponema pallidum* | b |
| *Proteus vulgaris* | a |
| *Klebsiella pneumoniae* | a |
| *Bacillus anthracis* | f |
| *Streptococcus pyogenes* | d |

| | |
|---|---|
| 4.75 | d. |
| 4.76 | d. |
| 4.77 | c. |
| 4.78 | d. |
| 4.79 | b. |
| 4.80 | d. |
| 4.81 | a. |
| 4.82 | c. |
| 4.83 | c. |
| 4.84 | c. |
| 4.85 | b. |
| 4.86 | a. |
| 4.87 | d. |
| 4.88 | d. |
| 4.89 | c. |
| 4.90 | d. |
| 4.91 | a. |
| 4.92 | a. |
| 4.93 | a. |
| 4.94 | c. |
| 4.95 | c. |
| 4.96 | d. |
| 4.97 | d. |

| | |
|---|---|
| 4.98 | c. |
| 4.99 | d. |
| 4.100 | d. |
| 4.101 | a. |
| 4.102 | c. |
| 4.103 | b. |
| 4.104 | d. |
| 4.105 | b. |
| 4.106 | d. |
| 4.107 | d. |
| 4.108 | a. |
| 4.109 | b. |
| 4.110 | a. |
| 4.111 | d. |
| 4.112 | c. |
| 4.113 | c. |
| 4.114 | b. |
| 4.115 | c. |

# Chapter 5

| | |
|---|---|
| 5.1 | F |
| 5.2 | T |
| 5.3 | T |
| 5.4 | T |
| 5.5 | F |
| 5.6 | T |
| 5.7 | T |
| 5.8 | T |
| 5.9 | T |
| 5.10 | T |
| 5.11 | F |
| 5.12 | T |
| 5.13 | F |
| 5.14 | ethics; law |
| 5.15 | codes of ethics; ethical theory |
| 5.16 | professional duty; patient right |
| 5.17 | decide; without coercion |
| 5.18 | paternalism |
| 5.19 | consequentialism |
| 5.20 | distributive justice |
| 5.21 | formalism |
| 5.22 | civil |
| 5.23 | negligence |
| 5.24 | physical contact |
| 5.25 | implied consent |
| 5.26 | discovery |
| 5.27 | respondeat superior |
| 5.28 | sustain life; relieve suffering |
| 5.29 | Good Samaritan Laws |

5.30
1. increasing sophistication of medical science and technology

2. concerns about limits on financial resources for health care
3. changes in society and its values and expectations
4. growing emphasis on the autonomy of the individual

5.31
1. the act must be within the scope of employment
2. the injury caused must be from an act of negligence

5.32
1. scope of professional practice
2. requirements and qualifications for licensure
3. exemptions
4. grounds for administrative action
5. creation of examination board and processes
6. penalties and sanctions for unauthorized practice

5.33
1. a description of the specific procedure and/or treatment
2. the medically significant risks involved
3. any available alternatives for care or treatment
4. the name(s) of those responsible for the procedure or treatment

5.34 d.
5.35 c.
5.36 a.
5.37 d.
5.38 d.
5.39 a.
5.40 c.
5.41 b.
5.42 b.
5.43 d.
5.44 c.
5.45 b.
5.46 b.
5.47 g; a; f; e; h; d; c; b

# Chapter 6

6.1

| | |
|---|---|
| greater than normal acid in the urine | aciduria |
| increase alkalinity in the blood | alkalemia |
| from the front to the back of the body | anteroposterior |
| an absence of spontaneous breathing | apnea |
| a small artery | arteriole |
| without symptoms | asymptomatic |
| the presence of bacteria in the blood | bacteremia |
| a slow heart rate (less than 60/min) | bradycardia |
| inflammation of the bronchi | bronchitis |
| visual examination of the bronchial tree | bronchoscopy |
| cancer–causing | carcinogenic |
| enlargement of the heart | cardiomegaly |
| of or pertaining to the ribs and diaphragm | costophrenic |
| difficulty in swallowing | dysphagia |
| difficult or labored breathing | dyspnea |
| a tracing of the heart's electrical activity | electrocardiogram |
| within the trachea | endotracheal |
| an increased number of eosinophils in the blood | eosinophilia |
| bleeding from the nose | epistaxis |
| outside a cell or cell tissue | extracellular |
| to withdraw a tube from the body | extubate |
| coughing up of blood from the respiratory tract | hemoptysis |
| the stoppage of bleeding | hemostasis |
| an accumulation of blood in the thorax | hemothorax |
| abnormal enlargement of the liver | hepatomegaly |
| excess carbon dioxide in the blood | hypercapnia |
| lower than normal glucose in the blood | hypoglycemia |
| a condition with decreased muscle tone | hypotonia |
| a deficiency of oxygen in the blood | hypoxemia |
| within the alveoli | intraalveolar |
| within a blood vessel | intravascular |
| a surgical incision into the abdomen | laparotomy |
| an abnormal decrease in white blood cells | leukocytopenia |
| toxic or destructive to a kidney | nephrotoxic |
| the presence of air in the thorax | pneumothorax |
| situated behind and to one side or the other | posterolateral |
| pus–producing | pyogenic |
| inflammation of the nose | rhinitis |
| an abnormally rapid rate of breathing | tachypnea |
| softening of the trachea | tracheomalacia |
| the procedure by which an incision is made into the trachea | tracheotomy |
| a narrowing of any blood vessel | vasoconstriction |

6.2

**acidemia** increased acid in the blood

**anaerobic** the ability to live without oxygen

**anemia** an abnormal condition characterized by a reduction in the number of circulating red blood cells or the amount of normal hemoglobin available to carry oxygen

**anesthetic** a drug or chemical substance that causes partial or complete loss of sensation

**asepsis** the absence of pathogenic microorganisms; the removal of pathogenic microorganisms or infected material

**asystole** the absence of a heartbeat

**atelectasis** an abnormal condition characterized by the collapse of lung tissue

**atrophy** a wasting or diminution of size or physiologic activity of a part of the body, especially muscle tissue, because of disease or other influences

**bacteriocidal** destructive to bacteria

**bradypnea** an abnormally slow rate of breathing

**bronchiectasis** an abnormal condition of the bronchial tree characterized by irreversible dilatation of the bronchial walls

**bronchiolitis** an acute infection of the lower respiratory tract characterized by inflammation of the bronchioles

**bronchoconstriction** narrowing of the bronchi due to contraction of their smooth muscle

**bronchopleural fistula** a direct communication between a bronchus and the pleural space

**capnograph** an instrument used in anesthesia, respiratory physiology, and respiratory care to produce a tracing, or capnogram, which shows the proportion of carbon dioxide in expired air

**cardiogenic** originating in or caused by the heart

**cerebrovascular** of or pertaining to the vascular system of the brain

**costochondral** of or pertaining to a rib and its cartilage

**cricothyrotomy** an incision into the larynx between the cricoid and thyroid cartilages

**cyanosis** bluish discoloration of the skin and mucous membranes caused by an excess of deoxygenated hemoglobin in the blood

**decongestant** of or pertaining to a substance or procedure that eliminates or reduces congestion or swelling

**decontamination** the process whereby contaminants are removed from objects, usually by simple physical means, such as washing

**diaphoresis** the secretion of sweat, especially the profuse secretion associated with an elevated body temperature, physical exertion, exposure to heat, and mental or emotional stress

**diuresis** increased formation and secretion of urine

**ectopic** situation in an unusual place, away from its normal location

**electromyography** the recording and study of the electrical properties of muscle

**embolization** the process by which an embolus forms and lodges in a branch of the vasculature

**empyema** an accumulation of pus in a body cavity, especially the pleural space

**endocarditis** inflammation of endocardium

**endogenous** growing within or arising from the body

**epigastric** of or pertaining to the epigastrium

**erythema** a redness of the skin due to capillary congestion

**erythrocythemia** an increase in the number of erythrocytes in the blood

**extrathoracic** outside the thorax

**fungicide** an agent destructive to fungi

**genitourinary** referring to the genital and urinary systems of the body, either the organ structures or functions or both

**hematopoiesis** the normal formation of blood cells in the bone marrow

**hemolysis** rupture of the red blood cells

**hyperinflation** a condition of maximum inflation

**hyperkalemia** greater than normal amounts of potassium in the blood

**hyperoxia** a condition of abnormally high oxygen tension in the blood

**hyperplasia** an increase in the size of a tissue or organ due to a growth in the number of cells present

**hyperpnea** deep breathing (usually associated with exercise)

**hypertrophy** an increase in the size of a tissue or organ due to a growth in the size of cells present

**hypochloremia** a decrease in the chloride level in the blood

**hypopnea** shallow breathing

**hypothermia** an abnormal condition in which the temperature of the body is well below normal

**hypoxia** an abnormal condition in which the oxygen available to the body cells is inadequate to meet their metabolic needs

**infiltrate** a fluid that passes through body tissues

**interstitial** of or pertaining to the interstitium, i.e., the extracellular space

**intramuscular** within a muscle; used commonly to refer to an injection method whereby a hypodermic needle is introduced into a muscle to administer a medication

**intrapleural** within the pleural "space"

**laryngoscopy** the process of viewing the larynx with a laryngoscope

**laryngospasm** an involuntary contraction of the laryngeal muscles resulting in complete or partial closure of the glottis

**lobectomy** a type of chest surgery in which a lobe of a lung is removed

**lymphadenopathy** of or pertaining to and disease of the lymph nodes

**midsternal** of or pertaining to the imaginary line vertically bisecting the sternum

**nocturia** excessive urination at night

**oliguria** a diminished capacity to form and pass urine

**orthopnea** an abnormal condition characterized by difficulty breathing in the lying or recumbent position

**oximeter** a device used to measure the saturation of blood hemoglobin with oxygen

**pericarditis** an inflammation of the pericardium of the heart

**pleurisy** a condition characterized by abnormal deposition of a fibrinous exudate on the pleural surface

**pneumonectomy** the surgical removal of all or part of a lung

**polycythemia** an abnormal increase in the number of erythrocytes in the blood

**radiolucent** of or pertaining to a substance or tissue that readily permits the passage of x–rays or other radiant energy

**sclerosis** any condition characterized by hardening of tissue, especially that due to hyperplasia of connective tissue

**septicemia** infection in which pathogens are present in the circulating blood stream

**tachycardia** an abnormally fast heart rate (greater than 100/min)

**thoracentesis** the surgical perforation of the chest wall and pleural space with a needle for the aspiration of fluid for diagnostic or therapeutic purposes or for the removal of a specimen for biopsy

**thoracotomy** a surgical opening into the thoracic cavity

**thrombolysis** the process by which thrombi are dissolved

**tracheostomy** an opening through the neck into the trachea, through which an indwelling tube may be inserted

**transbronchial** across the bronchi or bronchial wall, as in a transbronchial biopsy

**venule** a small vein

6.3

| | |
|---|---|
| ABG | arterial blood gas |
| a.c. | before meals |
| ad lib. | as desired |
| ADH | antidiuretic hormone |
| AFB | acid–fast bacillus |
| AP | anterior–posterior; anteroposterior |
| ARDS | adult respiratory distress syndrome |
| ASHD | arteriosclerotic heart disease |
| B.I.D., b.i.d. | twice a day |
| BP | blood pressure |
| c̄ | with |
| CA, Ca | cancer |
| CAD | coronary artery disease |
| CBC | complete blood count |
| CC | chief complaint |
| cc | cubic centimeter |
| CHF | congestive heart failure |
| COPD | chronic obstructive pulmonary disease |
| CPR | cardiopulmonary resuscitation |
| CSF | cerebrospinal fluid |
| CVA | cerebrovascular accident |
| CXR | chest x–ray; chest radiograph |
| /d | per day |
| Dx | diagnosis |
| ECG, EKG | electrocardiogram |
| GI | gastrointestinal |
| Gtt., gtt. | drops |
| GU | genitourinary |
| Gyn | gynecology |
| HCT, Hct | hematocrit |
| Hg | mercury |
| HGB, Hgb, Hb | hemoglobin |
| h.s. | at bedtime |
| IM | intramuscular |
| I.V., IV | intravenously |
| LAT, lat. | lateral |
| mcg | microgram |
| MI | myocardial infarction |
| NPO | nothing by mouth |
| od | once a day |
| OR | operating room |
| os | mouth |
| paren | parenterally |
| P.C., p.c. | after meals |
| PND | paroxysmal nocturnal dyspnea |
| P.O. | orally |
| p.r.n. | as required |
| q.d. | every day |
| q.h. | every hour |
| Q.I.D., q.i.d. | four times a day |
| qm | every morning |
| qn | every night |
| RBC | red blood cell; red blood count |
| Rx | prescription |
| s̄ | without |
| SOB | short(ness) of breath |
| Stat. | immediately |
| subcu., SC | subcutaneous |
| TB | tuberculosis |
| T.I.D., t.i.d. | three times a day |
| TPR | temperature, pulse, and respiration |
| UA | urinalysis |
| URI | upper respiratory infection |
| WBC | white blood cell; white blood count |

**6.4**

The alveolar pressure of carbon dioxide ($Paco_2$) equals the volume of carbon dioxide per minute ($\dot{V}co_2$) times the constant .863 divided by the alveolar gas volume per minute ($\dot{V}_A$).

**6.5**

The transpulmonary pressure ($P_L$) equals the difference between the pressure in the alveoli ($P_{alv}$) and the pressure in the pleural space ($P_{pl}$).

**6.6**

The volume of gas expired (exhaled) per minute ($\dot{V}_E$) equals the number of breathing cycles per minute (f) times the tidal volume ($V_T$).

**6.7**

The ratio of deadspace volume ($V_D$) to tidal volume ($V_T$) equals the pressure of carbon dioxide in the arterial blood ($Paco_2$) minus the average pressure of carbon dioxide in the expired air ($P\bar{E}co_2$) divided by the pressure of carbon dioxide in the arterial blood ($Paco_2$).

**6.8**

The volume flow of blood per minute ($\dot{Q}$) equals the volume of oxygen (consumed) per minute ($\dot{V}o_2$) divided by the difference in concentration of oxygen between the arterial and average (mixed) venous blood [$C(a - \bar{v})O_2$] times a constant (10).

**6.9**

The ratio of shunted blood flow per minute ($\dot{Q}s$) to capillary blood flow ($\dot{Q}_c$) equals the difference (–) between the end–capillary ($Cco_2$) and arterial concentration ($Cao_2$) of oxygen in the blood divided by the difference (–) between the end–capillary ($Cco_2$) and average venous concentration ($C\bar{v}o_2$) of oxygen in the blood.

**6.10**

a. 350 mm (millimeters)
b. 1000 m (micrometers)
c. 0.25 sec (seconds)
d. 0.10 L (liters)
e. 2400 ml (milliliters)
f. 4.55 L (liters)
g. 2650 gm (grams)
h. 0.60 kg (kilograms)
i. 10 mg (milligrams)
j. 0.035 gm (grams)
k. 2000 g (micrograms)

**6.11**

a. 185.93 cm (centimeters)
b. 24.13 cm (centimeters)
c. 7.28 in (inches)
d. 0.263 m (meters)
e. 240 cm (centimeters)
f. 6.07 ft (feet)
g. 13.78 in (inches)

**6.12**

a. 1825.36 gallons (US)
b. 623.04 L (liters)
c. 5.68 L (liters)
d. 243.57 ft$^3$ (cubic feet)
e. 0.66 gallons (US)
f. 0.92 ft$^3$ (cubic feet)
g. 100 cm$^3$ (cubic centimeters; cc)

**6.13**

a. 143.33 lb (pounds)
b. 83.99 kg (kilograms)
c. 1.13 oz (ounces)
d. 241 g (grams; gm)
e. 3.30 lb (pounds)
f. 2540 g (grams; gm)

**6.14**

a. 101357 Pa (Pascals)
b. 15169 kPa (kiloPascals)
c. 325 dynes/cm$^2$
d. 6.30 Pa (Pascals)

**6.15**

a. 11844 cal (calories)
b. 25.81 BTU
c. 209.30 J (Joule)
d. 25000 ergs (dyne–cm)
e. 0.685 J (Joule)

# Chapter 7

7.1   T
7.2   F
7.3   F
7.4   T
7.5   T
7.6   F
7.7   F
7.8   T
7.9   F
7.10  T
7.11  T
7.12  T
7.13  F
7.14  T
7.15  kinetic energy
7.16  equal to
7.17  thermal equilibrium
7.18  latent heat of fusion
7.19  hydrometer
7.20  poise
7.21  cohesion
7.22  vaporization
7.23  boiling point
7.24  water vapor pressure

7.25 absolute humidity

7.26 relative humidity

7.27 diffusion

7.28 triple point

7.29 critical temperature

7.30 increases; decreases

7.31 restore

7.32 dependability; lack of moving parts; minimal maintenance

7.33 wall attachment; Coanda

7.34
1. by heating the object
2. by performing work on the object

7.35
1. water vapor
2. molecular water
3. humidity

7.36 d.

7.37 c.

7.38 b.

7.39 c.

7.40 c.

7.41 a.

7.42 b.

7.43 d.

7.44 b.

7.45 d.

7.46 c.

7.47 c.

7.48 b.

7.49 c.

7.50 a.

7.51

| | °K | °C | °F |
|---|---|---|---|
| a. | 347 | 74 | 165 |
| b. | 293 | 20 | 68 |
| c. | 313 | 40 | 104 |
| d. | 330 | 57 | 135 |
| e. | 283 | 10 | 50 |
| f. | 307 | 34 | 93 |

7.52
a. 1006.40 gm/cm$^2$
b. 1044.48 gm/cm$^2$
c. 3017.52 gm/cm$^2$
d. 25.40 gm/cm$^2$

7.53
a. Bubble 1: 24000 dynes/cm$^2$
   Bubble 2: 48000 dynes/cm$^2$
   Bubble 3: 16000 dynes/cm$^2$
b. Bubble 2 exerts twice the pressure as bubble 1 because its radius is half as large; with the same radius as bubble 2, bubble 3 exerts less pressure due to its lower surface tension.

7.54
a.

| Air Sample # | Saturated Capacity (mg/L) | Percent Relative Humidity | Percent Body Humidity |
|---|---|---|---|
| 1 | 17.30 | 57.8% | 22.8% |
| 2 | 19.42 | 66.6% | 29.5% |
| 3 | 35.61 | 29.5% | 24.0% |
| 4 | 30.35 | 91.1% | 63.1% |
| 5 | 43.80 | 68.5% | 68.5% |

b. 58% relative humidity; 23% body humidity
c. 69% relative humidity; 69% body humidity

7.55
a. 50% oxygen + 50% nitrogen = 1.339 g/L
   95% oxygen + 5% carbon dioxide = 1.455 g/L
   90% oxygen + 10% carbon dioxide = 1.482 g/L
   20% oxygen + 80% carbon dioxide = 0.429 g/L
   30% oxygen + 70% carbon dioxide = 0.554 g/L
b. 80% helium/20% oxygen mixture (lowest density)
c. 10% carbon dioxide/90% oxygen mixture (highest density)

7.56
Monday :      757.7 mm Hg
Tuesday:      747.4 mm Hg
Wednesday:   738.0 mm Hg
Thursday:     742.6 mm Hg
Friday:       752.2 mm Hg

7.57

| | cm H$_2$O | kPa | mm Hg |
|---|---|---|---|
| a. | 40.00 | 3.97 | 29.44 |
| b. | 61.18 | 6.00 | 45.01 |
| c. | 163.08 | 15.96 | 120.00 |
| d. | 8.00 | 0.78 | 5.89 |
| e. | 35.69 | 3.50 | 26.25 |
| f. | 108.72 | 10.64 | 80.00 |

7.58
a. nitrogen:    589.50 mm Hg
   oxygen:      158.17 mm Hg
   argon:       7.02 mm Hg
   CO$_2$:      0.23 mm Hg
   TOTAL:       754.93 mm Hg
b. There must be other trace gases in the atmosphere.

7.59

| Percent Oxygen | $P_{O_2}$ |
| --- | --- |
| 21% | 149.3 |
| 40% | 287.2 |
| 70% | 491.4 |
| 100% | 713.9 |

7.60

| | | |
| --- | --- | --- |
| nitrogen: | 573 | 75.39% |
| oxygen: | 100 | 13.16% |
| carbon dioxide: | 40 | 5.26% |
| water vapor: | 47 | 6.18% |
| TOTALS: | 760 | 100.00% |

# Chapter 8

8.1  F
8.2  F
8.3  F
8.4  T
8.5  T
8.6  F
8.7  F
8.8  T
8.9  T
8.10  T
8.11  F
8.12  F
8.13  F
8.14  T
8.15  F
8.16  bits
8.17  fuzzy
8.18  integrated circuit (IC)
8.19  multitasking
8.20  Parallel processing
8.21  memory
8.22  byte
8.23  read only memory (ROM)
8.24  random access memory (RAM)
8.25  density
8.26  keyboard
8.27  mouse or trackball
8.28  ASCII
8.29  optical scanner
8.30  pixel
8.31  analog
8.32  printer
8.33  software (a program)
8.34  algorithm
8.35  batch file

8.36  spreadsheet
8.37  formulas
8.38  records
8.39  downloading
8.40  automatic error correction
8.41  c.
8.42  b.
8.43  d.
8.44  b.
8.45  d.
8.46  d.
8.47  b.
8.48  d.
8.49  b.
8.50  a.
8.51  c.
8.52  d.
8.53  d.
8.54  d.
8.55  b.
8.56  a.
8.57  b.
8.58  d.
8.59  d.
8.60  a.
8.61  d.
8.62  a.
8.63  b.
8.64  c.
8.65  b.
8.66  c.
8.67  d.
8.68  d.
8.69  c.
8.70  d.
8.71  a.
8.72  c.
8.73  d.
8.74  a.
8.75  b.
8.76  d.

# Chapter 9

9.1
   a. angle of Louis
   b. ribs
   c. costal cartilages
   d. manubrium
   e. body of sternum
   f. xiphoid process
   g. thoracic vertebrae

9.2
a. sternomastoid
b. pectoralis major
c. diaphragm
d. scalenus medius
e. internal intercostal
f. external intercostal
g. internal oblique
h. transverse abdominus

9.3
a. right carotid artery
b. right subclavian artery
c. innominate artery
d. aorta
e. left carotid artery
f. left subclavian artery
g. pulmonary artery

9.4
a. middle concha
b. hard palate
c. thyroid cartilage
d. cricothyroid membrane
e. eustachian tube
f. palatine tonsil
g. epiglottis

9.5
a. epiglottis
b. hyoid bone
c. arytenoid cartilage
d. thyroid cartilage
e. cricothyroid ligament
f. cricoid cartilage
g. trachea

9.6
a. alveolar macrophage
b. capillary
c. red blood cell
d. alveolar type II cell
e. pore of Kohn
f. alveolar type I cell

9.7
a.

| Right Lung | Left Lung |
| --- | --- |
| 1. apical RUL | 1. apical–posterior LUL |
| 2. posterior RUL | 2. apical–posterior LUL |
| 3. anterior RUL | 3. anterior LUL |
| 4. lateral RML | 4. superior lingular LUL |
| 5. medial RML | 5. inferior lingular LUL |
| 6. superior basal RLL | 6. superior basal LLL |
| 7. medial basal RLL | 7. anterior basal LLL |
| 8. anterior basal RLL | 8. anterior basal LLL |
| 9. lateral basal RLL | 9. lateral basal LLL |
| 10. posterior basal RLL | 10. posterior basal LLL |

b. the superior/inferior lingular segments of the left upper lobe

9.8  b.
9.9  d.
9.10  c.
9.11  c.
9.12  c.
9.13  d.
9.14  d.
9.15  d.
9.16  d.
9.17  c.
9.18  c.
9.19  d.
9.20  a.
9.21  b.
9.22  d.
9.23  d.
9.24  d.
9.25  a.
9.26  d.
9.27  d.
9.28  a.
9.29  d.
9.30  c.
9.31  d.
9.32  b.
9.33  a.
9.34  a.
9.35  d.

9.36 d.
9.37 c.
9.38 c.
9.39 d.
9.40 b.
9.41 d.
9.42 d.

# Chapter 10

10.1
  a. pulmonary artery
  b. left atrium
  c. pulmonary veins
  d. superior vena cava
  e. tricuspid valve
  f. right ventricle
  g. aorta
  h. orifices of coronary arteries
  i. interventricular septum
  j. papillary muscles
  k. left ventricle
10.2
  a. pulmonic valve
  b. aortic valve
  c. mitral (bicuspid) valve
  d. tricuspid valve
  e. anulus fibrosus
10.3
  a. sinoatrial (SA) node
  b. atrioventricular (AV) node
  c. bundle branches
  d. Purkinje fibers
  e. superior vena cava
10.4
  a. P wave
  b. QRS complex
  c. T wave
  d. P–R interval
  e. S–T segment
  f. Q–T segment
  g. T wave
  h. P wave
  i. P–R interval
  j. Q–T segment
  k. S–T segment
10.5
  a. a waves
  b. c waves
  c. exceeds
  d. drops below
  e. rise
  f. aortic; pulmonary

  g. aortic; mitral
  h. AV valves
  i. ventricular relaxation
  j. a–c–v wave sequence
10.6   c.
10.7   d.
10.8   c.
10.9   d.
10.10  b.
10.11  d.
10.12  a.
10.13  c.
10.14  a.
10.15  a.
10.16  d.
10.17  d.
10.18  a.
10.19  a.
10.20  d.
10.21  d.
10.22  b.
10.23  a.
10.24  d.
10.25  d.
10.26  c.
10.27  d.
10.28  d.
10.29  a.
10.30  c.
10.31  d.
10.32  b.
10.33  b.
10.34  d.

# Chapter 11

11.1
  a. total lung capacity
  b. inspiratory capacity
  c. resting tidal volume
  d. functional residual capacity
  e. inspiratory reserve volume
  f. expiratory reserve volume
  g. vital capacity
  h. residual volume
11.2
  a. mouth pressure ($P_{ao}$)
  b. alveolar pressure ($P_{alv}$)
  c. pleural pressure ($P_{pl}$)
  d. body surface pressure ($P_{bs}$)
  e. transrespiratory gradient ($P_{rs}$)
  f. transpulmonary gradient ($P_L$)

g. transthoracic gradient ($P_W$)

h. all, except the pressures at the airway opening and body surface (both normally equal to atmospheric pressure)

i. pleural pressure ($P_{pl}$)

j. the transrespiratory gradient ($P_{rs}$), or difference between the airway opening (mouth) and alveolar pressures

k. the transpulmonary gradient ($P_L$), or difference between the pleural and alveolar pressures

11.3  c.
11.4  d.
11.5  b.
11.6  d.
11.7  c.
11.8  a.
11.9  c.
11.10  d.
11.11  c.
11.12  d.
11.13  a.
11.14  d.
11.15  d.
11.16  c.
11.17  d.
11.18  b.
11.19  d.
11.20  d.
11.21  c.
11.22  d.
11.23  d.
11.24  d.
11.25  b.
11.26  a.
11.27  a.
11.28  d.
11.29  d.
11.30  d.
11.31  d.
11.32  d.
11.33  d.
11.34  b.
11.35  c.
11.36  b.
11.37  b.
11.38  c.
11.39
  a. 1: 0.14
     2: 0.22
     3: 0.11
     4: 0.09
     5: 0.56
     6: 0.05
  b. patients 1, 2, and 3

c. patients 4 and 6
d. patient 5

11.40
  a.

| Patient # | $C_L$ | $C_T$ | $C_{LT}$ |
|---|---|---|---|
| 1 | .20 | .10 | .067 |
| 2 | .05 | .20 | .040 |
| 3 | .15 | .03 | .025 |
| 4 | .05 | .08 | .030 |
| 5 | .12 | .25 | .080 |
| 6 | .30 | .15 | .100 |
| 7 | .25 | .32 | .140 |
| 8 | .01 | .01 | .005 |

  b. patients 2, 3, 4, and 8
  c. patient 2
  d. patient 3
  e. patients 4 and 8

11.41
  a.

| $\Delta P$ (cm $H_2O$) | $R_{aw}$ (cm $H_2O$/L/sec) |
|---|---|
| 5.00 | 8.57 |
| 8.50 | 4.25 |
| 3.80 | 2.85 |
| 20.00 | 26.67 |
| 15.00 | 12.00 |
| 10.00 | 10.91 |

  b. inspiratory airway resistance (because the pressures at the airway opening are greater than the alveolar pressures)

  c. The first three cases represent normal spontaneous inspiration ($P_{alv}$ is negative); the remaining three cases involve positive pressure applied to the airways (both $P_{ao}$ and $P_{alv}$ are positive).

11.42
  a. 1: 0.40
     2: 0.02
     3: 7.20
     4: 1.76
     5: 0.045
     6: 22.50
     7: 0.015
     8: 0.40
     9: .01

  b. Filling and emptying of a lung unit will be more rapid than normal if the compliance is decreased, the resistance is decreased, or both conditions exist, as evident in examples #2, 5, 7, and 9.

c. Filling and emptying of a lung unit will be slower than normal if the compliance is increased, the resistance is increased, or both conditions exist, as evident in examples #3, 4, and 6.

d. No, a normal time constant does not mean that the lung unit has normal compliance and resistance. In example #8, the compliance is lower than normal, but the resistance is higher than normal; this results in a normal time constant (normal rate of emptying and filling).

11.43

a.

| Case # | f | $V_T$ | $\mathring{V}_E$ | $V_D$ | $V_A$ |
|--------|-----|------|------|-----|------|
| 1 | 12 | 500 | 6000 | 150 | 4200 |
| 2 | 24 | 250 | 6000 | 150 | 2400 |
| 3 | 6 | 1000 | 6000 | 150 | 5100 |
| 4 | 12 | 500 | 6000 | 300 | 2400 |
| 5 | 12 | 650 | 7800 | 300 | 4200 |
| 6 | 40 | 150 | 6000 | 150 | 0 |

b. If the minute ventilation remains constant, increasing the frequency of breathing causes a decrease in the alveolar ventilation per minute. This is because the proportion of deadspace ventilation per minute increases with higher breathing frequencies.

c. If the minute ventilation remains constant, decreasing the frequency of breathing causes an increase in the alveolar ventilation per minute. This is because the proportion of deadspace ventilation per minute decreases at lower breathing frequencies.

d. If the frequency of breathing and minute ventilation remain constant, increasing the physiologic deadspace per breath ($V_{Dphys}$) will result in a decrease in alveolar ventilation per minute.

e. The only way a patient can maintain a normal alveolar ventilation with an increase in physiologic deadspace is to increase the minute ventilation by increasing the tidal volume (an increase in rate would only further increase deadspace per minute ventilation).

f. Rapid shallow breathing always results in a decrease in alveolar ventilation per minute.

g. No. As shown in cases #1, 2, 3, 4, and 6, the $V_E$ does not always indicate the level of alveolar ventilation. In all five of these cases, the minute ventilation is 6000 ml/min; however, the alveolar ventilation per minute varies from a low of 2400 ml/min to a high of 5100 ml/min.

11.44

| $V_T$ | $V_D/V_T$ | $V_{Dphys}$ |
|-------|-----------|-------------|
| 350 | .31 | 109 |
| 480 | .46 | 219 |
| 960 | .50 | 480 |
| 500 | .53 | 265 |
| 1100 | .62 | 677 |

# Chapter 12

12.1 c.
12.2 c.
12.3 c.
12.4 b.
12.5 b.
12.6 d.
12.7 d.
12.8 d.
12.9 a.
12.10 b.
12.11 b.
12.12 d.
12.13 b.
12.14 d.
12.15 d.
12.16 b.
12.17 b.
12.18 c.
12.19 d.
12.20 d.
12.21 b.
12.22 d.
12.23 d.
12.24 d.
12.25 c.
12.26 a.
12.27 b.
12.28 d.
12.29 c.
12.30 d.
12.31 d.
12.32 c.
12.33 d.
12.34 c.
12.35 d.
12.36 b.
12.37 b.
12.38 b.
12.39 d.

12.40
a. 1: 41 mm Hg
   2: 62 mm Hg
   3: 40 mm Hg
   4: 72 mm Hg
   5: 24 mm Hg
   6: 41 mm Hg
b. Case #1 represents normal values for a healthy 70–kg adult male.
c. If the alveolar ventilation remains constant, an increase in carbon dioxide production will result in an increase in the alveolar partial pressure of carbon dioxide ($P_{ACO_2}$).
d. When faced with an increase in metabolic rate, the body maintains normal levels of alveolar carbon dioxide ($P_{ACO_2}$) by increasing alveolar ventilation.
e. If the carbon dioxide production remains constant, a decrease in alveolar ventilation will cause the alveolar partial pressure of carbon dioxide ($P_{ACO_2}$) to rise above normal.
f. If the carbon dioxide production remains constant, an increase in alveolar ventilation will cause the alveolar partial pressure of carbon dioxide ($P_{ACO_2}$) to drop below normal.
g. The data for cases #2 and 4 are consistent with alveolar hypoventilation. In both cases, ventilation is insufficient to meet metabolic needs, resulting in a rise in the alveolar partial pressure of carbon dioxide ($P_{ACO_2}$).
h. The data for case #5 is consistent with alveolar hypoventilation. In this case, ventilation is in excess of metabolic needs, resulting in a rise in the alveolar partial pressure of carbon dioxide ($P_{ACO_2}$).

12.41
a. 1:  100 mm Hg
   2:  56 mm Hg
   3:  122 mm Hg
   4:  72 mm Hg
   5:  419 mm Hg
   6:  144 mm Hg
   7:  239 mm Hg
   8:  460 mm Hg
   9:  668 mm Hg
   10: 158 mm Hg
b. Case #1 represents normal values for a healthy young adult.
c. With the $P_B$ and $F_{IO_2}$ constant, a decrease in alveolar ventilation (increase in $Paco_2$) causes the $P_{AO_2}$ to fall (case #2); conversely, an increase in alveolar ventilation (decrease in $Paco_2$) causes the $P_{AO_2}$ to rise (case #3).

d. With the $F_{IO_2}$ and alveolar ventilation constant, the alveolar partial pressure of oxygen ($P_{AO_2}$) varies directly with changes in the barometric pressure, i.e., a decrease in $P_B$ results in a decrease in $P_{AO_2}$ (case #4); an increase in $P_B$ results in an increase in $P_{AO_2}$ (case #5).
e. The partial pressure of oxygen in the lungs and blood can be increased without increasing the $F_{IO_2}$ by increasing the ambient pressure above that at sea level. Case #5 demonstrates this effect.
f. Increasing the $F_{IO_2}$ breathed by healthy individuals results in an increase in the alveolar partial pressure of oxygen ($P_{AO_2}$). Cases #6, 7, 8, and 9 demonstrate this effect.
g. The alveolar partial pressure of oxygen is determined by both the $F_{IO_2}$ and ambient pressure. At pressures below normal atmospheric pressure (in this case about a third that at sea level), the resulting $P_{AO_2}$ is proportionately lower. Thus the astronauts breathe oxygen at a partial pressure just slightly above normal (158 mm Hg vs. 100 mm Hg).

12.42
a.

| Case # | Dis $O_2$ ml/dL | HbO$_2$ ml/dL | TOT $O_2$ ml/dL |
|--------|-----------------|---------------|-----------------|
| 1 | 30 | 19.50 | 19.80 |
| 2 | 12 | 14.67 | 14.79 |
| 3 | 25 | 20.10 | 21.98 |
| 4 | 30 | 9.75 | 10.05 |
| 5 | 60 | 9.75 | 10.35 |
| 6 | 15 | 20.44 | 20.59 |
| 7 | 30 | 2.01 | 2.31 |
| 8 | 40 | 7.50 | 16.62 |

b. Case #1 represents normal values for a healthy young adult.
c. When the hemoglobin concentration is normal, lowering the blood $Po_2$ below normal results in a large drop in total oxygen content (case #2). This is due mainly to a decrease in the percent saturation of hemoglobin with oxygen and the resulting decrease in chemically combined oxygen.
d. When the hemoglobin concentration is normal, raising the blood $Po_2$ above normal results in a small increase in total oxygen content (case #3). This is due mainly to an increase in the physically dissolved oxygen content.

e. A low blood $P_{O_2}$ decreases the total oxygen content more than a high $P_{O_2}$ raises it, i.e., the low $P_{O_2}$ has the greater impact. This is because most oxygen is carried in the blood in chemical combination with hemoglobin, which under normal circumstances is already almost 100% saturated. Therefore, increases in to the blood. However, decreases in the $P_{O_2}$ below normal decrease hemoglobin saturation with oxygen, thereby causing a large decrease in total oxygen contents.

f. Because most oxygen is carried in chemical combination with hemoglobin, a decrease in hemoglobin concentration always lowers the total oxygen content of the blood. Cases #4 and 5 demonstrate this effect.

g. Under normal atmospheric conditions and in the presence of low blood hemoglobin concentrations, increasing the $P_{O_2}$ will not significantly increase the total oxygen contents. This is because most oxygen is carried in the blood in chemical combination with hemoglobin, which under normal circumstances is already almost 100% saturated. Therefore, increases in the $P_{O_2}$ above the normal value of 100 mm Hg add little oxygen to the blood. Case #5 demonstrates this effect.

h. In case #7, the low Hb saturation explains the low total oxygen content. Based on these data, there must be a hemoglobin saturation abnormality. Clinical conditions that might explain this problem include elevated carboxyhemoglobin and methemoglobin level. Both result in displacement of oxygen from the hemoglobin molecule and a lower than normal saturation for a given $P_{O_2}$.

i. In case #8, the acceptable level of total oxygen content (16.6 ml/dL) is being achieved mainly by virtue of the large dissolved oxygen content. This large proportion of dissolved oxygen, in turn, is the result of the hyperbaric $P_{O_2}$—equivalent to about four times normal atmospheric pressure.

12.43

a.

| Case # | $C(a-\bar{v})O_2$ ml/dL | $Q_T$ L/min |
|---|---|---|
| 1 | 4.80 | 5.5 |
| 2 | 7.10 | 3.7 |
| 3 | 2.70 | 9.8 |
| 4 | 4.80 | 15.4 |
| 5 | 4.80 | 3.1 |

b. Given a constant oxygen consumption ($\dot{V}O_2$) and total arterial oxygen content ($CaO_2$), a drop in cardiac output results in a decrease in mixed venous oxygen content and an increase in the arterial–venous oxygen content difference (case #2). Conversely, with all else constant, an increase in cardiac output results in an increase in the mixed venous oxygen content and a decrease in the arterial–venous oxygen content difference (case #3).

c. In order for the mixed venous oxygen content and arterial–venous oxygen content difference to remain normal when the oxygen consumption increases, the cardiac output must increase proportionately. Case #3 demonstrates this effect.

d. A reduction in total oxygen consumption means that the heart can maintain normal oxygen delivery at lower cardiac outputs. Case #5 demonstrates this effect.

# Chapter 13

13.1  T
13.2  T
13.3  T
13.4  F
13.5  T
13.6  T
13.7  F
13.8  T
13.9  F
13.10  F
13.11  T
13.12  True solution
13.13  saturated
13.14  Dissociation
13.15  100
13.16  10–fold
13.17  increases; acidic
13.18  60; 50
13.19  1000; 1200
13.20  humidity deficit
13.21  700
13.22  1/6
13.23  Aldosterone
13.24  Chloride
13.25  bicarbonate
13.26  potassium
13.27  20:1
13.28  neuromuscular function
13.29
1. filtration and reabsorption of sodium
2. regulation of water excretion in response to changes in secretion of antidiuretic hormone (ADH)

13.30
1. vomiting
2. diarrhea
3. GI suctioning
4. fever
5. profuse sweating
6. renal diseases
7. bypasses upper airway

13.31
1. 135–145
2. 96–105
3. 22–26
4. 3.5–5.0
5. 4.50–5.25
6. 1.2–2.3

13.32
1. ionized
2. protein bound
3. anion complex

13.33  c.
13.34  b.
13.35  a.
13.36  a.
13.37  b.
13.38  d.
13.39  d.
13.40  d.
13.41  a.
13.42  a.
13.43  d.
13.44  c.
13.45  d.
13.46  b.
13.47  a.

13.48

| Total Solute Content in grams | Solute Content in mg/ml |
| --- | --- |
| a.  .10 | 10 |
| b.  .06 | 30 |
| c.  10 | 200 |
| d.  100 | 100 |

13.49

| pH | nanomole/L (nM/L) |
| --- | --- |
| a.  7.32 | 48 |
| b.  7.07 | 85 |
| c.  6.92 | 120 |
| d.  6.21 | 610 |
| e.  5.62 | 2400 |

# Chapter 14

14.1   F
14.2   T
14.3   F
14.4   T
14.5   F
14.6   T
14.7   F
14.8   T
14.9   F
14.10  T
14.11  T
14.12  T
14.13  T
14.14  T
14.15  T
14.16  T
14.17  F
14.18  T
14.19  T
14.20  T
14.21  T
14.22  carbon dioxide
14.23  24,000
14.24  lactic acid
14.25  1
14.26  3600–4800
14.27  protein amino acids
14.28  7.35–7.45
14.29  increases; decreases
14.30  base excess (BE)
14.31  anion gap
14.32  chemoreceptor
14.33  proprioceptors
14.34  c.
14.35  d.
14.36  b.
14.37  a.
14.38  d.
14.39  d.
14.40  a.
14.41  c.
14.42  d.
14.43  c.
14.44  b.
14.45  d.
14.46  d.
14.47  a.
14.48  a.
14.49  c.
14.50  c.

14.51  d.
14.52  b.
14.53  d.
14.54  d.
14.55  c.
14.56  d.
14.57  c.
14.58  c.
14.59  d.
14.60  b.
14.61  d.
14.62  c.
14.63  d.
14.64  a.
14.65  d.
14.66  d.
14.67  b.
14.68  c.
14.69
  1: 7.40
  2: 7.22
  3: 7.62
  4: 7.35
  5: 7.45
14.70

## Acid–Base Interpretation

a.  combined respiratory and metabolic acidosis
b.  within normal limits
c.  acute(uncompensated) metabolic alkalosis
d.  (fully) compensated respiratory alkalosis
e.  partially compensated metabolic acidosis
f.  (fully) compensated metabolic alkalosis
g.  acute (uncompensated) metabolic acidosis
h.  combined respiratory and metabolic alkalosis
i.  acute (uncompensated) respiratory acidosis
j.  partially compensated metabolic alkalosis
k.  acute (uncompensated) respiratory acidosis
l.  (fully) compensated metabolic acidosis
m.  acute (uncompensated) respiratory alkalosis
n.  (fully) compensated respiratory acidosis
o.  acute (uncompensated) respiratory alkalosis
p.  partially compensated respiratory alkalosis
q.  (fully) compensated respiratory acidosis
r.  partially compensated respiratory acidosis
s.  (fully) compensated respiratory alkalosis
t.  within normal limits

# Chapter 15

15.1  T
15.2  F
15.3  T
15.4  F
15.5  F
15.6  T
15.7  T
15.8  F
15.9  T
15.10  F
15.11  F
15.12  F
15.13  T
15.14  T
15.15  F
15.16  F
15.17  T
15.18  T
15.19  hypoxia
15.20  increase
15.21  right–to–left
15.22  unventilated
15.23  absolute anemia
15.24  5 gm/dL
15.25  increases
15.26  $C\bar{v}O_2$ or mixed venous oxygen content
15.27  Purulent
15.28
  1. the oxygen content of arterial blood is decreased
  2. cardiac output or perfusion is decreased
  3. dysoxia (histotoxic hypoxia)
15.29
  1. asphyxia
  2. airway obstruction
  3. blockage of alveoli (edema or exudate)
  4. abrupt cardiorespiratory failure
  5. acute hemorrhage
15.30  d.
15.31  d.
15.32  d.
15.33  b.
15.34  d.
15.35  d.
15.36  d.
15.37  b.
15.38  d.
15.39  a.
15.40  d.
15.41  d.
15.42  d.
15.43  a.

15.44 d.
15.45 d.
15.46 c.
15.47 d.
15.48 b.
15.49 c.
15.50 d.
15.51 c.
15.52 d.
15.53 d.
15.54 b.
15.55 a.
15.56 b.
15.57 d.
15.58 d.
15.59

a. 1. Reduced Blood Flow
   2. Hb Deficiency
   3. Dysoxia
   4. R–to–L Shunt
   5. Hypoventilation
   6. Low V/Q
   7. Diffusion Defect

b. One could differentiate hypoxemia due to a diffusion defect, right–to–left shunt, and V/Q imbalance by administering supplemental oxygen. With an increased $O_2$ concentration, the $Po_2$ of a patient with a diffusion defect (case #7) or V/Q imbalance (case #6) will improve markedly; the $Po_2$ of a patient with a right–to–left shunt will not (case #4).

c. In cases #4–7, arterial hypoxemia is present (reduced $Cao_2$), but the oxygen content of the mixed venous blood ($C\bar{v}o_2$) is normal. This is possible only if the blood flow (cardiac output) increases to maintain a normal oxygen delivery to the tissues.

d. If a patient has a normal $Pao_2$, $P(A-a)o_2$, and $Cao_2$ but is still suffering the effects of tissue hypoxia, there must be an abnormality in oxygen utilization by the tissues (dysoxia). Case #3 illustrates this effect.

e. Although the $C\bar{v}o_2$ is a good laboratory indicator of the presence or absence of tissue hypoxia, it can be misleading. Case #3 is a good example. Here the patient may be suffereing from hypoxia, but the $C\bar{v}o_2$ is higher than normal. This can be caused by abnormal oxygen utilization by the tissues, as in dysoxia.

# Chapter 16

16.1
   a. clavicle
   b. body of sternum
   c. costal angle
   d. manubrium of sternum
   e. manubriosternal junction
   f. xiphoid
   g. scapula
   h. spinous process of T10
   i. C7
   j. T1
   k. T10
16.2  T
16.3  T
16.4  T
16.5  T
16.6  T
16.7  F
16.8  T
16.9  T
16.10 F
16.11 F
16.12 T
16.13 F
16.14 T
16.15 F
16.16 F
16.17 F
16.18 F
16.19 T
16.20 F
16.21 T
16.22 work of breathing
16.23 right heart
16.24 3–4
16.25 oblique
16.26 6th; 8th
16.27 3–5
16.28 5–7
16.29 lightly
16.30 bronchial (or tracheal)
16.31 crackles or rales
16.32 pleural friction rub
16.33 lower left sternal
16.34 5
16.35 vasoconstriction
16.36 cor pulmonale
16.37
   1. inspection
   2. palpation
   3. percussion
   4. auscultation

16.38
1. bronchogenic carcinoma
2. chronic obstructive lung disease
3. chronic cardiovascular disease

16.39
1. tachycardia
2. hypertension
3. tachypnea
4. cyanosis
5. restlessness
6. confusion

16.40 d.
16.41 d.
16.42 d.
16.43 b.
16.44 d.
16.45 d.
16.46 c.
16.47 b.
16.48 c.
16.49 a.
16.50 c.
16.51 c.
16.52 a.
16.53 c.
16.54 c.
16.55 b.
16.56 d.
16.57 c.
16.58 d.
16.59 c.
16.60 b.
16.61 d.
16.62 d.
16.63 b.
16.64 b.
16.65 b.
16.66 c.
16.67 d.
16.68 d.
16.69 c.
16.70 a.
16.71 c.
16.72 d.
16.73 d.
16.74 b.

# Chapter 17

17.1 T
17.2 F
17.3 T
17.4 T
17.5 T
17.6 F
17.7 T
17.8 T
17.9 F
17.10 F
17.11 T
17.12 F
17.13 F
17.14 T
17.15 collateral
17.16 modified Allen test
17.17 femoral artery
17.18 kilopascal (kPa)
17.19 pain; anxiety
17.20 Gloves
17.21 oxygen; carbon dioxide
17.22 Spectrophotometry
17.23 Photoplethysmography
17.24 1–5 torr
17.25 b.
17.26 c.
17.27 a.
17.28 d.
17.29 d.
17.30 c.
17.31 b.
17.32 c.
17.33 b.
17.34 a.
17.35 a.
17.36 d.
17.37 c.

# Chapter 18

18.1
a. restrictive curve
b. obstructive curve
c. normal curve

18.2
a. $FEV_{0.5}$
b. $FEV_1$
c. $FEV_3$

18.3
a. obstructive curve
b. normal curve
c. restrictive curve

18.4 F
18.5 T
18.6 F

18.7   T
18.8   T
18.9   F
18.10  T
18.11  T
18.12  T
18.13  F
18.14  T
18.15  T
18.16  F
18.17  T
18.18  T
18.19  screening
18.20  airway resistance
18.21  compliance
18.22  80
18.23  10
18.24  7
18.25  airway collapse; air trapping
18.26  0.5 and 2.5
18.27  diffusing capacity of the lung (DL)
18.28  ventilation and perfusion scans
18.29  transpulmonary pressure; volume
18.30  closing volume (CV)
18.31  greater; less
18.32  d.
18.33  d.
18.34  c.
18.35  d.
18.36  d.
18.37  a.
18.38  a.
18.39  c.
18.40  d.
18.41  d.
18.42  b.
18.43  b.
18.44  c.
18.45  b.
18.46  c.
18.47  d.
18.48  d.
18.49  b.
18.50  c.
18.51  d.
18.52  d.
18.53  a.
18.54  a.
18.55  c.
18.56  a.
18.57  c.
18.58  d.
18.59  c.
18.60  c.
18.61  d.

18.62
a.

| Lung Volumes | %PRED |
| --- | --- |
| TLC | 98% |
| FRC | 102% |
| RV | 102% |
| VC | 105% |

Forced Vital Capacity

| | | | |
| --- | --- | --- | --- |
| FVC | 5.05 | 4.78 | 106% |
| $FEV_1$ | 4.10 | 3.95 | 104% |
| $FEV_1\%$ | 81% | 83% | |
| $FEF_{200-1200}$ | 8.05 | 7.97 | 101% |
| $FEF_{25-75}$ | 4.38 | 4.49 | 98% |

b. all values are within normal limits
c. normal pulmonary function test

18.63
a.

| Lung Volumes | %PRED |
| --- | --- |
| TLC | 76% |
| FRC | 73% |
| RV | 77% |
| VC | 78% |

Forced Vital Capacity

| | | | |
| --- | --- | --- | --- |
| FVC | 2.28 | 2.92 | 78% |
| $FEV_1$ | 1.75 | 2.23 | 78% |
| $FEV_1\%$ | 77% | 78% | |
| $FEF_{200-1200}$ | 4.32 | 4.48 | 97% |
| $FEF_{25-75}$ | 2.83 | 2.74 | 103% |

b. 1. all lung volumes are decreased
   2. the FVC and $FEV_1$ are decreased
   3. the $FEV_1\%$, $FEF_{200-1200}$, and $FEF_{25-75}$ are within normal limits
c. restrictive disorder

18.64
a.

| Lung Volumes | %PRED |
| --- | --- |
| TLC | 111% |
| FRC | 146% |
| RV | 185% |
| VC | 79% |

## Forced Vital Capacity

| FVC | 2.67 | 3.83 | 70% |
|---|---|---|---|
| $FEV_1$ | 1.67 | 2.64 | 63% |
| $FEV_1\%$ | 63% | 83% | |
| $FEF_{200-1200}$ | 3.89 | 6.01 | 65% |
| $FEF_{25-75}$ | 1.45 | 2.56 | 57% |

b. 1. the TLC is increased due mainly to an increased RV
   2. the VC is decreased
   3. all flow–related measures are decreased substantially
c. air trapping with pulmonary obstruction

18.65
  a.

| Lung Volumes | %PRED |
|---|---|
| TLC | 97% |
| FRC | 105% |
| RV | 106% |
| VC | 96% |

## Forced Vital Capacity

| FVC | 2.96 | 3.63 | 82% |
|---|---|---|---|
| $FEV_1$ | 2.55 | 2.88 | 89% |
| $FEV_1\%$ | 86% | 78% | |
| $FEF_{200-1200}$ | 4.33 | 5.45 | 79% |
| $FEF_{25-75}$ | 1.95 | 3.37 | 58% |

b. 1. all lung volumes are within normal limits
   2. the FVC and $FEF_{200-1200}$ are moderately reduced
   3. the $FEV_1\%$ is normal
   4. the $FEF_{25-75}$ is substantially reduced
c. peripheral airways obstruction

18.66
  a.

| Lung Volumes | %PRED |
|---|---|
| TLC | 73% |
| FRC | 86% |
| RV | 68% |
| VC | 77% |

## Forced Vital Capacity

| FVC | 3.51 | 5.07 | 69% |
|---|---|---|---|
| $FEV_1$ | 2.10 | 3.64 | 58% |
| $FEV_1\%$ | 60% | 83% | |
| $FEF_{200-1200}$ | 5.67 | 7.32 | 77% |
| $FEF_{25-75}$ | 2.32 | 3.47 | 67% |

b. 1. the TLC and RC are markedly reduced
   2. all flow–related measures are markedly reduced
c. combined restrictive and obstructive disorder

# Chapter 19

19.1  T
19.2  F
19.3  T
19.4  F
19.5  F
19.6  T
19.7  F
19.8  T
19.9  F
19.10  F
19.11  T
19.12  T
19.13  T
19.14  F
19.15  T
19.16  density
19.17  black
19.18  posterior–anterior or PA
19.19  one half
19.20  one half
19.21  2
19.22  hilum or mediastinum
19.23  anterior air space
19.24  congestive heart failure
19.25  mediastinum
19.26  pneumomediastinum
19.27  6th; 10th
19.28  lateral or apical lordotic
19.29  d.
19.30  d.
19.31  d.
19.32  c.
19.33  b.
19.34  a.
19.35  d.
19.36  c.
19.37  a.
19.38  b.

19.39  a.
19.40  d.
19.41  d.
19.42  c.
19.43  c.
19.44  a.
19.45  c; e; a; b; d

# Chapter 20

20.1   F
20.2   F
20.3   T
20.4   F
20.5   T
20.6   F
20.7   F
20.8   F
20.9   F
20.10  T
20.11  T
20.12  F
20.13  F
20.14  T
20.15  F
20.16  T
20.17  T
20.18  F
20.19  T
20.20  T
20.21  F
20.22  T
20.23  F
20.24  F
20.25  T
20.26  cephalosporin
20.27  erythromycin
20.28  droplet nuclei
20.29  10 mm
20.30  Amphotericin B
20.31  bullae
20.32  mast cells
20.33  status asthmaticus
20.34  kyphosis
20.35  positive airway pressure (CPAP)
20.36  respiratory pressures
20.37  Guillain–Barre syndrome
20.38  Tensilon (edrophonium)
20.39  muscular dystrophy
20.40  increase; decrease
20.41  thoracentesis
20.42  tension pneumothorax
20.43  vasodilator

20.44  adult respiratory distress syndrome, or ARDS
20.45  22
20.46  interstitium
20.47  bacteria/toxins
20.48  tissue ischemia
20.49  d.
20.50  b.
20.51  a.
20.52  b.
20.53  d.
20.54  b.
20.55  d.
20.56  a.
20.57  b.
20.58  c.
20.59  a.
20.60  c.
20.61  c.
20.62  a.
20.63  c.
20.64  c.
20.65  d.
20.66  a.
20.67  c.
20.68  d.
20.69  d.
20.70  a.
20.71  a.
20.72  d.
20.73  a.
20.74  d.
20.75  b.
20.76  d.
20.77  b.
20.78  c.
20.79  d.
20.80  d.
20.81  c.
20.82  a.
20.83  a.
20.84  b.
20.85  b.
20.86  d.
20.87  b; h; a; f; d; e

# Chapter 21

21.1   T
21.2   T
21.3   T
21.4   T
21.5   F
21.6   F

21.7  F
21.8  T
21.9  T
21.10  T
21.11  T
21.12  T
21.13  T
21.14  F
21.15  F
21.16  T
21.17  T
21.18  T
21.19  T
21.20  T
21.21  T
21.22  side effect
21.23  Half–life
21.24  liver
21.25  tolerance or tachyphylaxis
21.26  Potentiation
21.27  affinity
21.28  agonist
21.29  competitive
21.30  tone
21.31  adenyl cyclase
21.32  acetylcholine
21.33  sympathomimetic or adrenergic
21.34  parasympathomimetic or cholinergic
21.35  hypertonic saline
21.36  10 and 20
21.37  anticholinergic
21.38  water
21.39  0.45
21.40  Proteolytics
21.41  antiinflammatory
21.42  cromolyn sodium
21.43  Pentamidine; antiprotozoal
21.44
　1. formation of glucose from body protein
　2. depletion of bone calcium
　3. increase of fat production
　4. impairment of immunologic response
　5. reduction of inflammatory response
　6. elevation of blood pressure

21.45

| Sympathetic Nervous System | Parasympathetic Nervous System |
|---|---|
| a. Thoracolumbar | Craniosacral |
| b. Short | Long |
| c. Long, with many branches | Short, with many branches |
| d. Acetylcholine | Acetylcholine |
| e. Nicotinic | Nicotinic |
| f. Norepinephrine | Acetylcholine (acetylcholine at sweat glands, blood vessels of skeletal muscles) |
| g. Alpha, beta | Muscarinic |
| h. Fight or flight | Freed to breed |

21.46  d.
21.47  b.
21.48  c.
21.49  a.
21.50  d.
21.51  d.
21.52  a.
21.53  b.
21.54  d.
21.55  c.
21.56  a.
21.57  c.
21.58  d.
21.59  a.
21.60  a.
21.61  a.
21.62  c.
21.63  b.
21.64  d.
21.65
　a. 0.5%
　b. 0.1%
21.66

| Total Solute Content in grams | Solute Content in mg/ml |
|---|---|
| a. .050 | 10 |
| b. .060 | 30 |

21.67  1.0 mg/ml
21.68  0.50 ml
21.69  12.00%
21.70  0.143%
21.71  15.00 ml

# Chapter 22

22.1 F
22.2 T
22.3 T
22.4 F
22.5 F
22.6 F
22.7 F
22.8 F
22.9 T
22.10 T
22.11 T
22.12 T
22.13 T
22.14 F
22.15 T
22.16 F
22.17 F
22.18 T
22.19 T
22.20 T
22.21 hypoxemia
22.22 vagal stimulation
22.23 one half
22.24 resistance
22.25 bacterial growth
22.26 internal
22.27 curved or MacIntosh
22.28 2–3
22.29 auscultation
22.30 nasotracheal intubation
22.31 tracheoinnominate fistula
22.32 tincture of Benzoin
22.33
  1. hypoxemia
  2. cardiac arrhythmias
  3. hypotension
  4. atelectasis
  5. mucosal trauma
  6. contamination
  7. increased intracranial pressures
22.34
  1. sterile suction catheter with thumb port
  2. sterile glove(s)
  3. sterile basin
  4. sterile water or saline
  5. sterile water–soluble lubricating jelly
  6. adjustable suction source
  7. $O_2$ delivery system (manual resuscitator/mask)
22.35
  a. 3.0
  b. 3.5
  c. 5.0
  d. 6.5
  e. 8.0
  f. 9.0
22.36
  a. tongue
  b. vallecula
  c. epiglottis
  d. vocal cord
  e. glottis
  f. arytenoid cartilage
22.37 d.
22.38 c.
22.39 a.
22.40 c.
22.41 a.
22.42 d.
22.43 d.
22.44 b.
22.45 b.
22.46 b.
22.47 b.
22.48 c.
22.49 c.
22.50 b.
22.51 a.
22.52 d.
22.53 c.
22.54 d.
22.55 d.
22.56 c.
22.57 c.
22.58 d.
22.59 c.
22.60 d.
22.61 c.
22.62 a.
22.63 b.
22.64 d.
22.65 c.
22.66 a.
22.67 d.
22.68 b.
22.69 c.
22.70 c.
22.71 a.
22.72 b.
22.73 a.
22.74 b.
22.75 c.
22.76 b.

# Chapter 23

23.1 T
23.2 T
23.3 F
23.4 T
23.5 F
23.6 T
23.7 T
23.8 T
23.9 F
23.10 T
23.11 F
23.12 T
23.13 F
23.14 T
23.15 F
23.16 F
23.17 T
23.18 T
23.19 F
23.20 F
23.21 T
23.22 F
23.23 F
23.24 coronary heart disease
23.25 clinical death
23.26 8–10
23.27 head–tilt/chin–lift
23.28 18
23.29 1/3–1/4
23.30 15–30
23.31 15; 2
23.32 sinus arrhythmia
23.33 electronic pacemaker
23.34 compensatory pause
23.35 morphine sulfate
23.36 cardioversion
23.37 c.
23.38 a.
23.39 d.
23.40 c.
23.41 c.
23.42 b.
23.43 c.
23.44 d.
23.45 b.
23.46 a.
23.47 c.
23.48 a.
23.49 d.
23.50 a.
23.51 b.

23.52 b.
23.53 b.
23.54 b.
23.55 d.
23.56 c.
23.57 c.
23.58 d.
23.59 b.
23.60 c.
23.61 d.
23.62 d.
23.63 a.
23.64 a.
23.65 b.
23.66 c.
23.67 b.
23.68
   Rate: 150
   Rhythm: regular
   P Waves: present, normal
   P–R Interval: 0.12 sec
   QRS Complexes: normal (sec)
   Interpretation: sinus tachycardia
23.69
   Rate: 50–55
   Rhythm: markedly irregular
   P Waves: indistinguishable (wavy baseline)
   P–R Interval: indistinguishable
   QRS Complexes: normal
   Interpretation: atrial fibrillation
23.70
   Rate: 80
   Rhythm: regular
   P Waves: present, normal
   P–R Interval: 0.32 sec
   QRS Complexes: normal
   Interpretation: first–degree heart block
23.71
   Rate: 56
   Rhythm: regular except 3rd complex
   P Waves: present, normal (except 3rd complex)
   P–R Interval: 0.20 sec
   QRS Complexes: normal except 3rd complex
      (QRS = 0.14 with compensatory pause)
   Interpretation: premature ventricular contraction
      (PVC) underlying rhythm is sinus bradycardia
23.72
   Rate: 135–140
   Rhythm: regular
   P Waves: indistinguishable
   P–R Interval: indistinguishable
   QRS Complexes: 0.12
   Interpretation: ventricular tachycardia

# Chapter 24

24.1   T
24.2   F
24.3   F
24.4   T
24.5   F
24.6   F
24.7   F
24.8   T
24.9   F
24.10   F
24.11   99%
24.12   Solid State Oxygen Generators (SSOG)
24.13   100 L/min; 50 psig
24.14   95%
24.15   gray
24.16   yellow
24.17   filling density
24.18   vapor pressure
24.19   50 psig
24.20   reserve bank
24.21   critical temperature
24.22   vaporizer
24.23   patient safety
24.24   zone valves
24.25   impossible
24.26   low–pressure
24.27   Bourdon–type
24.28   multiple–stage
24.29   gravity
24.30   c.
24.31   b.
24.32   a.
24.33   c.
24.34   a.
24.35   c.
24.36   a.
24.37   b.
24.38   b.
24.39   b.
24.40   d.
24.41   c.
24.42   b.
24.43   b.
24.44   c.
24.45   d.
24.46   b.
24.47   d.
24.48   a.
24.49   b.
24.50   c.
24.51   c.

24.52   c.
24.53   d.
24.54   a.
24.55   c.
24.56   b.
24.57   d.
24.58   c.
24.59   c.
24.60   b.
24.61   d.
24.62

| Gas or Mixture | Cylinder Factor | Duration of Flow Hours | Minutes |
|---|---|---|---|
| oxygen | 3.14 | 9 | 49 |
| oxygen | 3.14 | 10 | 28 |
| oxygen | 2.41 | 44 | 11 |
| oxygen | .28 | 0 | 51 |
| oxygen | .28 | 0 | 16 |
| $O_2/CO_2$ | 3.84 | 8 | 6 |
| $O_2/CO_2$ | 2.94 | 3 | 11 |
| $O_2/He$ | 2.50 | 7 | 2 |
| $O_2/He$ | .23 | 0 | 31 |

24.63
  a. DOT specs/service pressure
  b. serial number
  c. ownership mark
  d. original hydrostatic test
  e. spinning process used
  f. retesting information
24.64
  a. ASSS connection
  b. DISS outlet
  c. large (H/K) cylinder
  d. PISS connection
  e. DISS outlet
  f. small (E) cylinder
24.65
  a. high–pressure (2200 psig) inlet valve
  b. cylinder pressure gauge
  c. high–pressure chamber
  d. ambient pressure chamber
  e. flexible diaphragm
  f. spring
  g. valve stem/seat
  h. gas outlet
  i. safety vent
  j. adjustable hand control

# Chapter 25

25.1   F
25.2   F
25.3   F
25.4   T
25.5   F
25.6   F
25.7   F
25.8   T
25.9   T
25.10  F
25.11  T
25.12  F
25.13  F
25.14  F
25.15  50–75
25.16  drops; rises
25.17  servo–controller
25.18  capillary action
25.19  hyperpyrexia
25.20  50; 70
25.21  stability
25.22  weight density
25.23  mass median diameter (MMD)
25.24  Deposition
25.25  hygroscopic
25.26  sedimentation rate
25.27  baffle
25.28  piezoelectric transducer
25.29  infection
25.30
  1. surface area between water and gas
  2. time gas and water are in contact
  3. temperature of both water and gas
25.31
  1. particle size and physical nature
  2. force of gravity
  3. kinetic activity of carrier gas
  4. inertial forces
  5. the pattern of ventilation
25.32  d.
25.33  d.
25.34  c.
25.35  b.
25.36  d.
25.37  a.
25.38  d.
25.39  d.
25.40  d.
25.41  d.
25.42  c.
25.43  b.

25.44  a.
25.45  b.
25.46  a.
25.47  d.
25.48  b.
25.49  b.
25.50  d.
25.51  b.
25.52  c.
25.53  a.
25.54  c.
25.55  d.
25.56  a.
25.57  c.
25.58  b.
25.59  b.
25.60  d.
25.61  c.
25.62  d.
25.63  c.
25.64  d.
25.65  d.
25.66  c.
25.67  b.

# Chapter 26

26.1   T
26.2   F
26.3   F
26.4   F
26.5   T
26.6   T
26.7   T
26.8   F
26.9   T
26.10  F
26.11  T
26.12  T
26.13  T
26.14  T
26.15  T
26.16  T
26.17  T
26.18  T
26.19  F
26.20  T
26.21  liters per minute; concentration
26.22  least
26.23  50 mm Hg
26.24  obstructed
26.25  24
26.26  free radicals

26.27 vasoconstriction
26.28 50–60
26.29 oxygen conserving devices
26.30 3–4
26.31 4–5
26.32 one–way valves
26.33 0.24; 0.40
26.34 air entrainment port
26.35 12; 15
26.36 oxygen hood
26.37 avoiding fires; sudden decompression
26.38 1.8
26.39 c.
26.40 b.
26.41 c.
26.42 d.
26.43 d.
26.44 a.
26.45 b.
26.46 d.
26.47 c.
26.48 b.
26.49 c.
26.50 b.
26.51 b.
26.52 a.
26.53 d.
26.54 d.
26.55 c.
26.56 b.
26.57 c.
26.58 c.
26.59 b.
26.60 a.
26.61 c.
26.62 b.
26.63 c.
26.64 a.
26.65 a.
26.66 d.
26.67 c.
26.68 b.
26.69 c.
26.70 d.

26.71

| | Estimated Insp Flow (L/min) | Estimated $F_{IO_2}$ |
|---|---|---|
| a. | 24 | .28 |
| b. | 30 | .32 |
| c. | 60 | .32 |
| d. | 14 | .38 |
| e. | 40 | .41 |
| f. | 12 | .41 |
| g. | 27 | .36 |

h. Yes. a and b.
i. Yes. c and d; f and g.
j. Yes. Patients h and i have the same minute ventilations and $O_2$ input flows but different $F_{IO_2}$s. This is because patient i has a proportionately longer inspiratory time and a lower inspiratory flow. With a lower inspiratory flow, less air dilutes the $O_2$, and the resulting $F_{IO_2}$ is higher.

26.72
  a. .45
  b. .53
  c. .51
  d. .34
  e. .80

26.73

| | Air/$O_2$ Ratio | Total Output Flow (L/min) |
|---|---|---|
| a. | .14:1 | 12.59 |
| b. | .61:1 | 19.35 |
| c. | 1.03:1 | 20.26 |
| d. | 1.72:1 | 21.79 |
| e. | 3.16:1 | 62.37 |
| f. | 4.64:1 | 33.86 |
| g. | 7.78:1 | 43.89 |
| h. | 10.29:1 | 45.14 |
| i. | 25.33:1 | 79.00 |

# Chapter 27

27.1 F
27.2 T
27.3 T
27.4 F
27.5 T
27.6 T
27.7 F
27.8 T
27.9 T
27.10 T

27.11  F
27.12  T
27.13  T
27.14  T
27.15  F
27.16  F
27.17  F
27.18  T
27.19  T
27.20  alveolar; pleural
27.21  rise/increase
27.22  5–6
27.23  pulmonary barotrauma
27.24  20; 25
27.25  hypoventilation; hypoxemia
27.26  increases/raises
27.27  pressure–cycled
27.28  valve
27.29  oxygen blender
27.30  15 ml
27.31  inspiratory capacity
27.32  flow x time
27.33  IPPB
27.34  resting volume/FRC
27.35  nasogastric tube
27.36  threshold
27.37  d.
27.38  d.
27.39  d.
27.40  b.
27.41  b.
27.42  d.
27.43  a.
27.44  d.
27.45  d.
27.46  a.
27.47  c.
27.48  d.
27.49  b.
27.50  c.
27.51  d.
27.52  a.
27.53  a.
27.54  c.
27.55  b.
27.56  c.
27.57  c.
27.58  c.
27.59  b.
27.60  d.
27.61  c.
27.62  c.
27.63  d.
27.64  b.

27.65
  a. 50 psig gas inlet
  b. venturi jet
  c. flow control valve
  d. clutch plates
  e. diaphragm
  f. sliding alignment valve
  g. magnets
  h. nebulizer
  i. exhalation valve
27.66
  a. compressor/pump
  b. pressure control
  c. Bennett valve
  d. system pressure gauge
  e. exhalation valve
  f. nebulizer
  g. nebulizer control

# Chapter 28

28.1   T
28.2   F
28.3   F
28.4   T
28.5   T
28.6   T
28.7   F
28.8   T
28.9   T
28.10  T
28.11  F
28.12  T
28.13  T
28.14  F
28.15  T
28.16  F
28.17  F
28.18  T
28.19  T
28.20  T
28.21  T
28.22  F
28.23  gravity
28.24  1 1/2 to 2 hours
28.25  16 to 18
28.26  tilt–table
28.27  30–40
28.28  diaphragm
28.29  Vibration
28.30  100 mm Hg
28.31  6th or 7th
28.32  peripheral

28.33 Chest compression
28.34 forced expiration technique (FET)
28.35 bronchiolar collapse
28.36 good
28.37 diaphragm
28.38 Lateral costal
28.39 inspiratory resistive
28.40 rate of flow
28.41 duration
28.42 dyspnea
28.43 supplemental oxygen
28.44
  1. to prevent secretion accumulation
  2. to improve secretion mobilization
  3. to promote efficient breathing
  4. to improve ventilation distribution
  5. to improve CP exercise tolerance
28.45
  a. 1. Anesthesia
     2. CNS depression
     3. Narcotic–analgesics
  b. 1. Pain
     2. Neuromuscular dysfunction
     3. Pulmonary restriction
     4. Abdominal restriction
  c. 1. Laryngeal nerve damage
     2. Artificial airway
     3. Abdominal muscle weakness
     4. Abdominal surgery
  d. 1. Airway compression
     2. Airway obstruction
     3. Abdominal muscle weakness
28.46
  a. 6
  b. 5
  c. 1
  d. 3
  e. 2
28.47 d.
28.48 c.
28.49 c.
28.50 b.
28.51 a.
28.52 d.
28.53 d.
28.54 d.
28.55 b.
28.56 a.
28.57 d.
28.58 a.
28.59 b.
28.60 d.
28.61 b.
28.62 b.

28.63 b.
28.64 c.
28.65 c.
28.66 c.
28.67 b.
28.68 b.
28.69 d.
28.70 b.
28.71 d.
28.72 a.
28.73 a.
28.74 a.
28.75 c.
28.76 b.
28.77 a.

# Chapter 29

29.1  T
29.2  F
29.3  T
29.4  F
29.5  T
29.6  F
29.7  T
29.8  F
29.9  T
29.10 T
29.11 T
29.12 F
29.13 F
29.14 F
29.15 F
29.16 T
29.17 T
29.18 T
29.19 $Pa_{O_2}$; $P(A - a)_{O_2}$
29.20 elevated $Pa_{CO_2}$
29.21 acute
29.22 chronic obstructive pulmonary disease (COPD)
29.23 refractory
29.24 transpulmonary
29.25 arterial pH
29.26 24; 28
29.27 35
29.28 10
29.29 350
29.30 24; 28
29.31 5; 10
29.32 obesity

29.33
1. chronic obstructive pulmonary disease (COPD)
2. asthma
3. cystic fibrosis
4. pneumonia
5. pulmonary emboli (thromboemboli, fat emboli, etc.)
6. interstitial/parenchymal lung diseases (e.g., fibrosis)
7. oxygen toxicity
8. pulmonary edema
9. ARDS

29.34
1. infections (viral, bacterial, fungal)
2. aspiration (gastric contents, near–drowning, hydrocarbons)
3. inhaled toxins (oxygen, smoke, chemicals)
4. lung contusion
5. chest trauma
6. radiation pneumonitis
7. postperfusion (cardiopulmonary bypass)
8. high altitude pulmonary edema

29.35

| Values | |
|---|---|
| Adult Normal | Ventilatory Support |
| a. 65–75 | < 10–15 |
| b. 12–20 | > 35 |
| c. 80–100 | < 20–30 |
| d. 5–6 | > 10 |
| e. 120–180 | < 20 |
| | < (2 x $\mathring{V}_E$) |
| f. 0.25–0.40 | > 0.60 |
| g. 35–45 | > 50–55 |
| h. 75–100 | < 50 (air); |
| (breathing air) | < 70 (mask $O_2$) |
| i. 25–65 | 350–450 |

29.36
a. 3
b. 1
c. 5
d. 2
e. 4

29.37 a.
29.38 b.
29.39 d.
29.40 a.
29.41 d.
29.42 d.
29.43 d.
29.44 b.
29.45 d.
29.46 d.
29.47 b.
29.48 d.
29.49 d.
29.50 a.
29.51 d.
29.52 b.
29.53 b.
29.54 b.
29.55 c.
29.56 a.
29.57 d.
29.58 d.
29.59 c.
29.60 b.
29.61 c.
29.62 c.
29.63 c.
29.64 a.
29.65 b.
29.66 b.
29.67 d.
29.68 c.

# Chapter 30

30.1 T
30.2 F
30.3 T
30.4 T
30.5 T
30.6 F
30.7 F
30.8 T
30.9 F
30.10 F
30.11 T
30.12 F
30.13 T
30.14 T
30.15 F
30.16 T
30.17 F
30.18 T
30.19 T
30.20 F
30.21 T
30.22 T
30.23 F
30.24 F

30.25 F

30.26 pressure

30.27 constant

30.28 cycling or trigger

30.29 sensitivity, patient–effort, or trigger level control

30.30 response time

30.31 Controlled ventilation

30.32 lung characteristics

30.33 driving pressure

30.34 limit

30.35 small

30.36 flow

30.37 expiration

30.38 greater

30.39 50

30.40
1. underwater columns
2. spring–loaded diaphragms or disks
3. balloon valves with preset internal pressures
4. reverse venturi devices
5. electromechanical valves

30.41
1. magnitude of applied positive pressure
2. nature of the inspiratory waveform
3. duration of positive pressure
4. duration of expiratory phase
5. nature of the expiratory phase

30.42
a. 6
b. 4
c. 1
d. 2
e. 5

30.43

| | CMV | IMV |
| --- | --- | --- |
| a. | prohibited | allowed |
| b. | patient may or may not determine rate (f) | above IMV rate patient controls rate and $V_T$ |
| c. | ventilator only | patient contributes to $\dot{V}_E$ |
| d. | minimal | patient must use muscles |
| e. | higher for given $\dot{V}_E$ | lower for given $\dot{V}_E$ |

30.44
a. 2.50
b. 4.80
c. 1.60
d. 1.20
e. 4.50

30.45 c.
30.46 b.
30.47 c.
30.48 c.
30.49 b.
30.50 c.
30.51 d.
30.52 d.
30.53 c.
30.54 b.
30.55 b.
30.56 d.
30.57 d.
30.58 d.
30.59 a.
30.60 c.
30.61 b.
30.62 b.
30.63 a.
30.64 c.
30.65 b.
30.66 d.
30.67 a.
30.68 a.
30.69 b.
30.70 b.
30.71 d.
30.72 d.
30.73 d.
30.74 a.
30.75 c.
30.76 c.
30.77 c.
30.78 b.
30.79 d.
30.80 d.
30.81 b.
30.82 d.
30.83 b.
30.84 d.
30.85 a.
30.86 c.
30.87 c.
30.88 c.
30.89 d.
30.90 d.

# Chapter 31

31.1   T
31.2   T
31.3   T
31.4   T
31.5   F
31.6   T
31.7   T
31.8   T
31.9   T
31.10  F
31.11  T
31.12  T
31.13  T
31.14  T
31.15  F
31.16  T
31.17  battery backup
31.18  eccentric wheel
31.19  output control
31.20  sensitivity
31.21  baseline
31.22  ramp
31.23  compress
31.24  d.
31.25  c.
31.26  b.
31.27  d.
31.28  c.
31.29  b.
31.30  b.
31.31  d.
31.32  a.
31.33  a.
31.34  b.
31.35  a.
31.36  c.
31.37  b.
31.38  a.
31.39  c.
31.40  b.
31.41  a.
31.42  d.
31.43  c.
31.44  a.
31.45  c.

# Chapter 32

32.1   T
32.2   T
32.3   T
32.4   F
32.5   T
32.6   F
32.7   T
32.8   F
32.9   T
32.10  F
32.11  T
32.12  T
32.13  T
32.14  F
32.15  F
32.16  1 1/2 to 2
32.17  0.5 to 1.5 cm $H_2O$
32.18  rectangular; sine–wave
32.19  35
32.20  25–30
32.21  healthy
32.22  minimal leak (MLT); minimal occluding volume (MOV)
32.23  $Paco_2$
32.24  pressure differential
32.25  a/A
32.26  refractory hypoxemia
32.27  34%
32.28  threshold
32.29  b.
32.30  c.
32.31  a.
32.32  a.
32.33  b.
32.34  d.
32.35  d.
32.36  b.
32.37  c.
32.38  a.
32.39  c.
32.40  d.
32.41  c.
32.42  d.
32.43  a.
32.44  d.
32.45  b.
32.46  c.
32.47  d.
32.48  d.
32.49  a.
32.50  b.

32.51  c.
32.52  a.
32.53  d.
32.54  a.
32.55  b.
32.56  a.
32.57  c.
32.58  b.
32.59  c.
32.60  c.
32.61  d.
32.62  b.
32.63  c.
32.64  d.

# Chapter 33

33.1  T
33.2  F
33.3  T
33.4  F
33.5  T
33.6  F
33.7  T
33.8  T
33.9  F
33.10  F
33.11  T
33.12  F
33.13  oxygenation; ventilation
33.14  2
33.15  electrocardiographic (ECG)
33.16  60; 100
33.17  physiologic shunt (QS/QT)
33.18  5; 7
33.19  2–3
33.20  65 and 75
33.21  15; 30
33.22  fatigue
33.23  24; 48
33.24  15
33.25  thermodilution
33.26
  a. 5
  b. 7
  c. 10
  d. 2
  e. 9
  f. 3
  g. 1
  h. 1
  i. 11
  j. 6
  k. 8

33.27  a.
33.28  a.
33.29  b.
33.30  b.
33.31  a.
33.32  c.
33.33  d.
33.34  a.
33.35  a.
33.36  d.
33.37  b.
33.38  a.
33.39  a.
33.40  d.
33.41  d.
33.42  d.
33.43  a.
33.44  a.
33.45  b.
33.46  b.
33.47  c.
33.48  d.
33.49  a.
33.50  d.
33.51  d.
33.52  b.
33.53  d.
33.54  b.
33.55  c.
33.56  a.
33.57  a.
33.58  c.
33.59  c.
33.60  c.
33.61  d.
33.62  d.
33.63  d.
33.64  c.
33.65  b.
33.66  a.
33.67  d.
33.68  a.
33.69  b.
33.70  c.
33.71  b.
33.72  c.
33.73  d.
33.74  d.
33.75  a.
33.76  d.
33.77  d.
33.78  d.
33.79  b.
33.80  d.
33.81  d.

33.82  b.
33.83  b.
33.84  b.
33.85
   a. normal
   b. excessive (hyperventilation)
   c. insufficient (hypoventilation)
   d. normal
33.86
   b. 1. resistance
      2. increased
      3. bronchospasm; increased secretions
   c. 1. compliance
      2. decreased
      3. pneumothorax; atelectasis
33.87
   a. normal pattern
   b. asynchronous breathing
   c. paradoxical breathing
33.88
   a. normal arterial pulse
   b. aortic insufficiency
   c. cardiogenic shock
   d. pulsus alternans/CHF
   e. bigeminy/PVCs
   f. paradoxus/cardiac tamponade
33.89
   a. right atrium
   b. right ventricle
   c. pulmonary artery
   d. PA wedge pressure

# Chapter 34

34.1   T
34.2   T
34.3   F
34.4   T
34.5   F
34.6   T
34.7   F
34.8   T
34.9   F
34.10  T
34.11  F
34.12  T
34.13  F
34.14  T
34.15  weaning
34.16  strength; endurance
34.17  40
34.18  1.5; 2.0
34.19  intermittent mandatory ventilation

34.20  5 to 10
34.21  COPD
34.22  b.
34.23  d.
34.24  d.
34.25  c.
34.26  b.
34.27  c.
34.28  c.
34.29  d.
34.30  d.
34.31  a.
34.32  c.
34.33  b.
34.34  a.
34.35  c.
34.36  b.
34.37  c.
34.38  d.
34.39  c.
34.40  b.
34.41  d.
34.42  b.
34.43  c.
34.44  d.
34.45  d.
34.46  c.
34.47  a.
34.48  b.
34.49  c.
34.50  d.
34.51  b.
34.52  d.
34.53  a.
34.54  c.

# Chapter 35

35.1   T
35.2   F
35.3   T
35.4   T
35.5   F
35.6   F
35.7   T
35.8   F
35.9   F
35.10  F
35.11  F
35.12  T
35.13  T
35.14  T
35.15  T

35.16  T
35.17  T
35.18  T
35.19  T
35.20  T
35.21  F
35.22  F
35.23  T
35.24  T
35.25  T
35.26  umbilical vein
35.27  fetal hemoglobin (HbF)
35.28  ductus arteriosus
35.29  5–6
35.30  40
35.31  6–7
35.32  40–60
35.33  2:1
35.34  38; 42
35.35  5
35.36  7
35.37  –60 to –80
35.38  depressed respiratory drive
35.39  0.2; 0.5
35.40  meconium aspiration syndrome
35.41  respiratory syncytial virus
35.42  ECMO or extracorporeal membrane oxygenation
35.43  Surfactant replacement therapy
35.44
   a. placenta
   b. umbilical vein
   c. ductus venosus
   d. foramen ovale
   e. ductus arteriosus
   f. umbilical arteries
35.45  b.
35.46  d.
35.47  d.
35.48  a.
35.49  b.
35.50  d.
35.51  d.
35.52  d.
35.53  d.
35.54  d.
35.55  c.
35.56  c.
35.57  d.
35.58  d.
35.59  d.
35.60  d.
35.61  d.
35.62  b.
35.63  c.

35.64  a.
35.65  c.
35.66  d.
35.67  d.
35.68  d.
35.69  c.
35.70  b.
35.71  b.
35.72  b.
35.73  c.
35.74  c.
35.75  d.
35.76  c.
35.77  a.
35.78  d.
35.79  c.
35.80  b.
35.81  c.
35.82  b.
35.83  c.
35.84  b.
35.85  d.
35.86  a.
35.87  a.
35.88  d.
35.89  b.
35.90  a.
35.91  b.
35.92  c.
35.93  d.
35.94  d.
35.95  c.
35.96  c.
35.97  d.
35.98  a.
35.99  d.
35.100 d.
35.101 d.
35.102 a.
35.103 b.
35.104 d.
35.105 c.
35.106 d.
35.107 b.
35.108 b.
35.109 a.
35.110 a.
35.111 c.

# Chapter 36

36.1   T
36.2   T
36.3   F
36.4   F
36.5   T
36.6   F
36.7   T
36.8   F
36.9   T
36.10  T
36.11  F
36.12  T
36.13  F
36.14  T
36.15  1/3
36.16  medical
36.17  outside
36.18  health protection
36.19  high–level wellness
36.20
  1. eating breakfast
  2. eating moderately and regularly
  3. not smoking
  4. engaging in exercise
  5. limiting alcohol
  6. sleeping 7–8 hours nightly
36.21
  1. physical health
  2. social health
  3. emotional health
  4. mental health
  5. spiritual health
  6. vocational health
36.22  d.
36.23  b.
36.24  c.
36.25  b.
36.26  d.
36.27  b.
36.28  c.
36.29  a.
36.30  d.
36.31  a.
36.32  d.
36.33  c.
36.34  b.
36.35  c.
36.36  a.
36.37  a.
36.38  c.
36.39  d.

36.40  c.
36.41  d.
36.42  a.
36.43  d.
36.44  a.
36.45  d.
36.46  b.
36.47  c.
36.48  d.
36.49  c.
36.50  d.
36.51  d.
36.52  d.
36.53  c.
36.54  d.
36.55  b.
36.56  a.
36.57  d.
36.58  d.
36.59  a.

# Chapter 37

37.1   T
37.2   F
37.3   F
37.4   T
37.5   F
37.6   T
37.7   T
37.8   F
37.9   F
37.10  F
37.11  F
37.12  T
37.13  T
37.14  T
37.15  T
37.16  F
37.17  T
37.18  T
37.19  F
37.20  T
37.21  rehabilitation
37.22  cope effectively
37.23  psychosocial
37.24  quality of life
37.25  Program deficiencies
37.26  lactate
37.27  anaerobic threshold
37.28  1.0
37.29  60–70%
37.30  200

37.31  stated program objectives
37.32  log or diary
37.33  twelve–minute walk
37.34  80
37.35  outpatient
37.36
1. control of respiratory infections
2. basic airway management
3. improvement in ventilation and cardiac status
4. improvement in ambulation and other physical activity
5. reduction in overall medical costs
6. reduction in hospitalizations
7. psychosocial support
8. occupational retraining and placement
9. family education, counseling, and support
37.37
1. 5  exercycles
2. 2  treadmills
3. 1  rowing machine
4. 2  upper extremity ergometers
5. 5  pulse oximeters
6. 1  emergency $O_2$ cylinder
7. bronchodilator medications
8. inspiratory resistance breather (1 each)
37.38

| Accepted Benefits | Unlikely Benefits |
| --- | --- |
| increased physical endurance | prolonged survival |
| increased maximum $O_2$ consumption | improved PFT values |
| increased performance with: | lowered pulmonary–artery pressure |
| decreased ventilation | improved ABG results |
| decreased $O_2$ consumption | improved blood lipids |
| decreased heart rate | change in muscle $O_2$ extraction |
| increased anaerobic threshold | change in step desat or apnea |

37.39  a.
37.40  b.
37.41  d.
37.42  b.
37.43  d.
37.44  c.
37.45  d.
37.46  a.
37.47  d.
37.48  d.
37.49  d.
37.50  a.

37.51  c.
37.52  c.
37.53  c.
37.54  b.
37.55  c.
37.56  c.
37.57  d.
37.58  c.
37.59  a.
37.60  d.
37.61  c.
37.62  c.
37.63  d.
37.64  a.
37.65  b.
37.66  d.
37.67  d.
37.68  d.
37.69  b.
37.70  c.
37.71  d.
37.72  d.
37.73  d.
37.74  c.
37.75  c.
37.76  b.

# Chapter 38

38.1   T
38.2   T
38.3   F
38.4   F
38.5   T
38.6   T
38.7   T
38.8   F
38.9   T
38.10  F
38.11  T
38.12  T
38.13  Medicare
38.14  24; 7
38.15  Health Care Financing Administration (HCFA)
38.16  12 months
38.17  –300
38.18  18–40
38.19  860
38.20  20; 25
38.21  344
38.22  5–8
38.23  greater than 90
38.24  0.25

38.25  3 months
38.26  patient
38.27  0.5
38.28  12–15 inches of Hg
38.29  activated glutaraldehyde
38.30
1. absence of severe dyspnea while on a ventilator
2. acceptable arterial blood gas results
3. inspired $V_IO_2s$ that are relatively low
4. psychological stability
5. evidence of developmental progress (children)
6. absence of life–limiting cardiac dysfunction/arrhythmias
7. no PEEP (if needed, 10 cm $H_2O$)
8. ability to clear secretions by cough or suction
9. a tracheostomy tube as opposed to an endotracheal tube
10. no readmissions expected for more than one month

38.31
1. mechanical ventilator and backup unit (if needed)
2. oxygen source
3. hospital bed
4. patient lift
5. portable suction
6. bag–valve–mask unit/portable resuscitator
7. disposable supplies (circuits, catheters, pads)
8. monitoring devices such as pulse oximeter
9. trach tubes and related care kits

38.32
1. finders' fees—practitioner payment for patient referrals
2. hiring hospital staff in return for patient referrals
3. paid consultation services ties to patient referrals
4. offering patients free services or cash to use a particular DME
5. offering patients free equipment to use a particular DME
6. offering to pay patients' electric bills if they use a particular DME

38.33  b.
38.34  d.
38.35  d.
38.36  d.
38.37  b.
38.38  c.
38.39  d.
38.40  b.
38.41  a.
38.42  d.
38.43  d.
38.44  d.

38.45  d.
38.46  d.
38.47  c.
38.48  b.
38.49  b.
38.50  d.
38.51  c.
38.52  d.
38.53  b.
38.54  b.
38.55  d.
38.56  d.
38.57  a.
38.58  d.
38.59  d.
38.60  a.
38.61  c.
38.62  d.
38.63  d.
38.64  d.
38.65  d.
38.66  d.
38.67  d.
38.68  d.
38.69  a.
38.70  c.
38.71  d.
38.72  b.
38.73  c.
38.74  a.
38.75  d.
38.76  d.